STUDY GUIDE TO SUBSTANCE ABUSE TREATMENT

A Companion to
*The American Psychiatric Publishing
Textbook of Substance Abuse Treatment,*
Fifth Edition

T0199908

STUDY GUIDE TO SUBSTANCE ABUSE TREATMENT

A Companion to
The American Psychiatric Publishing Textbook of Substance Abuse Treatment, Fifth Edition

Edited by

Philip R. Muskin, M.D.

Professor of Psychiatry,
Columbia University Medical Center;
Chief, Consultation-Liaison Psychiatry,
New York–Presbyterian Hospital/Columbia Campus;
Faculty, Columbia University Center for Psychoanalytic
Training and Research, New York, New York

If you would like to buy between 25 and 99 copies of this or any other American Psychiatric Publishing title, you are eligible for a 20% discount; please contact Customer Service at appi@psych.org or 800–368–5777. If you wish to buy 100 or more copies of the same title, please e-mail us at bulksales@psych.org for a price quote.

Manufactured in the United States of America on acid-free paper
19 18 17 16 15   5 4 3 2 1
First Edition

Typeset in Adobe's Palatino LT Std and Helvetica LT Std

American Psychiatric Publishing
A Division of American Psychiatric Association
1000 Wilson Boulevard
Arlington, VA 22209-3901
www.appi.org

Contents

Part I: Questions

CHAPTER 1

CHAPTER 2

CHAPTER 3

CHAPTER 4

CHAPTER 5

CHAPTER 6

CHAPTER 7

CHAPTER 8

CHAPTER 9

CHAPTER 10

CHAPTER 11

CHAPTER 12

Part II: Answer Guide

Contributors

Senior Contributor

Anna L. Dickerman, M.D.
Assistant Professor of Psychiatry, Weill Cornell Medical College; Assistant Attending Psychiatrist, Psychiatry Consultation-Liaison Service, New York-Presbyterian Hospital/Weill Cornell Medical Center, New York, New York

Lawrence Amsel, M.D., M.P.H.
Assistant Professor of Clinical Psychiatry, College of Physicians and Surgeons, Columbia University; Attending Psychiatrist, Columbia University Medical Center, New York, New York

Robert Boland, M.D.
Vice Chair for Education, Department of Psychiatry, Brigham and Women's Hospital, Boston, Massachusetts

Rachel A. Caravella, M.D.
Fellow in Psychosomatic Medicine, Columbia University Medical Center, New York, New York

Stephanie Cheung, M.D.
Assistant Professor of Psychiatry, Columbia University Medical Center, New York, New York

Eric D. Collins, M.D.
Associate Clinical Professor of Psychiatry, Columbia University of Physicians and Surgeons, New York, New York; Physician-in-Chief, Silver Hill Hospital, New Canaan, Connecticut

Elizabeth A. Evans, M.D.
Clinical and Research Fellow, Division on Substance Abuse, New York State Psychiatric Institute, New York, New York

Elena Friedman, M.D.
Assistant Professor of Psychiatry, Weill Cornell Medical College; Assistant Attending Psychiatrist, Consultation-Liaison Psychiatry Service, New York–Presbyterian Hospital/Weill Cornell Medical Center, New York, New York

Christina Kitt Garza, M.D.
Instructor in Psychiatry, Columbia University, New York, New York

Richard G. Hersh, M.D.
Associate Professor of Psychiatry, Columbia University Medical Center, New York, New York

Yael Holoshitz, M.D.
Clinical Fellow in Public Psychiatry Program, Columbia Psychiatry/New York State Psychiatric Institute, New York, New York

Meredith A. Kelly, M.D.
Fellow in Addiction Psychiatry, Columbia University Medical Center, New York, New York

Jon A. Levenson, M.D.
Associate Professor of Psychiatry, Columbia University Medical Center, New York, New York

John Luo, M.D.
Senior Physician Informaticist, UCLA Health; Professor of Psychiatry, David Geffen School of Medicine, University of California, Los Angeles, California

Philip R. Muskin, M.D.
Professor of Psychiatry, Columbia University Medical Center; Chief, Consultation-Liaison Psychiatry, New York–Presbyterian Hospital/Columbia Campus; Faculty, Columbia University Center for Psychoanalytic Training and Research, New York, New York

Nasir H. Naqvi, M.D., Ph.D.
Assistant Professor of Clinical Psychiatry, Department of Psychiatry, Columbia University, New York, New York

Sara Siris Nash, M.D.
Assistant Professor of Psychiatry, Columbia University Medical Center, New York, New York

Daniel P. Notzon, M.D.
Fellow in Substance Abuse Disorders, Columbia University Medical Center/New York State Psychiatric Institute, New York, New York

Sarah Richards Kim, M.D.
Fellow in Child and Adolescent Psychiatry, Division of Child and Adolescent Psychiatry, Columbia Psychiatry, New York, New York

Amy Rosinski, M.D.
Clinical Assistant Professor, Department of Psychiatry, University of Michigan Health System; Director, Consultation-Liaison Services, University Hospital, Ann Arbor, Michigan

Lisa S. Seyfried, M.D.
Assistant Professor, Department of Psychiatry, University of Michigan Health System; Section Director, Psychiatry Hospital Services, University Hospital, Ann Arbor, Michigan

Anna Skiandos, D.O.
Associate Director of Psychiatry; Substance Abuse Services at Project Renewal, New York, New York

Anne Skomorowsky, M.D.
Assistant Professor of Psychiatry, Columbia University Medical Center, New York, New York

Shilpa Srinivasan, M.D., DFAPA
Associate Professor of Clinical Psychiatry and Associate Training Director, Geriatric Psychiatry, Department of Neuropsychiatry, University of South Carolina School of Medicine, Columbia, South Carolina

Marcia L. Verduin, M.D.
Associate Dean for Students and Professor of Psychiatry, College of Medicine, University of Central Florida, Orlando, Florida

S. Robert Vorel, M.D., Ph.D.
Assistant Professor of Clinical Psychiatry, Columbia University Medical Center, New York, New York

Monique Yohanan, M.D., M.P.H.
Editor, *Behavior Health, MCG* (formerly Milliman Care Guidelines, now part of the Hearst Health Network)

Erin Zerbo, M.D.
Assistant Professor, Department of Psychiatry, Rutgers New Jersey Medical School; Attending Psychiatrist, University Hospital, Newark, New Jersey

Disclosure of Competing Interests

Shilpa Srinivasan, M.D., DFAPA, is a member of the American Board of Psychiatry and Neurology Geriatric Psychiatry Exam Committee (2013–present). **Monique Yohanan, M.D., M.P.H.,** is Editor of *Behavior Health, MCG* (formerly Milliman Care Guidelines, now part of the Hearst Health Network).

None of the rest of the contributors to this book have indicated competing interests to disclose during the year preceding manuscript submission.

Preface

This self-examination guide is a companion to, not a replacement of, reading *The American Psychiatric Publishing Textbook of Substance Abuse Treatment*, 5th Edition. Patients with substance-related and addictive disorders can present diagnostic and therapeutic challenges. The textbook will prepare readers to understand the epidemiology, neurobiology, psychology, and treatment of patients with substance-related and addictive disorders. Therefore, we have attempted to organize questions along those domains. As you work through this self-examination book, let it guide you to chapters in the textbook as a path to your self-education. Some questions will seem obvious or easy, and some questions will be quite difficult. We have endeavored to use the style of question writing found in certification examinations; however, this is not a board preparation book. The contributors to this book are a group of clinicians and educators with a broad range of experience and expertise who undertook the task of writing the questions. The contributors have graciously donated their share of the proceeds from this book to charitable foundations dedicated to mental health.

Philip R. Muskin, M.D., Editor

Part I

Questions

CHAPTER 1

Neurobiology of Addiction

1.1 Which of the following neurotransmitter systems plays a shared role in the binge/intoxication stage for all drugs of abuse?

A. γ-Aminobutyric acid (GABA).
B. Opioid.
C. Serotonin.
D. Dopamine.
E. Norepinephrine.

1.2 Which of the following behavioral phenomena is thought to be due to elevated brain reward thresholds during acute drug abstinence?

A. Increased craving.
B. Decreased tolerance.
C. Decreased control over drug seeking.
D. Increased negative motivational/affective state during acute abstinence.
E. Decreased arousal.

1.3 Which of the following brain areas or systems is most directly implicated in emotional dysregulation during the withdrawal/negative affect stage of addictive behavior?

A. Lateral habenula.
B. Mesolimbic dopamine system.
C. Hypothalamic-pituitary-adrenal (HPA) axis.
D. Prefrontal cortex.
E. Insula.

1.4 Which of the following brain areas or systems is most directly involved in executive control over incentive salience/preoccupation?

A. Prefrontal cortex.
B. Basolateral amygdala.
C. Hypothalamic-pituitary-adrenal (HPA) axis.
D. Ventral striatum.
E. Endogenous opioid system.

1.5   Which of the following is the correct sequence of physiological/molecular events leading to the synaptic plasticity that underlies addiction?

   A. Reduction in inhibitory G-protein levels → increased cyclic adenosine monophosphate (cAMP) levels → increased protein kinase A (PKA) activity→ cAMP response element binding protein (CREB) regulation of gene expression → synaptic plasticity.
   B. Increased cAMP levels → CREB regulation of gene expression→ reduction in inhibitory G-protein levels → increased PKA activity → synaptic plasticity.
   C. CREB regulation of gene expression → increased cAMP levels → reduction in inhibitory G-protein levels → increased PKA activity → synaptic plasticity.
   D. Increased PKA activity → increased cAMP levels → CREB regulation of gene expression → reduction in inhibitory G-protein levels → synaptic plasticity.
   E. Increased cAMP levels → reduction in inhibitory G-protein levels → CREB regulation of gene expression → increased PKA activity → synaptic plasticity.

CHAPTER 2

Genetics of Addiction

2.1 Which of the following statements best describes the genetic influences on the development of substance use disorders?

A. Substance use disorders follow recessive Mendelian patterns of inheritance.
B. Substance use disorders are inherited via risk alleles that require a gene-by-environment interaction.
C. Twin and adoption studies have demonstrated the heritability of certain substance use disorders.
D. Epidemiologic studies have shown that the development of substance use disorders is dependent on the interaction of risk alleles with socioeconomic status.
E. In determining the risk for developing a substance use disorder, genetic influences are considered roughly equivalent among most individuals.

2.2 From the evidence to date, which of the following statements about the heritability of alcohol and substance use disorders is most accurate?

A. Twin studies have estimated heritability of alcohol dependence, ranging from 50% to 60%.
B. Twin studies have shown that concordance rates for opioid and stimulant dependence are similar for monozygotic and dizygotic twin pairs.
C. Twin studies have estimated heritability of nicotine dependence, ranging from 80% to 90%.
D. The risk for developing alcohol and opioid use disorders has been correlated in twin studies.
E. Genetic influences for substance abuse in general, but not for specific drugs of abuse, have been demonstrated.

2.3 Which of the following statements about genetic susceptibility for developing alcohol dependence is most accurate?

A. Decreased metabolism of acetaldehyde increases risk for developing alcohol dependence.
B. Decreased alcohol dehydrogenase function increases risk for developing alcohol dependence.

C. Low level of response to alcohol has been shown to be protective against developing alcohol dependence in a genomewide linkage association study.
D. Increased risk for alcohol dependence has been mapped to an alcohol dehydrogenase gene cluster on chromosome 4q (*ADH4*).
E. *ADH4* codes for a subunit in the alcohol dehydrogenase gene cluster that mainly contributes to enzyme function in the liver and has little bearing on the risk of alcohol dependence.

2.4   Which of the following statements best describes the role of the *DRD2* locus in susceptibility to drug or alcohol dependence?

A. The *DRD2* locus codes for dopamine D$_2$ receptors and is a candidate gene for schizophrenia but not for susceptibility to drug or alcohol dependence.
B. Substantial evidence implicates the *DRD2* locus in the heritability of nicotine dependence.
C. Findings implicating the *DRD2* locus in nicotine dependence may be attributable to nearby loci on chromosome 11.
D. *DRD2* has been implicated in increased risk for alcohol dependence.
E. *DRD2* has been implicated in increased risk for opioid dependence.

2.5   Which of the following statements about susceptibility genes for substance dependence is most accurate?

A. A cluster of nicotinic receptor genes on chromosome 15 has been associated with number of cigarettes smoked per day and with lung cancer, but not with nicotine dependence.
B. Genomewide association studies have mapped susceptibility for nicotine dependence to a cluster of nicotinic receptor genes on chromosome 15.
C. The μ-opioid receptor gene *OPRM1* has been associated with opioid dependence but not with alcohol or other drug dependence.
D. *GABBRA2*, which codes for one of the four subunits of the γ-aminobutyric acid (GABA) receptor, has shown significant associations with large effect sizes on risk of alcohol dependence.
E. 5-HTTLPR, a rare polymorphism in the serotonin transporter gene, has been implicated in drinking and drug-taking behavior among adolescents and college students.

C H A P T E R 3

Epidemiology of Addiction

3.1 What is the most widely used illicit drug or drug class internationally?

A. Opioids.
B. Cocaine.
C. Alcohol.
D. Cannabis.
E. Stimulants.

3.2 Globally, epidemiological surveys consistently show that men are much more likely than women to have a substance use disorder. In the United States, use of which substance is associated with being a white female?

A. Cannabis.
B. Stimulant.
C. Alcohol.
D. Cocaine.
E. Nicotine.

3.3 The revisions introduced in DSM-5 were informed by epidemiological data gathered from large-scale nationally representative surveys. Which of the following statements about DSM-5 and addiction is *not* true?

A. The substance-related legal problems symptom continues to have clinical utility in determining diagnostic thresholds.
B. Abuse and dependence have been combined into a single disorder of graded severity (substance use disorder).
C. Craving is now recognized as a key clinical feature of substance use disorders.
D. Cannabis withdrawal is now a recognized syndrome.
E. Prevalence rates of substance use disorders in the United States may change when DSM-5 criteria are used.

3.4 Large epidemiological surveys suggest that nearly a quarter of alcohol users will become alcohol dependent at some point in their lives. Which of the following is *not* associated with the transition from alcohol use to dependence?

A. Male gender.
B. Being black rather than white.
C. Older age.
D. Family history of substance use disorders.
E. Presence of comorbid disorders.

3.5 Epidemiological surveys are informative about who becomes addicted to substances. In developed countries, having an alcohol use disorder is associated with which of the following?

A. Being male, young, unmarried, and of high socioeconomic status.
B. Being male, older, unmarried, and of low socioeconomic status.
C. Being male, older, married, and of high socioeconomic status.
D. Being male, older, married, and of low socioeconomic status.
E. Being male, young, unmarried, and of low socioeconomic status.

CHAPTER 4

Cross-Cultural Aspects of Addiction

4.1 The term *ethnicity* refers to which of the following?

 A. People from diverse cultures who share a common background.
 B. The sum total of a group's life ways.
 C. The comparison of characteristics across culture groups.
 D. Distinct groupings within a culture.
 E. The cumulative social learning process.

4.2 Confounding variables are commonly noted to affect prevalence estimates comparing the impact of addiction between ethnic groups. In which of the following studies would it be important to account for differences in *age distribution*?

 A. A survey of alcohol consumption in Mexican women presenting to a family practice clinic.
 B. A survey of high school students looking at differences in cannabis use between ethnic groups.
 C. A survey comparing alcohol use in Hawaiian residents born in Asia with those born in Hawaii.
 D. A survey examining the prevalence of substance use disorders in Native Americans compared with non–Native Americans.
 E. A survey of drug use in Hispanic persons born in the Unites States versus those born outside the United States.

4.3 Which of the following terms can be applied to a grouping resulting from a specific addiction, such as one might find in a crack house?

 A. Culture.
 B. Subculture.
 C. Background.
 D. Ethnicity.
 E. Cross-cultural.

4.4 The clinical formulation of culture has traditionally been associated with which of the following?

A. Norm conflict.
B. Normative versus deviant behavior.
C. Socially prescribed use.
D. Cultural change.
E. Culture-bound syndromes.

4.5 Culturally sensitive care can be delivered through all of the following models, and each model has its own challenges. Which model runs the risk of marginalization?

A. Evidence-based manualized interventions.
B. Separate services.
C. Cultural consultation model.
D. Sensitized melting pot approach.
E. Individualized strategy.

CHAPTER 5

Science in the Treatment of Substance Abuse

5.1 By the early 1920s, most of the opioid detoxification clinics were closed. Which of the following was an important factor in this change?

A. Detoxification was not a common treatment for opioid addiction at the beginning of the twentieth century.
B. The clinics were deemed a failure because the patients did not become abstinent.
C. There were numerous treatments other than detoxification available for the treatment of opiate addiction.
D. Physicians could safely prescribe maintenance opioids independently of these clinics.
E. Most state governments discontinued their reimbursement of these clinics.

5.2 Many well-known substance abuse treatment programs have historically expressed nonacceptance of medications as treatment options to prevent relapse. Which of the following best accounts for this decision?

A. There are limited medications available for this purpose.
B. Treatment programs are unaware of the potential benefit of these medications.
C. Medication use conflicts with their treatment philosophy.
D. There is insufficient research to support the use of these pharmacological approaches.
E. Medications are not cost-effective for the health care system.

5.3 Why is detoxification the *most* common form of treatment for substance use disorders?

A. Detoxification provides long-term benefit for patients with substance use disorders.
B. Detoxification makes the patient more comfortable and therefore more likely to comply with longer-term treatment.
C. Detoxification represents the best use of limited resources.

D. Detoxification alone is a highly effective treatment for substance use disorders.

E. Detoxification is covered by most insurance programs, even state Medicaid programs.

5.4 Which of the following best describes the position taken by the Central Council of Alcoholics Anonymous (AA) regarding individuals who are taking physician-prescribed treatment medications for substance dependence?

A. Individuals who are taking naltrexone, but not methadone or buprenorphine, are permitted to attend and speak freely at all AA meetings.

B. Use of physician-prescribed treatment medications is permitted.

C. Individuals taking physician-prescribed treatment medications are not permitted to attend any AA meetings.

D. Individuals taking any physician-prescribed treatment medications are permitted to attend and speak freely at all AA meetings.

E. The Central Council of AA has no position on this issue.

5.5 Why have some clinicians denied that naltrexone is effective in patients with alcohol use disorder?

A. Naltrexone does not reliably produce long-term abstinence from alcohol; rather, it reliably produces a reduction in heavy drinking.

B. Studies have shown that naltrexone treatment leads to greater dropout rates from treatment.

C. Opioid receptor antagonists such as naltrexone are not approved in countries outside of the United States.

D. There is no evidence that opioid receptors are relevant in the reward pathway associated with addiction to alcohol.

E. Naltrexone has no effect on drinking patterns in patients with alcohol use disorder.

5.6 Which of the following best accounts for why there has been little motivation for pharmaceutical companies to pursue medications to treat substance use disorders?

A. The existing drugs have showed little success in preventing relapse.

B. Medications already available are used so little.

C. Medications to treat substance use disorders do not reduce costs.

D. Medications to treat substance use disorders do not reduce emergency visits.

E. Because of the Affordable Care Act, insurance will not pay for medications for the treatment of substance use disorders.

CHAPTER 6

Assessment of the Patient

6.1 Which of the following interview questions is most likely to make a patient feel comfortable during an initial interview?

A. How long have you been addicted to cocaine?
B. Why do you use cocaine?
C. Is anyone else in your family addicted?
D. What brought you to see me today?
E. Have you ever been to a hospital because of your cocaine use?

6.2 Which of the following substances requires inpatient detoxification?

A. Marijuana.
B. Nicotine.
C. Benzodiazepines.
D. Cocaine.
E. Amphetamines.

6.3 Which of the following patients has a substance-induced mental disorder?

A. A 16-year-old boy who began drinking to cope with social anxiety.
B. A 31-year-old man who developed auditory hallucinations 2 years after cessation of cocaine use.
C. A 30-year-old woman who complains of depressed mood after 2 years of near-daily marijuana use.
D. A 77-year-old man with a history of daily alcohol use who experiences disorientation and visual hallucinations 3 days after his last drink.
E. A 21-year-old woman who developed depressed mood and suicidal thoughts 1 week after using cocaine for the first time.

6.4 Which of the following medical problems is least likely to be related to alcohol dependence?

A. Cerebellar degeneration.
B. Peripheral vascular disease.

C. Cardiomyopathy.
D. Pancreatitis.
E. Aspiration pneumonia.

6.5   Which of the following is true regarding the use of collateral informants when obtaining a substance use history?

A. Contact with collateral informants should occur only with written permission from the patient.
B. There is no role for the involvement of collateral informants in treatment planning and recovery.
C. Patients are most likely to maintain abstinence if collateral informants are not involved in treatment.
D. Collateral informant interviews are unlikely to provide helpful information.
E. Collateral informants should not be asked about the patient's substance use, as this violates patient confidentiality.

CHAPTER 7

Screening and Brief Intervention

7.1   For which of the following patients does evidence support the use of screening and brief intervention (SBI)?

     A. A patient seeking treatment for moderate alcohol use disorder.
     B. A patient seen in an emergency department for chest pain following cocaine use.
     C. A patient seen in a primary care clinic for an annual physical.
     D. A patient who presents for treatment of a panic attack following cannabis use.
     E. A patient who has been arrested for driving under the influence.

7.2   Which of the following screening tools is most useful for brief screening?

     A. Alcohol Use Disorders Identification Test (AUDIT-C).
     B. Alcohol, Smoking and Substance Involvement Screening Test (ASSIST).
     C. CAGE questionnaire.
     D. Michigan Alcoholism Screening Test (MAST).
     E. Drug Abuse Screening Test (DAST).

7.3   Which of the following problem drinkers is in the *precontemplative* stage of change?

     A. A 40-year-old man who recently started drinking after 2 years of abstinence.
     B. A 66-year-old woman who has decided to stop drinking.
     C. A 42-year-old man who attends Alcoholics Anonymous weekly and has been sober for 3 years.
     D. A 27-year-old woman who has experienced blackouts when drinking but denies having a problem with alcohol.
     E. A 39-year-old man who has entered a 28-day rehabilitation program.

7.4 A patient states that one reason he drinks during the day is because he does not want family and friends to see his hands shake. Which of the following responses exemplifies the technique of reflective listening?

A. "I am concerned that you are putting yourself at risk by drinking during the daytime."
B. "You should tell your family about your drinking."
C. "You are embarrassed about your tremor."
D. "Do you think that other people will notice your tremor?"
E. "Let's set a goal that you will not drink during the daytime."

7.5 Which of the following is a proven effect of brief intervention (BI) for patients with alcohol use?

A. Reductions in motor vehicle crashes.
B. Reduction in mortality.
C. Reduction in emergency room utilization.
D. Reduction in risky drinking by 10% at 1 year.
E. Reduction in risky drinking by 10 drinks per week.

7.6 Which of the following patients would be considered a "risky" drinker?

A. A 45-year-old man who consumes 12–14 grams of ethanol 7 times a week.
B. A 35-year-old woman who drinks four 12-ounce beers a day.
C. A 68-year-old man who drinks 2 ounces of 80-proof liquor every other day.
D. A 50-year-old man who drinks 12 ounces of wine over the course of a weekend.
E. A 22-year-old woman who drinks a glass of wine every day.

CHAPTER 8

Patient Placement Criteria

8.1 Which of the following is an example of placement matching?

A. You determine that your patient is suitable for motivational enhancement therapy.
B. You determine that your patient is not suitable for naltrexone treatment.
C. You determine that your patient is suitable for family therapy.
D. You determine that your patient requires intensive outpatient care.
E. You determine that your patient should be transferred to another provider.

8.2 As part of the evaluation and treatment of a 47-year-old married real estate agent with alcohol use disorder, you recommend that his spouse and teenage children attend Alanon and Alateen, respectively. This is an example of which of the following American Society of Addiction Medicine (ASAM) Patient Placement Criteria (PPC) assessment dimensions?

A. Family history of psychiatric illness.
B. Health insurance status.
C. Patient demographics.
D. Recovery environment.
E. Participation in self-help recovery groups.

8.3 As the treating psychiatrist, you engage a 49-year-old patient with alcohol use disorder in a therapeutic discussion of the pros and cons of his alcohol use. To which American Society of Addiction Medicine (ASAM) Patient Placement Criteria (PPC) assessment dimension does this correspond?

A. Acute intoxication and/or withdrawal potential.
B. Biomedical conditions and complications.
C. Emotional, behavioral, or cognitive conditions and complications.
D. Readiness to change.
E. Recovery environment.

8.4   Which of the following is an American Society of Addiction Medicine (ASAM) Patient Placement Criteria (PPC) basic treatment level?

  A. Early intervention.
  B. Intensive outpatient/partial hospitalization.
  C. Student health services.
  D. Emergency room detoxification.
  E. Peer support groups.

8.5   Which of the following tools is used to evaluate the American Society of Addiction Medicine (ASAM) Patient Placement Criteria (PPC) assessment dimension of acute intoxication or withdrawal as part of a multidimensional patient assessment?

  A. CAGE questionnaire.
  B. Alcohol Use Disorders Identification Test-C (AUDIT-C).
  C. Clinical Institute Withdrawal Assessment for Alcohol Scale—Revised (CIWA-Ar).
  D. Drug Abuse Screening Test (DAST).
  E. Michigan Alcoholism Screening Test (MAST).

CHAPTER 9

"Recovery" in Chronic Care Disease Management

"Disease Control" in Substance Use Disorders

9.1 Recent federal legislation will promote changes in the way that substance abuse is treated. Which of the following is the most accurate statement about these changes?

A. The Wellstone and Domenici Mental Health Parity and Affordable Addiction Equity (MHPAE) Act of 2009 requires physicians to report patients who drink and drive, and thus put others at risk, to an appropriate law enforcement agency.
B. The Patient Protection and Affordable Care (PPAC) Act of 2010 requires all health care plans to offer prevention screening and brief interventions to detect and reduce medically harmful substance abuse.
C. The MHPAE Act requires that care for substance abuse be administered only by professionals who are trained substance abuse specialists.
D. The PPAC Act pertains only to patients who self-identify as having substance abuse problems.
E. Taken together, the MHPAE Act and the PPAC Act will aid in getting substance abuse patients out of primary care and into specialty addiction clinics.

9.2 Which of the following statements most accurately describes the chronic care management (CCM) model?

A. The CCM model involves a multidisciplinary team approach focused on tracking disease status with the goal of relapse prevention.
B. The CCM model prevents the suboptimal outcomes that can derive from patients managing their own care.
C. Although more effective than traditional episodic-reactive approach, the CCM model is costlier and often resented by patients.

D. The recovery model is incompatible with the CCM model and will need to be abandoned because the CCM model is implemented more widely.

E. The CCM model is applicable to type 2 diabetes and rheumatologic disorder because those illnesses involve patient self-management to an important degree.

9.3 Although there are multiple differing definitions of *recovery*, the definitions share some common elements. Which of the following most accurately describes the common elements?

A. Some definitions use the term *abstinence* and others use the term *sobriety*; however, all definitions agree that the term *recovery* applies only to individuals who have stopped using illicit substances.

B. Current definitions of *recovery* include adherence to a 12-step approach as a necessary condition.

C. All definitions recognize that *recovery* describes an outcome of behavior change.

D. Recovery involves a process of behavior change that includes improved health and well-being.

E. Recovery requires abstinence; thus a patient may improve while taking medication, the use of medications, however, precludes being in recovery.

9.4 Which of the following best describes the study by Dawson et al. (2005) examining diagnostic transitions among adults with self-reported alcohol dependence?

A. Abstinence is an effective but not prevalent method of achieving disease control in alcohol-dependent individuals.

B. Only 18% of the total sample of subjects who had prior alcohol dependence were in remission for the past year.

C. Those individuals in the study who were previously treated for alcohol dependence (an indication of a more severe illness) had significantly higher rates of total abstinence than the rest of the total sample.

D. Abstinence is the only method of achieving stable remission from alcohol dependence.

E. Those who had been previously treated were unlikely to still have a diagnosis of alcohol dependence.

9.5 The Look AHEAD (Action for Health in Diabetes) study (Gregg et al. 2012), although focusing on adults with type 2 diabetes, has elements analogous to those in the recovery approach to substance abuse. Which of the following best describes the comparison between these studies?

A. Weight loss was an important outcome variable in the Look AHEAD study, and reduction in alcohol intake also contributes to weight loss.

B. In the Look AHEAD study, the intensive lifestyle intervention (ILI) involved changes in lifestyle supported by individual and group counseling analogous to those supported in a 12-step recovery program.

C. In both the ILI intervention and the recovery approach, individual counseling served to ensure that patients take their prescribed medication.
D. In the ILI intervention, patients only showed improvement if they increased their medication intake over the 4 years of the study.
E. The ILI intervention involved weight loss and exercise, which cannot be compared with the behavior changes required in the recovery approach to substance use.

CHAPTER 10

Neurobiology of Alcohol Use Disorder

10.1 In which of the following brain regions is neural activity both correlated with cue-induced alcohol craving and reduced by successful treatments?

A. Ventral striatum/nucleus accumbens.
B. Ventral tegmental area.
C. Orbitofrontal cortex.
D. Anterior cingulate cortex.
E. Amygdala.

10.2 Which of the following acute effects of alcohol is a phenotypic marker of alcoholism risk?

A. High rewarding/euphoric effects.
B. Low neural excitability.
C. Low sedative-ataxic effects.
D. Low behavioral disinhibition.
E. High anxiolytic effects.

10.3 Which of the following is linked to allelic variation of the *OPRM1* gene?

A. Degree of sedative-ataxic effects of alcohol.
B. Level of alcohol cue-induced neural activity within the ventral striatum/nucleus accumbens.
C. Level of impulsivity caused by alcohol.
D. Level of tolerance to alcohol.
E. Level of alcohol-induced dopamine release within the ventral striatum/nucleus accumbens.

10.4 Which of the following physiological processes is thought to be most directly involved in the acute withdrawal syndrome that occurs upon cessation of heavy drinking?

  A. Downregulation of adrenergic neurotransmission.
  B. Rebound hyperactivity of glutamatergic neurotransmission.
  C. Increased γ-aminobutyric acid (GABA)–ergic tone.
  D. Dopamine receptor downregulation in the nucleus accumbens.
  E. Hypothalamic-pituitary-adrenal (HPA) downregulation.

10.5 The binding of corticotropin-releasing hormone (CRH) to which of the following brain regions leads to increased behavioral reactivity to stress after cessation of heavy alcohol use?

  A. Amygdala complex.
  B. Ventral striatum/nucleus accumbens.
  C. Anterior pituitary.
  D. Lateral hypothalamus.
  E. Periaqueductal gray matter.

CHAPTER 11

Treatment of Alcohol Intoxication and Alcohol Withdrawal

11.1 Which of the following laboratory assays would be best to utilize during alcohol treatment if your goal is to detect heavy alcohol use and monitor drinking status?

A. Alanine aminotransferase (ALT).
B. γ-Glutamyl transpeptidase (GGT).
C. Aspartate aminotransferase (AST).
D. Carbohydrate-deficient transferrin (CDT).
E. Ethyl glucuronide (EtG).

11.2 A 65-year-old patient with a history or delirium tremens is on your service for management of alcohol withdrawal. If the patient's withdrawal is left untreated, when might you expect to see symptoms of delirium tremens emerge?

A. 0–1 days from last drink of alcohol.
B. 2–4 days from last drink of alcohol.
C. 5–7 days from last drink of alcohol.
D. 6–8 days from last drink of alcohol.
E. 8–10 days from last drink of alcohol.

11.3 You admit a 40-year-old patient with alcohol use disorder to your service. To manage his withdrawal, you would like to use a symptom-triggered approach (versus fixed multiple daily dosing). Which one of the following should you use to assess the severity of alcohol withdrawal symptoms?

A. CAGE questionnaire.
B. Clinical Institute Withdrawal Assessment for Alcohol–Revised (CIWA-Ar).
C. Alcohol Use Disorders Identification Test (AUDIT).
D. Michigan Alcoholism Screening Test (MAST).
E. Addiction Severity Index (ASI).

11.4 To prevent precipitation of Wernicke's encephalopathy in a patient with alcohol use disorder, thiamine should be administered *before* which of the following?

A. Glucose.
B. Magnesium.
C. Potassium.
D. Phosphate.
E. Folate.

11.5 You are discussing treatment options for alcohol detoxification with a patient who tells you he prefers outpatient detoxification to inpatient. After reviewing his history, you tell him that you do *not* recommend outpatient treatment of alcohol withdrawal. Which of the following in his history most led you to recommend inpatient treatment?

A. He was arrested a few years ago for assault and public intoxication.
B. He prefers to drink beer over hard liquor.
C. He has a history of alcohol withdrawal seizures.
D. He smokes one pack of cigarettes per day.
E. He smokes marijuana 3–4 times per week.

CHAPTER 1 2

Neurobiology of Stimulants

12.1 A 33-year-old woman with a decade-long history of cocaine use tearfully states that she wants nothing more than to reconcile with her ex-husband, have more visits with her children, and get a job. However, she never spends much time on these goals before she prostitutes herself in order to use again. She knows she is making bad decisions, but when faced with a choice between feeling good quickly from cocaine *versus* possibly feeling good later upon achieving a goal, she always chooses the high. What is the term for this decision-making tendency related to chronic stimulant use?

A. Delayed discounting.
B. Tolerance.
C. Cue-induced drug seeking.
D. Dependence.
E. Stimulant-induced drug seeking.

12.2 Methamphetamine and cocaine have similar properties, but methamphetamine is more neurotoxic because of which feature that cocaine lacks?

A. Interference of dopamine reuptake.
B. Promotion of dopamine release.
C. Short-lasting effect.
D. Faster metabolism.
E. Prolonged increase in dopamine that does not habituate.

12.3 N-methyl-D-aspartate (NMDA) antagonists prevent both dopaminergic and serotonergic neurotoxicity, suggesting these medications could decrease methamphetamine toxicity by interference with which NMDA receptor-binding neurotransmitter?

A. Dopamine.
B. Serotonin.
C. Glutamate.
D. Norepinephrine.
E. γ-Aminobutyric acid (GABA).

12.4 Which γ-aminobutyric acid (GABA)–modulating medication was found to *decrease* relapse in cocaine users?

A. Gabapentin.
B. Baclofen.
C. Vigabatrin.
D. Tiagabine.
E. Topiramate.

12.5 What would the expected presentation be for a longtime methamphetamine user who abruptly discontinues use?

A. Diarrhea.
B. Nausea.
C. Depression.
D. Dysautonomia.
E. Pain.

CHAPTER 13

Clinical Management: Cocaine

13.1 Which of the following agonist approaches to the treatment of cocaine addiction, when combined with contingency management, has been shown to *reduce* cocaine use more effectively than either treatment alone or placebo?

A. D-Amphetamine.
B. Methylphenidate.
C. Modafinil.
D. Bupropion.
E. Disulfiram.

13.2 Which of the following medications targeting neuroadaptations to chronic cocaine use, when combined with amphetamine salts, has been shown to *reduce* cocaine use compared with placebo?

A. *N*-acetyl cysteine (NAC).
B. Vigabatrin.
C. Topiramate.
D. Lofexidine.
E. Doxazosin.

13.3 Chronic cocaine use produces which of the following neurochemical changes?

A. Increased postsynaptic dopamine receptors in cocaine users.
B. Increases in dopamine transporter in acutely abstinent cocaine abusers relative to control subjects.
C. Increases in D_2 dopamine receptor binding in detoxified cocaine users relative to control subjects.
D. Increased cerebral blood flow and cortical perfusion among chronic cocaine users.
E. Deficits in attention without a change in working memory.

13.4 For which of the following cognitive enhancers, compared with placebo, have studies demonstrated improvements in sustained attention, reduction in cocaine-positive urine specimens, and fewer self-reports of cocaine use?

A. Varenicline.
B. Modafinil.
C. Amphetamines.
D. Glutamate agonists.
E. Galantamine.

13.5 Which of the following treatment modalities can be most effectively combined with pharmacotherapies to improve treatment outcomes significantly for individuals with cocaine addiction?

A. Contingency management.
B. Standard counseling.
C. Twelve-step facilitation (TSF).
D. Cognitive-behavioral therapy (CBT).
E. Methadone maintenance.

CHAPTER 14

Clinical Management: Methamphetamine

14.1 When compared with cocaine, methamphetamine (MA) exhibits which of the following important differences in neuronal effects?

A. MA induces intracellular dopamine-containing vesicles to dock with the cell membrane and leak dopamine into the synaptic cleft.
B. Although cocaine blocks reuptake of dopamine from the synaptic cleft, MA does not.
C. MA has a short half-life and duration of action—barely exceeding 60 minutes.
D. MA exerts its primary action at the dopamine transporter to increase extracellular dopamine.
E. MA decreases the cytoplasmic concentration of dopamine, thus reducing the levels of dopamine oxidation products in the cytoplasm and limiting the neurotoxicity of MA.

14.2 The police bring a 27-year-old man with a history of anxiety and cannabis dependence to the emergency room with new-onset paranoid delusions and acute agitation. A friend provides history that the patient was smoking methamphetamine (MA) for the prior 2 days. To manage the patient's toxicity, including the agitation, which of the following would be the most appropriate intervention?

A. Administer emetics and gastric lavage.
B. Initiate dialysis.
C. Avoid attempting to talk with the patient.
D. Administer haloperidol combined with lorazepam in repeated doses over a 12-hour observation period.
E. Avoid the use of atypical antipsychotics.

14.3 Which of the following is a problem uniquely experienced by adult MA-dependent women associated with their methamphetamine (MA) use?

A. Over 70% of adult MA-dependent women report histories of physical and sexual abuse and are more likely than men to present for treatment with greater psychological distress.

31

B. In one sample of all MA-dependent women, 45% showed serological evidence of hepatitis C infection.

C. Rates of HIV seroprevalence are threefold higher among MA-using women compared with those who do not use MA.

D. Over 63% of women seeking substance abuse treatment reported MA as their primary drug of choice.

E. Women show higher dropout rates and more MA use during treatment than men.

14.4 The Matrix Model, a blended treatment approach that has shown efficacy for treatment of methamphetamine (MA) use disorders, incorporates which of the following components?

A. Contingency management, individual psychoeducation, group psychodynamic therapy, and 12-step program participation.

B. Motivational interviewing, contingency management, acceptance and commitment therapy, and 12-step facilitation (TSF).

C. Motivational interviewing, family therapy, TSF, and 12-step program participation.

D. Community reinforcement and family therapy, contingency management, individual psychodynamic psychotherapy, and motivational interviewing.

E. Individual and group cognitive-behavioral therapy (CBT), family education, motivational interviewing, and 12-step program participation.

14.5 There are no medications that are approved by the U.S. Food and Drug Administration (FDA) for the treatment of methamphetamine (MA) addiction. Which of the following lists drugs with only positive results from clinical trials in human beings demonstrating reduced stimulant use/prevention of relapse to MA or amphetamine-type stimulants (ATSs)?

A. Citicoline, naloxone, and bupropion.

B. Topiramate, lobeline, and aripiprazole.

C. Mirtazapine, naltrexone, and bupropion.

D. MA vaccine, naloxone, and modafinil.

E. γ-Vinyl-γ-aminobutyric acid (GVG), methylphenidate, aripiprazole.

CHAPTER 15

Hallucinogens and Club Drugs

15.1 A patient would most likely seek acute medical attention for which of the following symptoms after ingesting a classic hallucinogen?

A. Hallucinations.
B. Dysphoria.
C. Panic.
D. Nausea/vomiting.
E. Palpitations.

15.2 Which of the following hallucinogens or club drugs is considered to be a drug of dependence/addiction?

A. Lysergic acid diethylamide (LSD).
B. Psilocybin.
C. Methylenedioxymethamphetamine (MDMA).
D. Ketamine.
E. Mescaline.

15.3 You are performing a psychiatric evaluation on a 31-year-old male who has been using lysergic acid diethylamide (LSD) on a regular basis for several years. Which of the following chief complaints would you be most likely to encounter as a result of his chronic hallucinogen use?

A. Depression.
B. Insomnia.
C. Flashbacks.
D. Memory deficits.
E. Psychosis.

15.4 A 22-year-old woman presents to the medical emergency department with friends after she complained to them of chest pain at a party. She admits to taking some sort of "pill" around 2 hours prior to presentation. In the emergency department, she tells staff members that she "is in love with them" and wanders into other patients' rooms, trying to hug them. Her pupils are dilated, blood pressure is 180/100, and pulse is 120. Her affect is euphoric, and she exhibits no motor impairment. Which substance did the patient most likely ingest?

A. Phencyclidine (PCP).
B. Dextromethorphan.
C. *Salvia divinorum*.
D. Ketamine.
E. Methylenedioxymethamphetamine (MDMA).

15.5 Methylenedioxymethamphetamine (MDMA) has been found to have benefit for which of the following conditions?

A. Major depressive disorder.
B. Posttraumatic stress disorder (PTSD).
C. Chronic pain.
D. Alcohol dependence.
E. Anxiety associated with terminal illness.

CHAPTER 16

Tobacco Use Disorder

16.1   What pharmacological properties make nicotine addictive and promote the maintenance of nicotine dependence?

   A. Nicotine-induced symptomatic relief lasts many hours.
   B. Nicotine concentrations in the brain decline rapidly.
   C. Nicotine is metabolized slowly by the liver.
   D. Chronic nicotine exposure increases stress tolerance.
   E. Nicotine desensitizes the hypothalamic-pituitary-adrenal (HPA) pathway.

16.2   Your patient tells you that she smokes cigarettes. According to the U.S. Preventive Services Task Force recommendations, what should you do next?

   A. Assess her level of motivation to quit.
   B. Assist her with medication and counseling.
   C. Advise her to quit.
   D. Assess the severity of her physical dependence.
   E. Assess her triggers and social supports.

16.3   What does motivational interviewing entail?

   A. Asking questions designed to elicit client's own incentives for behavior change.
   B. Providing information about community resources that can help with abstinence.
   C. Educating the client about the consequences of ongoing use.
   D. Informing the client about the benefits of quitting.
   E. Discussing advantages and side effects of different medication options.

16.4   Which psychosocial intervention helps individuals quit tobacco by promoting increased awareness of bodily sensations, acceptance of craving symptoms, and uncoupling of cravings and linked positive reinforcements?

   A. Motivational interviewing.
   B. Learning About Healthy Living.
   C. Nicotine Anonymous.
   D. Mindfulness.
   E. Cognitive-behavioral therapy (CBT).

16.5   Which nicotine replacement therapy (NRT) has the highest abuse liability?

   A. Transdermal patch.
   B. Gum.
   C. Lozenge.
   D. Inhaler.
   E. Nasal spray.

16.6   You have a patient with schizophrenia and tobacco use disorder, treated with olanzapine and quetiapine. You have recently prescribed varenicline and nicotine replacement therapy (gum), and the patient was able to quit smoking. The patient reports increased sedation, hypersomnia, dizziness, and dry mouth. What would be the best course of action to take with this patient?

   A. Increase the nicotine replacement therapy dose because these symptoms are consistent with nicotine withdrawal.
   B. Discontinue nicotine replacement therapy because it is increasing olanzapine and quetiapine levels.
   C. Discontinue varenicline because these symptoms are side effects of varenicline.
   D. Decrease quetiapine dose because discontinuation of tobacco increased quetiapine levels.
   E. Decrease olanzapine dose because discontinuation of tobacco increased olanzapine levels.

CHAPTER 17

Benzodiazepines and Other Sedatives and Hypnotics

17.1 The weight of evidence suggests that all sedative hypnotics as well as alcohol interact with which receptor?

A. β_1-Adrenergic.
B. Histamine$_1$ (H$_1$).
C. Serotonin 1A (5-HT$_{1A}$).
D. γ-Aminobutyric acid type A (GABA$_A$).
E. Serotonin 2A (5-HT$_{2A}$).

17.2 For benzodiazepines, which of the following adverse effects is most likely to persist even after several years of daily administration?

A. Lethargy.
B. Memory impairment.
C. Weakness.
D. Dizziness and falls.
E. Ataxia.

17.3 Physiological dependence to benzodiazepines occurs in approximately half of patients who have received daily medication for which length of time?

A. 1 week.
B. 2 weeks.
C. >1 month.
D. >2 months.
E. >4 months.

17.4 A 36-year-old woman with generalized anxiety disorder is being treated with lorazepam, 0.5 mg twice daily. She has no other medical or psychiatric history and is taking no other medications. She initially experiences a good effect, but on a 6-month follow-up visit, she tells her physician that she recently had to take extra tablets beyond what is prescribed to achieve symptom relief. Her doctor's investigation at this point should first focus on which of the following possible explanations for her complaint?

A. Nonadherence.
B. Drug diversion.
C. Misdiagnosis.
D. Substance use disorder.
E. Pseudoaddiction.

17.5 A 52-year-old man with a history of sedative-hypnotic use disorder and comorbid panic disorder presents to a hospital seeking detoxification from alprazolam. He has been taking the drug daily for the past year at dosages as high as 12 mg/day. He has no other medical problems and is physically healthy on examination. He appears motivated for detoxification albeit fearful of side effects and admits that in the past he has left detoxification facilities prematurely because of a worsening of his anxiety symptoms. Which of the following first steps would be most helpful to successfully detoxify this patient?

A. Begin a rapid taper of alprazolam.
B. Rapidly cross-taper the patient to clonazepam.
C. Very slowly taper the alprazolam.
D. Slowly infuse flumazenil.
E. Discontinue alprazolam and begin oxazepam.

17.6 Which of the following best describes the evidence supporting the use of long-acting benzodiazepines for maintenance treatment of patients with sedative, hypnotic, or anxiolytic use disorder who have been unsuccessful at remaining abstinent?

A. No peer-reviewed literature exists to support or refute benzodiazepine maintenance treatment.
B. Maintenance treatment is not an effective way to treat most substance use disorders.
C. Treatment with maintenance benzodiazepines usually leads to a worsening of substance use disorders.
D. Outside of uncontrolled trials, there is little empirical evidence to support this approach.
E. Clonazepam maintenance has comparable efficacy to methadone treatment for opioid use disorder.

17.7   A 26-year-old patient has successfully detoxified from diazepam after 5 years of daily use. The patient currently denies withdrawal symptoms but reports continued craving for the drug. Outside of the substance use disorder, the patient has no other medical or psychiatric diagnoses. Which of the following is a first-line treatment for helping this patient maintain the gains achieved during detoxification and attain sustained, long-term abstinence?

A. Carbamazepine.
B. Behavioral therapy.
C. Flumazenil.
D. Oxazepam.
E. Imipramine.

CHAPTER 18

Treatment of Anabolic-Androgenic Steroid–Related Disorders

18.1 Which drug is often combined with anabolic-androgenic steroids (AASs) to reduce undesirable side effects?

A. Furosemide.
B. Probenecid.
C. Human growth hormone.
D. Tamoxifen.
E. Thyroid hormone.

18.2 Which of the following is the most likely physical exam finding associated with anabolic-androgenic steroid (AAS) use in men?

A. Male-pattern baldness.
B. Prostatic hypertrophy.
C. Testicular atrophy.
D. Hepatomegaly.
E. Hypertension.

18.3 Which of the following psychotropic medications is *most* appropriate for treating muscle dysmorphia, a form of body dysmorphic disorder seen in users of anabolic-androgenic steroids (AASs)?

A. Fluoxetine.
B. Bupropion.
C. Lithium.
D. Amphetamine.
E. Haloperidol.

18.4. Which of the following laboratory abnormalities is most reliably found in men using anabolic-androgenic steroids (AASs)?

    A. Elevated high-density lipoprotein (HDL) cholesterol.
    B. Elevated luteinizing hormone (LH).
    C. Elevated testosterone level.
    D. Decreased testosterone level.
    E. Increased red blood cell (RBC) count.

18.5 A 42-year-old man comes to your office reporting new onset of anhedonia, low mood, poor concentration, decreased sex drive, and fatigue. He admits that 1 week ago, he abruptly stopped using anabolic-androgenic steroids (AASs). What would the best treatment strategy be for you and your endocrinologist colleague to address the patient's complaints?

    A. Start fluoxetine, and reevaluate symptoms in 4–6 weeks.
    B. Start testosterone, then in 1 month discontinue the testosterone and start clomiphene.
    C. Start naltrexone to reduce hedonic effects in the event of relapse.
    D. Start clomiphene and human chorionic gonadotropin (HCG), with the addition of testosterone depending on level.
    E. Start testosterone, then in 1 month discontinue the testosterone and start HCG.

CHAPTER 19

Neurobiology of Opiates and Opioids

19.1   A cancer patient with painful bony lesions has been getting prescriptions for oxy-codone from her oncologist for the pain. She reports to her oncologist that for 2 months her 8/10 pain would go down to 3/10 with the prescribed dose, but recently, she found she was getting less and less relief with that same dose. She tried an increased dose, and the pain went down to 3/10. She now worries about running out of medication too quickly. Which best describes the phenomenon?

   A. Withdrawal.
   B. Abuse.
   C. Dependence.
   D. Addiction.
   E. Tolerance.

19.2   How long can a newly abstinent, seriously heroin-dependent person expect to experience the most intense signs and symptoms of withdrawal?

   A. 6–12 hours.
   B. 48–96 hours.
   C. Weeks to months.
   D. More than 1 year.
   E. The signs and symptoms can be expected to persist even while receiving maintenance treatment.

19.3   What kind of neuron tonically inhibits dopaminergic neurons in the ventral tegmental area (VTA) and is of main importance in opioid addiction?

   A. Dopaminergic.
   B. γ-Aminobutyric acid (GABA)–ergic.
   C. Cholinergic.
   D. Noradrenergic.
   E. Serotonergic.

19.4 Which medication or category of medication is made from the opium poppy?

    A. Opiate.
    B. Opioid.
    C. Methadone.
    D. Fentanyl.
    E. β-Endorphin.

19.5 The stress-responsive hypothalamic-pituitary-adrenal (HPA) axis is profoundly disrupted by heroin addiction and normalized by maintenance treatment with which substance?

    A. Naltrexone.
    B. Naloxone.
    C. Metyrapone.
    D. Methadone.
    E. Adrenocorticotropic hormone (ACTH).

CHAPTER 20

Opioid Detoxification

20.1 Which one of the following objective signs is consistent with opioid intoxication rather than opioid withdrawal?

A. Constricted pupils.
B. Dilated pupils.
C. Diarrhea.
D. Lacrimation.
E. Rhinorrhea.

20.2 You admit a 25-year-old patient for opioid detoxification. He tells you he is using five bags of heroin intravenously per day. Approximately how many hours after his last heroin use would you expect withdrawal to begin?

A. 3–5 hours.
B. 4–6 hours.
C. 8–12 hours.
D. 13–17 hours.
E. 36–72 hours.

20.3 You are teaching a medical student about buprenorphine. The medical student asks you why there are two forms of buprenorphine (buprenorphine alone and buprenorphine combined with naloxone). What do you tell her about the purpose of the naloxone in the combination formulation?

A. To allow one to check blood levels.
B. To deter intravenous abuse.
C. To make it more safe in overdose.
D. To enhance the oral bioavailability.
E. To increase the half-life.

20.4 A 35-year-old woman presents to the emergency room in opioid withdrawal. What is the largest *initial* dose of methadone that you can safely give to her?

A. 10 mg.
B. 20 mg.

C. 30 mg.
D. 40 mg.
E. 50 mg.

20.5 What is one potential advantage of a clonidine-naltrexone opioid detoxification compared with either methadone taper or clonidine detoxification?

A. Reduction in time to detoxification.
B. Higher patient acceptance.
C. Less need for medical monitoring.
D. Fewer staff required.
E. Less precipitated withdrawal.

CHAPTER 21

Methadone and Buprenorphine Maintenance

21.1   What distinguishes methadone from prior treatments for opioid dependence?

A. Strong *N*-methyl-D-aspartate (NMDA) antagonism.
B. Efficacy.
C. Lack of respiratory depression.
D. Predictable half-life.
E. Mostly renal excretion.

21.2   In treatment of opioid addiction, methadone exerts its therapeutic effect via which pharmacological mechanism?

A. Withdrawal suppression.
B. *N*-methyl-D-aspartate (NMDA) agonism.
C. μ-Receptor antagonism.
D. Decreased cross-blockade.
E. Long-lasting analgesia.

21.3   In the United States, methadone treatment for opioid dependence is usually provided in which type of setting?

A. Substance abuse psychiatrists' offices.
B. Pain management clinics.
C. Inpatient substance abuse rehabilitation units.
D. Outpatient substance abuse rehabilitation units.
E. Opioid treatment programs.

21.4   Which of the following correlates with better outcomes in methadone treatment for opioid dependence?

A. Gradual methadone dose reduction over time.
B. Lower daily maintenance dosing.
C. Higher methadone blood levels.

D. Nonpharmacological treatment.

E. Decreased availability of methadone take-home doses.

21.5   What is one of the most common adverse effects of methadone maintenance therapy?

A. QTc prolongation.

B. Constipation.

C. Decreased sweating.

D. Cognitive impairment.

E. Poor psychomotor performance.

21.6   What is the mechanism of action of buprenorphine?

A. Short-acting opioid antagonism.

B. Long-acting opioid agonism.

C. Mixed opioid agonism-antagonism.

D. Long-acting γ-aminobutyric acid (GABA) agonism.

E. Positive allosteric modulation of GABA.

21.7   Who can prescribe buprenorphine for opioid dependence in the United States?

A. Opioid treatment programs only.

B. General psychiatrists anywhere in the world.

C. Physicians with special training and a special Drug Enforcement Administration number.

D. Physicians who are board certified in addiction psychiatry with a regular Drug Enforcement Administration number.

E. Physicians who have treated at least 30 patients with buprenorphine under supervision.

21.8   You start a patient on buprenorphine and the patient complains of anxiety, insomnia, nausea, and diaphoresis. What would be the best course of action to take?

A. Do not do anything differently because these symptoms are unlikely to be related to the medication.

B. Stop buprenorphine because these symptoms are the side effects of the medication and will not improve.

C. Increase the dose of buprenorphine to increase the opioid agonism and improve the symptoms.

D. Wait a few days or decrease the starting dose to minimize opioid withdrawal.

E. Add a benzodiazepine for anxiety and insomnia.

CHAPTER 22

Opioid Antagonists

22.1 What medication acts exclusively as a nonselective opioid antagonist, with no opioid agonist properties?

A. Methadone.
B. Naloxone.
C. Naltrexone.
D. Buprenorphine.
E. Clonidine.

22.2 Naltrexone's effect on hypothalamic-pituitary-adrenal (HPA) and hypothalamic-pituitary-gonadal (HPG) activity may account for what adverse response in some patients upon treatment initiation?

A. Nausea.
B. Insomnia.
C. Anxiety.
D. Headache.
E. Appetite disturbances.

22.3 What accounts for approximately half of the deaths of heroin users in the United States?

A. Liver failure.
B. Malnutrition.
C. Cardiac arrhythmia.
D. Overdose.
E. Stroke.

22.4 In addition to supportive care, what is the treatment of choice in acute opioid overdose?

A. Naloxone.
B. Naltrexone.
C. Clonidine.
D. General anesthesia.
E. Benzodiazepines.

22.5 Compared with those who discontinue opioid agonist treatment, individuals who discontinue opioid antagonist treatment are at much greater risk for what outcome, cited by experts as a reason that antagonist treatment is "unacceptable"?

A. Relapse and overdose.
B. Depression and suicide.
C. Cognitive impairment.
D. Social stigmatization.
E. Panic attacks.

CHAPTER 23

Neurobiology of Marijuana

23.1   After consumption of marijuana, which of the following symptoms is most likely to persist?

   A. Impairment in motor coordination.
   B. Appetite stimulation.
   C. Increase in sociability.
   D. Altered perception of time.
   E. Heightened sensitivity of stimuli.

23.2   Which of the following acute symptoms is a person most likely to experience when smoking hash oil compared with marijuana?

   A. Increased craving for marijuana.
   B. Sensitivity to colors.
   C. Decreased appetite.
   D. Paranoid thoughts.
   E. Altered perception of time.

23.3   Which of the following is a DSM-5 criterion for marijuana withdrawal?

   A. Apathy.
   B. Increased appetite.
   C. Craving.
   D. Sleep difficulty.
   E. Tachycardia.

23.4   Which of the following is a rationale for the illicit use of JWH-018 as an alternative to marijuana?

   A. Ability to activate both CB_1 and CB_2 cannabinoid receptors.
   B. Psychotropic effects.
   C. Low potency.
   D. Numerous therapeutic utilities.
   E. Chemical structures that are almost identical.

23.5   Why was the clinical development of rimonabant stopped?

A. CB_1-antagonist effects in human subjects.
B. Similarity to nabilone.
C. Propensity to produce CB_1-agonist psychotropic side effects.
D. Propensity to worsen lipid profiles and insulin resistance in humans.
E. Weight gain.

CHAPTER 24

Treatment of Cannabis Use Disorder

24.1 The synthetic cannabinoids such as K2 and Spice generally have which of the following characteristics?

A. They are partial agonists at CB_1 and CB_2 cannabinoid receptors and are less potent than Δ^9-tetrahydrocannabinol (Δ^9-THC).
B. They are full agonists at CB_1 and CB_2 receptors but are less potent than Δ^9-THC.
C. They are partial agonists at CB_1 and CB_2 receptors with similar potency to Δ^9-THC but have a greater risk of adverse effects.
D. They are full agonists at CB_1 and CB_2 receptors and are more potent than Δ^9-THC, with a greater risk of adverse effects.
E. They are full agonists at CB_1 and CB_2 receptors and have few adverse effects.

24.2 The reinforcing effects of cannabis are attributable to which of the following neurochemical properties?

A. Decreased activity of dopamine neurons in the ventral tegmental area.
B. Decreased extracellular dopamine in the nucleus accumbens.
C. Dopamine release in the ventral striatum.
D. Serotonin release in the ventral striatum.
E. Enhanced synaptic plasticity in the nucleus accumbens.

24.3 Which of the following statements about cannabis withdrawal is most accurate?

A. Cannabis withdrawal may include increased appetite and weight gain.
B. Cannabis withdrawal may include hypersomnia.
C. Cannabis withdrawal is driven by a compensatory upregulation of the endocannabinoid system.
D. Cannabis withdrawal does not affect any neurotransmitter systems other than the endocannabinoid system.
E. Cannabis withdrawal is alleviated by marijuana use or dronabinol administration.

24.4   Psychotherapeutic interventions for the treatment of cannabis use disorder have been shown to have which of the following effects?

A. Cognitive-behavioral therapy (CBT) and motivational enhancement therapy (MET) may be potentiated when combined with contingency management (CM) strategies.
B. Longer treatments reduce marijuana use more than brief treatments.
C. For adolescents, more resource-intensive family treatments are superior to other psychotherapeutic interventions in reducing use.
D. Twelve-step facilitation (TSF) is likely to improve treatment efficacy.
E. Long-term abstinence rates achieved by individuals participating in CM alone are higher than those achieved by individuals receiving other psychotherapy treatments.

24.5   Which of the following is a finding of randomized controlled trials (RCTs) studying medications for the treatment of cannabis use disorder?

A. *N*-Acetylcysteine (NAC) and gabapentin have been shown to reduce marijuana use.
B. Dronabinol has been shown to reduce marijuana use.
C. Bupropion has been shown to minimize marijuana withdrawal symptoms.
D. Divalproex sodium has been shown to reduce marijuana use.
E. Nefazodone has been shown to reduce marijuana use, but not marijuana withdrawal symptoms.

CHAPTER 25

Psychodynamic Psychotherapy

25.1 The clinician considering implementation of psychodynamic and psychoanalytic theory in the treatment of addiction would do so based on which of the following?

   A. Universal support among theorists for a major role for psychodynamic and psychoanalytic theory in addiction treatment.
   B. Awareness that psychodynamic treatment of addiction is not efficacious for patients with comorbid borderline personality disorder and alcohol use disorders.
   C. Awareness that psychodynamic treatment of addiction is not efficacious for patients with comorbid major depression and alcohol use disorders.
   D. Awareness that psychodynamic theory cannot be of use to individuals in 12-step programs.
   E. Awareness that psychodynamic theory can be of use in individual and group rehabilitation settings.

25.2 The self-medication hypothesis of substance use is based on which of the following?

   A. Freud's early psychoanalytic observations of cocaine-using patients.
   B. Observations over the past 30 years of dual-diagnosis patients' specific substance choice.
   C. The use of cocaine to counter patients' feelings of rage and aggression.
   D. The use of opioids to counter patients' feelings of depressive anergic restlessness.
   E. The use of alcohol to prevent the tolerance of loving or aggressive feelings.

25.3 The application of psychodynamic theory to the treatment of substance abuse includes which of the following?

   A. Modification of the traditional psychoanalytic approach to avoid patient regression.
   B. Postponement of 12-step group participation until the psychodynamic treatment is completed.
   C. Focus on childhood history to the exclusion of the patient's current conflicts.

D. The requirement that one psychodynamic theory be used exclusively with any single patient.

E. Avoidance of discussion of the therapist-patient relationship.

25.4 Which one of the following is a clear indication for individual psychodynamic psychotherapy for a patient with addiction?

A. Active use of substances.
B. Severe organicity.
C. Psychosis.
D. Antisocial personality.
E. Social phobia associated with avoidance of groups.

25.5 Which of the following is true about the use of group treatment for patients in addiction treatment?

A. Group therapies, including Alcoholics Anonymous or Narcotics Anonymous, are not indicated for patients in individual psychotherapy.
B. Group treatments can help defuse powerful negative transferences that can develop in individual psychotherapy.
C. Only exploratory, not supportive, psychotherapy groups are of use to patients in addiction treatment.
D. Patients seeking abstinence should attend substance abuse groups only.
E. The 12-step groups should be avoided when a patient's primary therapist is not available.

25.6 Exploration of defenses commonly seen in patients with addictions supports which of the following?

A. Higher-level defenses are always encountered initially in the treatment of patients with addiction.
B. Higher-level defenses often emerge with time and treatment in recovery from addiction.
C. The alcoholic patient ignoring the effects of liver damage is using intellectualization as a defense.
D. The alcoholic patient curious about the effects of liver damage is using splitting as a defense.
E. Higher-level defenses such as reaction formation preclude noncompliance in the treatment of patients with addiction.

25.7 Treatment outcome research for patients with addiction supports which of the following?

A. Standardized treatment for all addiction patients.
B. Postponement of treatment for comorbid conditions until substance use disorders are in full remission.
C. Mandatory participation in 12-step programs and individual psychotherapy.

D. Avoidance of Alcoholics Anonymous participation because of a possible association with higher substance-related health care costs.

E. Significant health care cost savings resulting from investment in substance abuse treatment.

25.8 Neurobiology studies informing the role of psychotherapy in the treatment of addiction have suggested which of the following?

A. Psychotherapy can be understood as a controlled form of learning in the context of the therapeutic relationship.

B. Environmental signals, including those from psychotherapy, have no effect on the plasticity of the brain.

C. Neuroimaging studies have shown that psychotherapy has no influence on biological activity in the brain.

D. Psychotherapy is not indicated with addiction patients, as the acute and chronic reinforcing effects of drug addiction lead to enhancement of voluntary control.

E. Cognitive-behavioral psychotherapy for patients with addiction discounts the functional characteristics of the individual patient's brain.

25.9 Which of the following is true regarding the treatment of patients with comorbid personality disorders?

A. Alcoholism and drug abuse are rare in patients with personality disorders.

B. Treatments targeting alcohol abuse only were more effective than treatments targeting maladaptive behavioral and interpersonal patterns.

C. An acute substance-induced personality change is easily distinguished from personality disorder symptoms.

D. Addiction patients with narcissistic traits or personality disorder are not treatable.

E. Psychotherapy with patients with borderline personality disorder and addiction requires an emphasis on structure and limit setting.

25.10 The course of addiction recovery for patients treated with psychodynamic psychotherapy will include which of the following?

A. An immediate acceptance of an addiction diagnosis at the outset of individual psychotherapy.

B. A high level of motivation for addiction treatment maintained throughout the treatment process.

C. No need for 12-step program participation or additional psychotherapy after achieving abstinence.

D. Relapse prevention, which can include laboratory tests or family meetings.

E. Less emphasis on patient confidentiality if the patient is forced into treatment by an employer or probation office.

CHAPTER 26

Cognitive-Behavioral Therapies

26.1   Cognitive-behavioral therapy (CBT) treatments have a number of theoretical sources and empirical roots in the psychological literature. Which of the following is the most accurate statement about these sources and roots?

A. Drug use behaviors are learned through their association with the positively re-inforcing (reward) properties of the substances themselves, and thus operant conditioning is important in creating a therapy to counter these behaviors.
B. As reinforcement learning is the basis of substance abuse according to the CBT approach, other risk factors such as family history or personality traits are incidental and not relevant to the treatment.
C. CBT must incorporate an understanding of unconscious conflicts, as described in the psychoanalytic literature, if it is to be effective in eliminating root causes of substance use.
D. Albert Ellis and Aaron Beck emphasized a purely behavioral approach to therapy that was later challenged for its narrow focus.
E. Drug related cues or stimuli are related to drug craving only in those individuals who have a genetic vulnerability, and thus are not relevant to CBT for substance use.

26.2   Which of the following is the most accurate description of the "sleeper effect" phenomenon described by Carroll et al. (1994)?

A. Individuals receiving desipramine reported less insomnia, and this was seen to be a mediator of overall improvement.
B. After a clinical treatment trial for substance abuse ended, individuals receiving cognitive-behavioral therapy (CBT) continued to further reduce their frequency of substance abuse.
C. Individuals receiving CBT maintained their clinical improvement over the following year, as measured by frequency of cocaine use.
D. CBT combined with lifestyle changes, including exercise and improved sleep hygiene, showed a better response rate than CBT alone.
E. Baseline circadian abnormalities, especially with day-night reversal, predicted poorer outcome.

26.3 Multiple clinical trials conducted by Carroll and her team at Yale over a 20-year period focused on cognitive-behavioral therapy (CBT) treatment for substance abuse. Which of the following is the *most* accurate statement about these studies?

A. The series of studies was marked by a progressively larger effect size for CBT over comparison or control conditions.
B. In these studies, when CBT was conducted to rigorous standards of adherence, subjects showed an equivalent improvement independent of the subject's baseline substance use.
C. Although CBT was more effective than supportive clinical management, all subjects who demonstrated skill acquisition achieved equivalent improvement.
D. Those receiving CBT did better than those receiving interpersonal therapy (IPT), but disulfiram was no better than placebo.
E. Although skill acquisition was strongly associated with long-term reduction in cocaine use, subjects' compliance with homework exercises did not significantly correlate with improved outcomes.

26.4 Cognitive-behavioral therapy (CBT) has been shown to be an effective treatment for substance abuse. Which of the following is the *most* accurate description of the therapeutic approach used in CBT?

A. Framing the role of the therapist as the expert on substance-related disorders and in charge of the therapy aids patients in developing confidence that the therapist can help them reduce their substance use.
B. Patients are helped to identify the large issues in their lives and avoiding focusing on smaller decisions.
C. The key defining features of CBT are functional analysis of drug use and an emphasis on skill training.
D. Patients receive training to improve their relationships by focusing on the needs of others in their lives and reducing their own assertiveness.
E. CBT is most effective when the patient defines the focus of sessions depending on patient's emotions in the "here and now."

26.5 A trial evaluating training methods for CBT demonstrated which of the following training methods in cognitive-behavioral therapy (CBT) to be the most efficacious for clinicians?

A. Review of the National Institute on Drug Abuse (NIDA) CBT manual only.
B. Review of the NIDA CBT manual plus access to a Web-based training site.
C. Participation in a didactic seminar plus review of the NIDA CBT manual.
D. Participation in a didactic seminar plus supervision from a CBT trainer.
E. Access to CBT manual plus completion of three CBT cases.

CHAPTER 27

Motivational Enhancement

27.1 A 46-year-old obese man with recently diagnosed hypertension, a 20-year history of a cocaine use disorder, and erectile dysfunction is evaluated in the emergency room for chest pain shortly after using $250 worth of cocaine intranasally. His symptoms rapidly resolve, and the evaluating physician attempts to counsel him about the dangers of ongoing cocaine use, offering a referral for substance abuse treatment. The patient appears disinterested, thanks the doctor for saving his life, and asks to be discharged, saying, "I just pushed it a little too far this time." In which of the "stages of change" does the patient appear to be regarding his cocaine use?

A. Precontemplation.
B. Contemplation.
C. Planning.
D. Action.
E. Maintenance.

27.2 Motivational interviewing (MI) and motivational enhancement therapy (MET) techniques could have adverse effects for which of the following patients?

A. An intravenous heroin user with no desire to stop using despite a recent diagnosis of endocarditis.
B. A two-pack-per-day smoker worried about the health effects of cigarettes but fearful of weight gain.
C. A 42-year old-woman with bipolar I disorder and several recent medical admissions for alcohol withdrawal.
D. A 52-year-old man with a severe alcohol use disorder recently discharged from a detox unit who presents with his wife seeking observed disulfiram treatment.
E. A 45-year-old artist and daily marijuana user who insists he needs the drug to be creative.

27.3 A 36-year-old woman who uses vaporized marijuana five or six times per day presents to your office seeking treatment for anxiety after she quit her job due to "unmanageable stress." When asked about her substance abuse, she states that she would like to quit but fears that any new job she might get would require preemployment drug testing and that she "cannot fathom" cutting down or stopping marijuana because her anxiety will "skyrocket." Which of the following intervention statements would be *best to make next,* in keeping with the principles of motivational interviewing?

A. "Many patients with drug addiction have a history of traumatic experiences. Have you ever witnessed a horrifying incident or been a victim of violence or abuse?"
B. "Perhaps you use marijuana because you cannot tolerate negative emotions."
C. "Marijuana can reduce motivation; it seems like it is really holding back your life."
D. "Clearly, marijuana is making your symptoms worse, but you still are resistant to stopping it. What do you make of that?"
E. "So you'd like to stop using because of how it is holding you back professionally, but you find yourself really paralyzed by anxiety, and marijuana seems to be the only thing you've tried that has ever helped with it?"

27.4   What is the *most* important difference between motivational enhancement (ME) and contingency management (CM) interventions for substance use disorders?

A. ME interventions do not provide rewards for abstinence from drugs or alcohol.
B. ME interventions are ineffective for opioid use disorders.
C. ME interventions seek to elaborate internal motivations or contingencies that are self-sustaining.
D. The benefits of ME interventions are relatively constant over time.
E. ME interventions are only effective for drug users in the precontemplation stage.

27.5   Screening, Brief Intervention, and Referral to Treatment (SBIRT) interventions for hazardous alcohol use may be *less* effective for which of the following subgroups of the general population?

A. Patients in a primary care clinic.
B. Women.
C. Dual-diagnosis patients.
D. Patients in general practice settings.
E. Adolescents.

CHAPTER 28

Twelve-Step Facilitation

An Adaptation for Psychiatric Practitioners and Patients

28.1   A 35-year-old patient in treatment for social phobia recently reveals his long history of heavy alcohol use (as many as eight drinks per drinking day, 3–4 days per week). He started attending Alcoholics Anonymous (AA) meetings two or three times per week. He reports that he struggles to engage in the sessions and feels like the other attendees' problems are "way more serious" than the difficulties he has experienced as a result of drinking. What is the *best next step* to take with this patient?

   A. Start the patient on gabapentin to augment the pharmacological treatment of his social phobia.
   B. Confront the patient about his minimization of his alcoholism and how it reduces his chances for recovery.
   C. Re-explore the patient's current motivation to achieve sobriety and help to identify obstacles to feeling comfortable in the 12-step setting.
   D. Provide education about AA, including that participants are not required to speak during meetings.
   E. Emphasize the importance to the patient of identifying an AA sponsor to help him deal with the difficulties he is experiencing at meetings.

28.2   A 22-year-old patient who identifies as an atheist has attended a few Alcoholics Anonymous (AA) meetings to address his severe alcohol abuse but is concerned about their incorporation of spirituality and use of the word "God," because he feels this is inconsistent with his own beliefs. What would be the best intervention to make next?

   A. "The experience from many years in AA is that without a spiritual awakening, people aren't really able to quit drinking for good."
   B. "If you feel that it is too big a stumbling block, we can try to find a meeting with people who have the same questions about this that you do."
   C. "This model has really worked for people; you should trust the people there who have been able to stop drinking."

D. "It's not meant to be taken literally; think of it as a symbol for your struggle to quit drinking."

E. "You seem resistant to thinking about what has been happening in your life in a different way even though you haven't been able to stop drinking on your own."

28.3 A 36-year-old woman with a severe alcohol use disorder and bipolar I disorder (three past hospitalizations for mania) has started attending Alcoholics Anonymous (AA) meetings. She is trying to identify a sponsor. Which of the following traits in a sponsor might be most beneficial for this patient?

A. A sponsor with a co-occurring psychiatric disorder.
B. A sponsor with many years of sobriety and experience in AA.
C. A sponsor willing to regularly speak with you about the patient by phone.
D. A sponsor with similar sociodemographic characteristics to the patient.
E. A sponsor who continues to attend meetings at a high frequency.

28.4 Which of the following is the primary goal of 12-step facilitation (TSF) for patients struggling with substance abuse?

A. To explore past traumas that might affect current substance use.
B. To replace 12-step group treatment for patients who cannot tolerate a group setting.
C. To facilitate attendance and productive utilization of 12-step meetings.
D. To illustrate the role of using substances in self-medicating psychiatric symptoms of participating patients.
E. To address the shortcomings of the 12-step model as regards the management of co-occurring psychiatric illness.

28.5 A 44-year-old man with a 4-month history of depression and alcohol dependence has been attending Alcoholics Anonymous (AA) meetings two or three times per month. He stopped going to meetings, citing his continued drinking as evidence that "meetings don't work." What would be the most appropriate response to this patient?

A. "AA isn't for everybody; people tend to know soon whether it will work for them or not."
B. "This shows that you need more intensive treatment for your drinking."
C. "I won't continue to treat you if you don't make a commitment to abstinence."
D. "Maybe the real issue is your depression leading you to drink."
E. "You're right, you've continued to drink despite going to some meetings, but it seems like it has been difficult to attend meetings at the frequency that might really help you."

CHAPTER 29

Contingency Management

29.1 The parents of a 17-year-old high school student who lives with them want to address his marijuana use through contingency management (CM). Which CM intervention is most effective to help curb this patient's marijuana use?

    A. Home drug testing and rewarding negative test results with gift certificates.

    B. Drug testing in a specialized laboratory and rewarding negative test results with gift certificates.

    C. Contingent upon positive test results, sending a deterrent letter to the patient's school stating that he will withdraw from school because he is a "junkie."

    D. Paying $10 cash for every negative test result.

    E. Confronting the patient about the negative consequences of his marijuana use.

29.2 What is an effective target of contingency management (CM) treatment as demonstrated by research studies?

    A. Doing homework assignments in cognitive-behavioral therapy (CBT).

    B. Looking for a job.

    C. Finding a sober friend.

    D. Entering treatment.

    E. Going to an Alcoholics Anonymous meeting.

29.3 What learning principle best applies to contingency management (CM) interventions?

    A. Intermittent reinforcement.

    B. Negative reinforcement.

    C. Positive reinforcement.

    D. Aversive conditioning.

    E. Response substitution.

29.4 Which substance use disorder is most suitable for contingency management (CM) intervention?

    A. Cocaine, because there currently is no specific pharmacotherapy.
    B. Alcohol, because the monitored administration of disulfiram (Antabuse) introduces a specific contingency between drinking and an immediate negative consequence.
    C. Nicotine, because in contrast to other substance use disorders, there are only limited immediate severe negative consequences to smoking cigarettes; introducing voucher incentives immediately contingent upon nonsmoking is therefore particularly effective in smoking cessation.
    D. Marijuana, because the teenage onset of this disorder sets the particularly favorable stage for CM intervention of the patient's home and family milieu as settings of incentives of drug abstinence.
    E. CM is an evidence-based effective treatment for a variety of substance use disorders, including stimulants, alcohol, nicotine, and marijuana.

29.5 A company decides to adopt a contingency management (CM) strategy to curb alcohol use among its employees. Given that most employees who drink alcohol also smoke cigarettes, which is the best target for the CM intervention?

    A. Alcohol, because there is no clinically significant relationship between alcohol use and smoking cigarettes.
    B. Abstinence from all substances to avoid *substitution,* namely, increased smoking to compensate for stopping drinking.
    C. Abstinence from all substances, which is the usual recommendation, despite lack of clear research evidence.
    D. Smoking, because smoking and drinking are related and smoking cessation is the easier-to-achieve goal given the current climate of laws against smoking and the presence of smoking detectors.
    E. CM interventions of substance use disorders are ineffective in company settings because of conflicting interests, including patient confidentiality and employees' fear of repercussion due to treatment failure.

CHAPTER 30

Network Therapy

30.1 Which of the following is most likely to contribute to the effectiveness of network therapy in the treatment of substance use disorders?

  A. Resolution of conflicts in the patient's interpersonal relationships.
  B. Confrontation of the patient's addiction by concerned relatives and friends.
  C. Education of network members about substance use disorders to better understand and help the patient.
  D. Intervention by therapist and network members to facilitate treatment engagement.
  E. The availability of greater social supports to the patient.

30.2 What psychotherapeutic treatment modality best characterizes network therapy?

  A. Group therapy.
  B. Family therapy.
  C. Individual therapy.
  D. Twelve-step facilitation.
  E. Intervention.

30.3 What is a contraindication for network therapy for alcohol use disorder?

  A. Unwillingness to stop drinking.
  B. Inability to stop drinking.
  C. Inability to comply with outpatient detoxification.
  D. Simultaneous attendance of Alcoholics Anonymous meetings.
  E. Unwillingness to accept reduced controlled drinking ("harm reduction") as treatment goal.

30.4 What is an important difference between network therapy and group therapy for substance use disorders?

  A. Network members network outside therapy sessions; group members do not.
  B. Groups, but not networks, have a therapist.
  C. Group members use the group therapy sessions for their own treatment; network members do not use the network for their own treatment.

D. Group sessions take place in the therapist's office; network sessions take place in the patient's home.

E. Reduced controlled drinking (harm reduction) is a treatment goal in network therapy but not in group therapy.

30.5 Which other treatment modality is not combined with network therapy?

A. Cognitive-behavioral therapy (CBT), because cognitive therapy is too technical for network members.

B. Contingency management (CM), because network members cannot be expected to provide incentives for abstinence to the patient.

C. Twelve-step facilitation (TSF), because this is self-help treatment rather than professional help.

D. An intervention, because the role of network members is to support the patient in achieving abstinence, not to confront the patient's unwillingness to go into treatment.

E. Motivational enhancement (ME), because network therapy is not effective if patients are ambivalent.

CHAPTER 31

Group Therapy

31.1 Which of the following is true about group therapy in patients with substance use disorders (SUDs)?

A. Group therapy is primarily used in inpatient and residential settings.
B. Group therapy is only indicated for patients without co-occurring psychiatric disorders.
C. Group therapy may be problematic for use in managed care settings.
D. Group therapy is not helpful for the symptoms and adverse effects that are the consequences of substance abuse.
E. Group psychotherapy is the psychosocial treatment of choice for most patients with SUDs.

31.2 Which of the following is *not* true about the etiology and treatment of substance use disorders (SUDs)?

A. SUDs are rarely familial.
B. Cultural factors such as ethnic identification are important to address in treatment.
C. Substance abuse groups deal with many domains, including developmental, medical, and sociocultural.
D. The etiology of SUDs is multifactorial.
E. Group psychotherapy may include both cognitive-behavioral therapy (CBT) and relapse prevention.

31.3 Which of the following statements is *not* true about patient selection for group therapy for substance use disorders (SUDs)?

A. Significant cognitive deficits are a contraindication.
B. Patients with severe antisocial personality disorder require a specialized group structure.
C. Preparatory sessions are not necessary before group entry to assess suitability.
D. In general, suicidal or homicidal patients are not suitable for group therapy.
E. Acute psychotic illness is a contraindication.

31.4   Which of the following statements about successful group leaders is *incorrect*?

A. Role of the group leader is active within the group process.
B. Successful leader attributes include compassion, empathy, and a sense of humor.
C. Most of group content is focused on early childhood-parental dynamics.
D. Leader techniques include supportive confrontation and the creation of an empathic holding environment.
E. Integrity and humility are critical leader attributes.

31.5   Which of the following statements about different types of groups is *incorrect*?

A. Self-help and 12-step groups are a core part of group therapy for addiction.
B. Several models emphasize progression of group members from one phase of treatment to the next.
C. Groups often include a cognitive-behavioral focus.
D. Longer duration of groups predict increased abstinence.
E. Group therapy for substance use disorders (SUDs) is primarily employed in residential settings.

CHAPTER 32

Family Therapy

32.1 Several large-scale studies have determined which factor to be the predominant influence in getting individuals with substance use disorders to seek treatment?

A. Legal mandate.
B. Family pressure.
C. Primary medical doctor.
D. Pressure from employer.
E. Financial concerns.

32.2 What family treatment model applies strategic-structural-behavioral–based (SSBB) methods with additional focus regarding systems external to the family, such as the school, legal, employment, mental health, and health system realms?

A. Multidimensional Family Therapy (MDFT).
B. Functional Family Therapy (FFT).
C. Transitional Family Therapy (TFT).
D. Brief Strategic Family Therapy (BSFT).
E. INternational CAnnabis Need for Treatment (INCANT).

32.3 In addition to supporting abstinence via a *daily sobriety contract*, what is the other main component of Behavioral Couples Therapy (BCT)?

A. Focusing on systems external to the couple.
B. Conducting therapy in the family home.
C. Taking an intergenerational approach.
D. Using relationship-focused interventions.
E. Employing enactment (i.e., practicing a new behavior within session).

32.4 In strategic-structural-behavioral–based (SSBB) models, the term *reframing* is used to describe what therapeutic process?

A. Determining what resources may be called upon to effect positive change in a family.
B. Altering family interactions to that keep the family and identified patient from making significant change.

C. Practicing a new pattern of behavior within session.

D. Forming therapeutic alliances.

E. Redefining a problem or dysfunctional pattern in a more positive way.

32.5   The role of genetics is thought to be most pronounced in which substance use disorder?

A. Marijuana.

B. Opiates.

C. Alcohol.

D. Cocaine.

E. Amphetamines.

CHAPTER 33

Inpatient Treatment

33.1 Why is it recommended that patients with co-occurring substance use disorders (SUDs) and psychiatric disorders receive treatment in an integrated inpatient setting?

    A. There is less stigmatization.
    B. It provides better cost containment.
    C. It reduces treatment dropout rates.
    D. It is generally more effective.
    E. There are better patient satisfaction ratings.

33.2 What are the defining characteristics of the Minnesota Model?

    A. Structured cognitive-behavioral therapy (CBT) and relapse prevention techniques.
    B. A medical model of addiction and significant physician involvement.
    C. 12-step philosophy and many counselors who are in recovery themselves.
    D. An algorithm for medical detoxification of alcohol and opioid use disorders.
    E. A contingency management (CM) program where patients earn increasing responsibility.

33.3 What is the evidence base regarding the outcome of inpatient treatment?

    A. Several randomized controlled trials found abstinence rates of 50%–60%.
    B. Several uncontrolled studies found abstinence rates ranging from 25% to 60%.
    C. No randomized controlled studies have been done, and so no estimate can be made.
    D. Several case-control cohorts found abstinence rates ranging from 25% to 60%.
    E. Case reports and anecdotal data indicate abstinence rates ranging from 50% to 60%.

33.4 Studies have shown that individuals who are married, educated, employed full-time and who have strong family support tend to have a better prognosis after inpatient treatment. You are seeing a 24-year-old single female cocaine user who does not have good family support. She has been unable to stop using cocaine despite intensive outpatient treatment. How should her demographic data influence your decision to recommend an inpatient treatment setting?

A. Strongly—you should not recommend inpatient treatment because she is unlikely to have a good outcome.

B. Strongly—you should not recommend inpatient treatment because she lacks the social support necessary to ensure adherence to aftercare.

C. Strongly—you should not recommend inpatient treatment because she is young and therefore less likely to agree with the program's philosophy.

D. Not at all—you should recommend inpatient treatment because she has been unable to stop using in a less restrictive setting.

E. Not at all—you should recommend inpatient treatment because she does not have good family support.

33.5 What has integrating employment into treatment, such as an employer mandating an employee to treatment, been shown to improve?

A. Substance-related outcomes.
B. Work-related outcomes.
C. Substance- and work-related outcomes.
D. Substance-related outcomes but not work-related outcomes.
E. Work-related outcomes but not substance-related outcomes.

CHAPTER 34

Therapeutic Communities

34.1 The therapeutic community (TC) approach has been summarized by the phrase "community as method." What does this mean?

A. Staff members act as "rational authorities" to establish standards for communal living and interdependence.
B. The primary therapeutic modality is group therapy sessions, which are led by staff and peers in recovery.
C. Individuals learn to use the activities and elements of the community as a vehicle for self-change.
D. A community of staff and peers creates a framework to transform negative conditioned responses into positive responses.
E. Individuals are provided with basic essentials and a social structure so they can concentrate on recovery.

34.2 What are the four interrelated areas upon which the therapeutic community (TC) perspective is built?

A. Personhood, social learning theory, vocational therapy, and self-help groups.
B. Self-help groups, staff as role models, peer guidance, social hierarchy.
C. The social context, the family structure, the disease model, the moral model.
D. Personality structure, the substance use disorder, coping skills, social support.
E. The substance use disorder, the individual, the recovery process, right living.

34.3 Both peers and staff can act as role models in a therapeutic community (TC). What are two main concepts that illustrate the therapeutic approach of these role models?

A. Role models organize therapeutic-educative activities and manage privileges.
B. Role models set expectations and assess how individuals are progressing.
C. Role models reinforce social hierarchy and act as one-on-one counselors.
D. Role models "act as if" and display responsible concern.
E. Role models confront individuals and mediate conflicts.

34.4 What characteristics are commonly found in substance abusers enrolled in a therapeutic community (TC)?

A. Absence of conflict with family members.
B. Significant psychosocial dysfunction.
C. Some college education and a history of employment.
D. Relatively minor legal history.
E. Lack of psychiatric comorbidity.

34.5 What has been a consistent research finding among therapeutic community (TC)
participants?

A. Longer retention in treatment is correlated with better posttreatment outcomes.
B. Treatment completion shows no improvement in employment.
C. Participation in a TC does not alter criminal activity.
D. TCs are an effective and cost-effective treatment for all substance abusers.
E. Enrollment alone in a TC is correlated with improved psychosocial functioning.

CHAPTER 3 5

Community-Based Treatment

35.1 A 22-year-old man is referred to the CPEP (comprehensive psychiatric emergency program) at 1 A.M. on Saturday morning by the emergency department attending after having been evaluated for right wrist pain. He fell down a flight of subway steps, fracturing his wrist. He states that he had gone out drinking that evening and "got wasted" after consuming about four beers and three shots of liquor over the course of the evening. He reports his tolerance was lower than he expected. He minimizes the extent of his injury because he has fractured his nondominant hand and reports that he typically doesn't drink this much and only "parties like this" about every other month. What is the *next best* clinical step regarding this patient's alcohol use?

    A. Recommend inpatient detox because of his excessive consumption.
    B. Assess for at-risk drinking behavior.
    C. Assess for an alcohol use disorder.
    D. Refer client to the closest Alcoholics Anonymous (AA) meeting held that Sunday morning in his neighborhood.
    E. Provide patient with a follow-up appointment at an outpatient substance abuse clinic.

35.2 What is an important first step in a brief intervention for at-risk drinkers who are ambivalent about stopping their use?

    A. Admission to inpatient detox.
    B. Insisting on attending specialized treatment.
    C. Referral to 12-step recovery program.
    D. Allying with the patient in setting goals and agreeing on a plan.
    E. Referral to a 28-day alcohol rehabilitation center.

35.3 What was the clinical significance of CASASARD?

    A. Intensive case management (ICM) clients were significantly more likely to have completed treatment, be abstinent from substances, and be employed than those who received the usual screening and referral to treatment.

B. Drug courts showed significant reduction in drug and alcohol use and improved family relationships.

C. Brief motivational interviewing techniques increase tobacco quit rates 2%–8% as compared with brief advice.

D. In substance-abusing individuals, approaches using therapeutic communities, psychosocial rehabilitation, 12-step program, and enhancement of supportive relationships are all successful.

E. Adding a family-based treatment component to a family treatment drug courts (FTDC) program has also been shown to improve the chances that an at-risk child will remain in the family.

35.4   An individual with severe alcohol disease and multiple DWIs (driving while intoxicated) has been referred to a drug treatment court. What outcome can this individual most likely expect?

A. Regularly scheduled weekly or twice-weekly urine drug screens.

B. Judicial hearings every 6 months.

C. Gifts for negative urine toxicologies.

D. Referral to a program expected to last 3–4 years.

E. An interlock device that must be worn to monitor blood alcohol concentration (BAC).

35.5   You are evaluating a married 32-year-old woman, currently employed full-time as an administrative assistant for treatment services, after three of her close friends and supportive husband have called to express concern regarding her drug and alcohol use. She has cocaine and an alcohol use disorder. According to guidelines published by the American Society of Addiction Medicine, your patient requires intensive outpatient treatment. What type of service meets these criteria?

A. A program that requires 20 hours of intensive outpatient services.

B. A program that requires 9 hours of intensive outpatient services.

C. A partial hospitalization program, because she has both an alcohol use disorder and a cocaine use disorder.

D. Twelve-step recovery meetings without any other substance abuse treatment, because of her full-time employment.

E. A program with more immediate access to medical and psychiatric services.

CHAPTER 36

History of Alcoholics Anonymous and the Experiences of Patients

36.1 As of 2011, what is the most common means of referral to Alcoholics Anonymous (AA)?

A. Self-referral.
B. Referral by a health care provider.
C. Referral by another AA member.
D. Referral by court order.
E. Referral by family.

36.2 According to the latest Alcoholics Anonymous (AA) survey, what is the most common length of sobriety among AA members?

A. Not sober and actively drinking.
B. Less than 1 year of sobriety.
C. 1–5 years of sobriety.
D. 5–10 years of sobriety.
E. More than 10 years of sobriety.

36.3 During an Alcoholics Anonymous (AA) meeting, a member tells his story to the group in attendance, putting emphasis on the effect of alcohol in his life, how he got sober, and what he is doing now to stay sober. What type of AA meeting was this member most likely attending?

A. Speaker meeting.
B. Step meeting.
C. Discussion meeting.
D. Open meeting.
E. Closed meeting.

36.4   Which of the following is one of the 12 steps of Alcoholics Anonymous (AA)?

A. The only requirement for AA membership is a desire to stop drinking.
B. Anonymity is the spiritual foundation of all our traditions.
C. We admitted we were powerless over alcohol.
D. Our common welfare should come first.
E. Every AA group ought to be fully self-supporting.

36.5   Which of the following is a common personal reaction to Alcoholics Anonymous (AA) that deters participation?

A. "I'm afraid I won't be able to get sober."
B. "I don't want to speak up in groups."
C. "I'd rather do this on my own."
D. "I can't identify with that group."
E. "I'm afraid of being judged."

CHAPTER 37

Psychological Mechanisms in Alcoholics Anonymous

37.1 Which 12-step cognition at the end of 12-step therapy treatment significantly predicts increased abstinence at 12-month follow-up?

A. Powerlessness over alcohol.
B. Belief in loss of control over drinking.
C. Belief in a higher power.
D. Disease attribution.
E. Commitment to Alcoholics Anonymous (AA) and to abstinence.

37.2 According to Project MATCH, how did the rates of abstinence at 12-month follow-up differ among patients assigned to cognitive-behavioral therapy (CBT), motivational enhancement therapy (MET), and 12-step facilitation (TSF)?

A. CBT clients reported the highest rate of abstinence.
B. MET clients reported the highest rate of abstinence.
C. TSF clients reported the highest rate of abstinence.
D. TSF clients reported higher rates of abstinence relative to CBT clients but not to MET clients.
E. None of the groups reported a significant higher rate of abstinence relative to the other two groups.

37.3 Which cognitive shift did patients who participated in 12-step therapy have in common with those who underwent cognitive-behavioral therapy (CBT) according to the Finney et al. (1998) study?

A. Endorsement of the disease model of alcoholism.
B. Alcoholic identity.
C. Goal of abstinence.
D. Self-efficacy to remain abstinent.
E. Increase in positive expectancies surrounding the use of substances.

37.4 Which specific psychological mechanism is one of the most important and well-studied causal mechanisms explaining substance use behavior change among 12-step program members?

A. Self-efficacy.
B. Acquiring a sponsor.
C. Spirituality.
D. Powerlessness over alcohol.
E. Motivation for drinking reduction.

37.5 Increased Alcoholics Anonymous (AA) attendance has been associated with reduction in which of the following negative affect states?

A. Anger.
B. Resentment.
C. Depression.
D. Selfishness.
E. Narcissism.

37.6 Which of the following is *not* true of the research regarding Alcoholics Anonymous (AA) and spirituality?

A. In Project MATCH, 27.6% of outpatient clients who attended AA meetings during the 12 weeks of treatment reported having had a spiritual awakening as a result of their AA attendance.
B. Spirituality is uniformly discussed in mainstream AA meetings regardless of differences in perceived AA group social dynamics.
C. Spirituality is measured by asking only about the extent that God is discussed in meetings.
D. Exposure to AA is associated with increased spirituality.
E. Gains in spiritual practices among AA members are a significant predictor of later abstinence.

37.7 A practitioner should consider *not* adopting which of the following measures in clinical practice with substance abusing patients?

A. Develop familiarity with the *Alcoholics Anonymous* text ("big book").
B. Experience firsthand the environment and fellowship of Alcoholics Anonymous (AA) by attending several closed meetings.
C. Routinely assess patients' prior experience with self-help groups.
D. Negotiate AA attendance at several meetings for some patients.
E. Develop strategies that entail arranging for a current AA member to speak with the patient and arrange to take the patient to a meeting.

CHAPTER 38

Outcomes Research on Twelve-Step Programs

38.1 Which of the following statements regarding 12-step mutual-help organizations (MHOs) is true?

A. There is extensive randomized-control trial evidence to support their efficacy.
B. They extend the benefits of professionally delivered treatment for substance use disorders.
C. The magnitude of benefit is significantly lower than that achieved with professional intervention efforts.
D. People with dual diagnoses are unlikely to benefit from attendance.
E. They are most beneficial as a short-term adjunct to outpatient professional intervention efforts.

38.2 Twelve-step facilitation is a professionally delivered intervention designed to support engagement with 12-step mutual-help organizations (MHOs) such as Alcoholics Anonymous (AA). Which of the following patient characteristics is most important to consider when deciding whether to provide a standard or intensive referral to a 12-step group?

A. Age.
B. Gender.
C. Spiritual beliefs.
D. Prior experience with 12-step groups.
E. Comorbid psychiatric diagnosis.

38.3 Which cognitive 12-step mutual-help organization (MHO) mechanism of change is most strongly associated with recovery in adolescents?

A. Enhanced self-efficacy.
B. Identifying coping strategies.
C. Motivation for abstinence.
D. Increased religiosity.
E. Reduction in anger.

38.4 Twelve-step mutual-help organization (MHO) participation has been associated with which of the following?

A. Increased health care costs.
B. Increased patient reliance on professional services.
C. An abstinence rate one-third lower than that achieved by patients treated in cognitive-behavioral therapy (CBT) programs.
D. Improved outcomes in adults, but not in adolescents.
E. Helping individuals change their social networks in support of recovery.

38.5 A 56-year-old man is convicted of driving under the influence and ordered to attend Alcoholics Anonymous (AA) as a requirement of sentencing. He drinks 7–10 alcoholic beverages per week and has no prior arrests for driving while intoxicated. Which of the following aspects of AA is most likely to be helpful to this person's recovery?

A. Increase in spiritual practices.
B. Increased confidence in ability to abstain in high-risk social situations in which alcohol is present.
C. Decreasing self-efficacy.
D. Increased ability to cope with negative affect.
E. Helping patients maintain current social networks.

CHAPTER 39

Women and Addiction

39.1 How prevalent are substance use disorders (SUDs) in women as compared with men?

A. The prevalence of SUDs is the same for men and women.
B. The prevalence of SUDs is higher in women as compared with men.
C. The prevalence of SUDs is higher in men as compared with women.
D. The prevalence of SUDs is higher in men only for certain substances.
E. The prevalence of SUDs is higher in women only for certain substances.

39.2 Which psychiatric comorbidity is more likely to occur in men with substance use disorders (SUDs) than in women?

A. Anxiety.
B. Depression.
C. Eating disorders.
D. Borderline personality disorder.
E. Attention-deficit/hyperactivity disorder.

39.3 What is the "telescoping" effect of substance use disorders (SUDs) in women?

A. Women have significantly more medical, psychiatric, and adverse social consequences as a result of their addiction.
B. Women advance more slowly than men from initial substance use to regular substance use.
C. Women have generally fewer years and smaller quantities of use at treatment entry and therefore have less severe disorders.
D. Women appear less vulnerable than men to the development of adverse medical consequences of addiction.
E. Women and men have very similar courses of SUD illness progression.

39.4   What is the relationship between temporal onset of substance use disorders (SUDs) and comorbid psychiatric disorders in women?

A. Women rarely have a primary mental health disorder that precedes the onset of an SUD.
B. Women with major depressive disorder are less likely than men to develop alcohol dependence.
C. Women usually develop SUD and other psychiatric disorders concurrently.
D. Women receiving treatment for SUDs are likely to have histories of physical or sexual abuse.
E. Women with eating disorders are unlikely to go to develop a SUD.

39.5   What is an important consideration in the treatment of women with substance use disorders (SUDs)?

A. Women-focused treatments have better outcomes.
B. Pharmacological treatments lead to better outcomes in women.
C. Addressing psychiatric comorbidities leads to better outcomes.
D. Pregnant women should not receive pharmacological treatments.
E. Sociocultural factors are not frequently barriers to treatment.

CHAPTER 40

Perinatal Substance Use Disorders

40.1 Which common psychiatric disorder or medical condition has the highest prevalence rate during pregnancy?

A. Depression.
B. Gestational diabetes.
C. Preeclampsia.
D. Tobacco use.
E. Alcohol use.

40.2 Among all drugs of misuse, which ones have the most conclusive evidence indicating that prenatal exposure results in negative maternal, fetal, and later development outcomes?

A. Alcohol and tobacco.
B. Cannabinoids and cannabis.
C. Hallucinogens and cocaine.
D. Inhalants and amphetamines.
E. Illicit and prescription opioids.

40.3 What treatment is recommended, because of its efficacy and safety profile, for treatment of nicotine use disorder in pregnant women?

A. Nicotine replacement transdermal (NRT) patch.
B. Voucher-based reinforcement therapy.
C. Nicotine replacement inhalers.
D. Bupropion.
E. Varenicline.

40.4   What is the appropriate recommendation to give to a pregnant woman using opioids regarding breastfeeding her baby?

   A. Women using opioids should try to stop using all substances cold turkey and not be placed on agonist therapy.
   B. Breastfeeding is prohibited for women using prescribed opioids.
   C. Breastfeeding is recommended for opioid-agonist–maintained women who are not using other drugs, unless there are medical contraindications.
   D. Pregnant women with opioid use disorders should be treated with the opioid antagonist naltrexone.
   E. Pregnant women with opioid use disorders are not eligible for treatment with buprenorphine.

40.5   Exposure to which substance during pregnancy typically does *not* produce neonatal abstinence syndrome (NAS) or a formal withdrawal syndrome in newborns?

   A. Percocet.
   B. Methadone.
   C. Fluoxetine.
   D. Nicotine.
   E. Methamphetamine.

CHAPTER 41

Adolescent Substance Use Disorders: Epidemiology, Neurobiology, and Screening

41.1 Current use of which illicit substance has been increasing among adolescents, after a prior period of decline?

A. Cocaine.
B. Heroin.
C. Marijuana.
D. Nicotine.
E. Phencyclidine (PCP).

41.2 Developmental patterns in which brain regions lead to particular vulnerability for substance use disorders during adolescence?

A. Curvilinear development of the striatum.
B. Linear development of the striatum.
C. Curvilinear development in the prefrontal cortex.
D. Linear development of the sensory and motor cortices.
E. Neuronal pruning in the sensory and motor cortices.

41.3 Which of the following screening tools for substance use disorders has low sensitivity in adolescents?

A. Screening, brief intervention, and referral to treatment (SBIRT).
B. Alcohol Use Disorders Identification Test (AUDIT).
C. Problem Oriented Screening Instrument for Teenagers (POSIT).
D. CRAFFT (mnemonic acronym for key words **C**ar, **R**elax, **A**lone, **F**orget, **F**riends, and **T**rouble).
E. CAGE questionnaire.

41.4 What is the relationship between adolescent report of substance use, parental report, and urine drug screens?

A. Greater than 95% of youths reporting no cannabis use will have negative urine toxicology.
B. Less than 50% of youths reporting cannabis use have positive urine toxicology.
C. Greater than 99% of teens reporting cannabis use will have positive urine toxicology.
D. Parent reports are more consistent with results of urine toxicology than youth reports.
E. Greater than 50% of youths reporting no cannabis use will have positive urine toxicology.

41.5 Which of the following questions is included in the CRAFFT screening interview for substance use disorders in teens?

A. Have you ever been in a car crash when the driver was intoxicated?
B. Do you ever use alcohol or drugs to relax, feel better about yourself, or fit in?
C. Do you use alcohol or drugs at social gatherings or parties?
D. Are you concerned that anyone in your family is using too much alcohol or drugs?
E. Did you ever forget to do something after using alcohol or drugs?

CHAPTER 4 2

Adolescent Substance Use Disorders: Transition to Substance Abuse, Prevention, and Treatment

42.1 What percentage of adolescents who use cannabis progress to use of additional illicit substances?

A. 5%.
B. 10%.
C. 25%.
D. 50%.
E. 66%.

42.2 Drug abuse prevention programs that limit drug use during which developmental period are most likely to lead to long-term beneficial effects?

A. 10–13 years.
B. 14–17 years.
C. 18–21 years.
D. 22–25 years.
E. 26–29 years.

42.3 What strategy has been shown to be most effective in reducing alcohol and drug consumption in teens?

A. Enhancing public advisory campaigns.
B. Increasing cost.
C. Intensifying legal consequences.
D. Mandating school-based educational programs.
E. Implementing self-esteem building programs.

42.4 Of the treatment modalities studied for substance use disorders in the Cannabis Youth Treatment Study (Dennis et al. 2004), which modality was associated with a significantly different outcome than the other modalities?

A. Motivational enhancement was found to be effective only when followed by 10 cognitive-behavioral therapy (CBT) sessions.
B. Individual CBT without a family psychoeducational intervention was ineffective.
C. The 12-session individual community reinforcement approach led to no significant reduction in rates of cannabis abuse.
D. The 12-week family therapy was the only condition that was followed by sustained results.
E. Multidimensional family therapy was almost three times more expensive than the other treatment modalities included in the study.

42.5 What is a limiting factor in most studies on treatment outcomes in substance use disorders in teens?

A. Treatment outcomes tend to focus on completion of programs rather than maintenance of gains.
B. Treatment outcomes are limited by lack of appropriate research participants.
C. Treatment outcomes are limited by difficulty consenting minors to participate in research.
D. Low relapse rates lead to low power in treatment outcome studies.
E. Poor availability of effective interventions for the adolescent population limit treatment outcome studies.

42.6 What is the primary rationale for determining whether to include aftercare in the treatment plan for adolescents following the completion of a substance abuse treatment program?

A. Aftercare interventions do not affect outcomes if the treatment program was effective.
B. Multiple aftercare personal sessions are required to maximize treatment outcomes.
C. Poor treatment responders are unlikely to benefit from further aftercare interventions.
D. Brief phone aftercare intervention is as efficacious as individual aftercare sessions.
E. Targeting aftercare to teens who relapse is an economical strategy to ration limited resources.

CHAPTER 43

Psychiatric Consultation in Pain and Addiction

43.1 Which of the following risk assessment screeners is most helpful in predicting which patients will ultimately be discharged form opioid treatment because of aberrant drug-related behaviors?

A. Screener and Opioid Assessment for Patients With Pain—Revised (SOAPP-R).
B. Pain Medication Questionnaire (PMQ).
C. Opioid Risk Tool (ORT).
D. Semistructured clinical interview by a psychologist trained in assessing aberrant behavior in the chronic pain patient.
E. DSM criteria for substance use disorder.

43.2 A chronic pain management specialist discovers that his patient is chewing controlled-release morphine. Which of the following is the most likely explanation for this behavior?

A. The patient is experiencing inadequate pain relief.
B. The patient is abusing the morphine for reasons other than pain relief.
C. The patient has run out of medication and is trying to make his pills last longer by breaking them into smaller pieces.
D. The patient is borrowing medication from someone else.
E. The patient is attempting to justify the continued use of morphine to his physician.

43.3 A psychiatrist is treating a patient with chronic back pain, which is treated by a pain practitioner with opioids. The psychiatrist prescribes benzodiazepines on an as-needed basis for anxiety. The psychiatrist drafts a treatment agreement with the patient stating that requests for benzodiazepine refills may not occur over the phone. Which of the following terms best describes this therapeutic technique?

A. Interval dispensing.
B. Risk assessment.
C. Boundary setting.

D. Contingency dispensing.

E. Collaboration with pain practitioner.

43.4 Which of the following is a common feature in the care of patients who are ultimately referred to a mental health professional for assessment of aberrant drug-related behavior?

A. A clear pain diagnosis with workable pain differential.

B. Formal risk assessment, including detailed personal and family drug and alcohol history.

C. Presence of numerous prior treatment agreements.

D. Problems with limits and boundary settings associated with the original prescription of controlled substances.

E. Lack of patient concern around symptom relief.

43.5 Which of the following is an appropriate action for the prescriber to take when a patient disagrees about the quantity of controlled substances to be dispensed?

A. Clear communication and documentation of the prescriber's reasoning.

B. Prescription of whatever the patient requests in order to reduce discomfort at all costs.

C. Revision of the treatment agreement in order to facilitate the patient's request.

D. Immediate and complete elimination of the use of controlled substances.

E. Omission of this disagreement from the medical record in order to protect the patient from legal ramifications.

CHAPTER 44

Prevention of Prescription Drug Abuse

44.1 Which prescription drug or class of drugs was most abused among twelfth-grade students?

    A. Adderall.
    B. Vicodin.
    C. Dextromethorphan-containing cough medications.
    D. Tranquilizers.
    E. Sedatives.

44.2 Which class of prescription drugs is most commonly abused among persons age 12 and older?

    A. Analgesics.
    B. Tranquilizers.
    C. Stimulants.
    D. Sedatives.
    E. Cough medications.

44.3 In which age group are females more likely to have abused prescription drugs relative to males?

    A. Adolescents (ages 12–17).
    B. Young adults (ages 12–25).
    C. Adults (ages 26–45).
    D. Middle-aged adults (ages 45–65).
    E. Older adults (ages 65 and older).

44.4 What is the strongest predictor of opioid misuse in chronic pain patients?

    A. Age.
    B. Gender.
    C. Disability.

D. Measures of socioeconomic status.

E. Previous alcohol or cocaine abuse.

44.5   In treatment samples studied, how do heroin abusers differ from prescription opioid abusers?

A. Heroin abusers have higher levels of benzodiazepine use.

B. Heroin abusers have higher levels of depression.

C. Heroin abusers have lower levels of chronic pain.

D. Heroin abusers are more likely to be involved in psychiatric treatment.

E. Heroin abusers have fewer family problems and less income from illegal sources.

44.6   Which prescription stimulant is most commonly abused by students?

A. Adderall.

B. Ritalin.

C. Concerta.

D. Metadate.

E. Strattera.

44.7   How do individuals who engage in nonmedical use of prescription stimulants differ from those who engage in nonprescription use of opioids?

A. Increased abuse of stimulants is associated with the increase in prescribing of stimulants, whereas increased abuse of opioids is not associated with increased prescribing of opioids.

B. There is a perception that because prescription stimulants are medical substances they are safe, whereas this perception does not exist for prescription opioids.

C. Abuse of prescription stimulants may be particularly apparent in friends and peers of persons with attention-deficit/hyperactivity disorder (ADHD), because of diversion, rather than in individuals with the disorder themselves, as occurs with opioids.

D. Abuse of prescription stimulants is concentrated in older adults, whereas abuse of prescription opioids is mostly concentrated in adolescents and young adults.

E. There are no gender differences associated with abuse of prescription stimulants, whereas there are well-documented gender differences in the abuse of opioids.

44.8   Which strategy to combat prescription drug abuse has the most limited data to suggest efficacy in reducing harm from prescription drug abuse?

A. Family-based drug abuse prevention approaches.

B. Treatment for addiction, such as buprenorphine for opioid addiction.

C. Community distribution of naloxone to high-risk individuals and interested friends and family members.

D. Take-back programs for patients to discard used prescriptions.

E. Controlled substance tracking and monitoring.

CHAPTER 45

HIV/AIDS and Hepatitis C

45.1 Which of the following statements concerning the epidemiology of hepatitis C virus (HCV) is *incorrect*?

A. HCV prevalence is highest for those born between 1945 and 1965.
B. HCV is most efficiently transmitted through exposure to infected blood, either through unscreened donors or by drug injection.
C. Long-term injection drug–using individuals have a high prevalence of HCV infection.
D. Provision of both primary and secondary prevention efforts and improving linkage to care can reduce the burden of HCV infection.
E. HIV co-infection dramatically triples the risk of liver disease, liver failure, and liver-related deaths from HCV.

45.2 Which of the following sources accounts for the majority of chronic infections from hepatitis C virus (HCV)?

A. Sexual transmission.
B. Unscreened blood product transfusion.
C. Perinatal exposure.
D. Injection drug use.
E. Occupational exposure.

45.3 Which of the following statements concerning primary prevention of new infections from either HIV or hepatitis C virus (HCV) is *not* true?

A. Community-based outreach can be an effective prevention strategy.
B. Substance abuse treatment constitutes an effective prevention technique.
C. Comprehensive prevention strategies include syringe programs.
D. Longer duration of exposure to methadone maintenance treatment (MMT) has not been associated with greater prevention benefits.
E. Substance abuse treatment that leads to reduced alcohol use is expected to have a role in secondary prevention of alcohol-related exacerbation of HIV and/or HCV infection.

45.4 Which of the following antiretroviral medications used for HIV infection is associated with the adverse side effects of anxiety, depression, suicidal ideation, confusion, and hallucinations?

A. Efavirenz.
B. Zidovudine.
C. Ritonavir.
D. Lopinavir.
E. Nevirapine.

45.5 Which of the following neuropsychiatric complications associated with hepatitis C virus (HCV) infection is most problematic in the management of HCV-infected patients?

A. Fatigue.
B. Lack of mental clarity.
C. Depression from chronic HCV.
D. Ribavirin-associated neuropsychiatric disturbance.
E. Interferon-alpha-associated neuropsychiatric disturbance.

CHAPTER 46

Substance Use Disorders Among Physicians

46.1 When a diagnosis of substance use disorder in a physician patient is being considered, which of the following is true?

A. Reports of alcohol on the breath cannot be related to diabetes mellitus.
B. Thyroid disease symptoms cannot be confused with substance use disorder symptoms.
C. Physicians cannot have attention-deficit/hyperactivity disorder (ADHD).
D. Psychiatric disorders such as bipolar disorder or depression should be on the differential diagnosis.
E. Physicians cannot have psychotic disorders.

46.2 Which of the following is true of the presenting signs and symptoms of physician substance misuse?

A. The signs of substance misuse are always specific and therefore easily identified.
B. Changes in sleep cannot reflect substance misuse.
C. Changes in weight cannot reflect substance misuse.
D. Needle marks, bruises, or bandages can reflect substance misuse.
E. Physicians are not likely to conceal symptoms reflecting their substance misuse.

46.3 Which of the following is true about the epidemiology of substance use among physicians in the United States?

A. The rate of substance use disorders is higher in the general population than among physicians.
B. Anesthesiologists and emergency medicine physicians are at higher risk for substance use disorders than other physicians.
C. Pediatricians and surgeons are at higher risk for substance use disorders than other physicians.
D. Anesthesiologists tend to use more benzodiazepines when misusing drugs than other types of substances.
E. Emergency medicine physicians tend to use more opioids when misusing drugs than other types of substances.

46.4 The "FRAMER" acronym for the principles of directive interventions recommended for clinicians treating substance-misusing physicians includes which of following?

A. Always conduct interventions in public places.
B. Never include a second clinician when conducting an intervention.
C. Begin all interventions with a threat to take a way a clinician's medical license.
D. Do not conduct an intervention with a physician who is intoxicated.
E. Any intervention should be at least 3 months after a sentinel incident of substance misuse.

46.5 Which of the following is accurate regarding the prognosis for physicians with substance use disorders?

A. Physicians treated for substance use disorder have a rate of treatment success of 10%.
B. Physicians treated for substance use disorders have a rate of treatment success comparable to that reported for general treatment populations.
C. The low cost of failure for physicians with substance use disorders may contribute to the treatment success rate.
D. The low reward for maintaining sobriety for physicians with substance use disorders may contribute to the treatment success rate.
E. Highly structured treatment and relapse prevention programs may explain the rates of treatment success for physicians with substance use disorders.

46.6 Which of the following regarding treatment for physicians with substance use disorders is true?

A. Caduceus groups are designed specifically for spouses of physicians with substance use disorders.
B. Physicians are never referred to 12-step groups because of concerns of confidentiality.
C. Health insurance will always cover the cost of residential treatments for physicians with substance use disorders.
D. Treatment of physicians with substance use disorders is not supported by extensive research.
E. Physicians with substance use disorders are always treated as outpatients given the stigma of residential treatment.

CHAPTER 47

Substance Use Issues Among Lesbian, Gay, Bisexual, and Transgender People

47.1 Which of the following statements about substance use in gay men and lesbians is true?

A. Research has demonstrated a genetic link between substance use and homosexuality.
B. Homophobia and antigay bias have contributed to substance use in gay men and lesbians.
C. The process of coming out results in internalization and pride in one's identity and can decrease the likelihood of substance use.
D. Substance use facilitates a link between sexual activity and intimacy, especially in gay men.
E. Gay men and lesbians with internalized homophobia are more likely to seek treatment for their substance use than are gay men and lesbians without internalized homophobia.

47.2 Which of the following is the optimal treatment approach for substance use in gay men and lesbians?

A. Clinicians should prescribe 12-step programs, such as Alcoholics Anonymous, as the optimal treatment for most gay men and lesbians with substance abuse problems.
B. Treatment should focus primarily on the substance of choice.
C. Abstinence, sobriety, and recovery are the primary focus of substance abuse treatment in gay men and lesbians.
D. Evaluation of internalized homophobia and the patient's state of self-acceptance is critical in effective treatment of substance abuse in gay men and lesbians.
E. Effective clinical treatment of substance abuse in gay men and lesbians requires that the men and women in question have publically "come out."

47.3   What best characterizes substance-associated risks faced by gay men and lesbians?

A. Domestic violence is often connected with substance use and is highly reported in the gay and lesbian communities.
B. Most gay men are unaware of safe sex practices and are especially unlikely to learn them if under the influence of substances.
C. Alcohol and drug use can significantly affect health maintenance in gay men and lesbians with HIV.
D. "Reparative therapies" describe attempts to treat substance use specifically associated with the gay and lesbian community.
E. "Survivor sex" details sex-for-pay encounters seen in homeless gay and lesbian youths and is rarely associated with drug or alcohol use.

47.4   Which of the following statements about suicidality in gay men and lesbians is true?

A. Suicidal thinking and attempts occur in gay men and lesbians at comparable rates with heterosexual individuals.
B. Suicidal thinking and attempts in gay men and lesbians occur less frequently than in heterosexual individuals.
C. Suicidal thinking and attempts in gay men and lesbians occur more frequently than in heterosexual individuals, but rates of mood disorders in gay men and lesbians are lower than in heterosexual individuals.
D. Suicidal thinking and attempts in gay men and lesbians occur more frequently than in heterosexual individuals, with increased suicidality in older individuals.
E. Suicidal thinking and attempts in gay men and lesbians occur more frequently than in heterosexual individuals, with increased suicidality in adolescents and young adults.

47.5   Which statement best characterizes the use of methamphetamine?

A. The use of methamphetamine has been linked to increased risk of contracting HIV.
B. Methamphetamine use/abuse is found almost exclusively in gay men.
C. Risk of methamphetamine use in the gay community is found equally among different racial and ethnic groups.
D. Most methamphetamine use among gay men occurs at home.
E. Methamphetamine use decreases social anxiety, facilitating increased sexual experiences.

CHAPTER 48

Minorities

48.1 A 25-year-old Asian American graduate student experiences severe flushing, nausea, and dysphoria after consuming two shots of whiskey. Which of the following genetic mechanisms is the most likely cause of his reaction?

A. Cytochrome P450 isoenzyme 1A2 ultrarapid metabolizer status.
B. Serotonin transporter gene polymorphism.
C. Aldehyde dehydrogenase (ALDH2) isoenzyme deficiency.
D. Tyrosine hydroxylase deficiency.
E. Methyl tetrahydrofolate reductase deficiency.

48.2 Sacramental ingestion of peyote cactus in the Native American Church is an example of which of the following?

A. Generational change.
B. Norm conflict.
C. Inadequate ensocialization.
D. Culturally prescribed use.
E. Disenfranchised groups.

48.3 Which of the following racial/ethnic groups has the highest alcoholic liver cirrhosis mortality rates?

A. White.
B. Black.
C. Hispanic.
D. Asian.
E. Pacific Islander.

48.4 A 19-year-old college freshman is brought to the local emergency department in an obtunded state. He had been at a frat party and consumed a case of beer in less than 2 hours. Which of the following cultural risk factors does his drinking represent?

A. Technological changes.
B. Pathogenic use patterns.
C. Inadequate ensocialization.

D. Disenfranchised groups.

E. Generational change.

48.5 By providing white and black addictions counselors with education about models of healing preferred by Native American patients receiving treatment in that program, which of the following perceived barriers to care can be ameliorated?

A. System barriers.

B. Family barriers.

C. Staff member barriers.

D. Patient barriers.

E. Community barriers.

CHAPTER 49

Testing to Identify Recent Drug Use

49.1   What is most drug testing used to detect?

A. Recent use of drugs and alcohol.
B. Dependence.
C. Intoxication.
D. Impairment.
E. Addiction.

49.2   A 25-year old man is pulled over while driving and found to have a blood alcohol concentration of 0.11. He pleads no contest to a charge of driving under the influence. As a condition of probation, he is required to abstain from alcohol use and to submit to follow-up testing. Which testing strategy is most appropriate for determining his abstinence from alcohol?

A. Blood alcohol level.
B. Urine alcohol level.
C. Urine test for ethyl glucuronide (EtG).
D. Saliva testing.
E. Breath alcohol testing.

49.3   How are most drug and alcohol tests confirmed?

A. By the laboratory that conducted the test.
B. By a sample donor's admission of recent use.
C. By the manufacturer of the test kit.
D. By on-site (not laboratory based) confirmation tests.
E. By a certified medical review officer.

49.4   Which of the following tests for drugs of abuse is most vulnerable to cheating?

A. Blood.
B. Urine.
C. Hair.

D. Saliva.

E. Sweat patches.

49.5   Which of the following is true of hair biomarker tests?

A. Result in lower positive test rates for drug use versus urine testing.

B. Can be used to distinguish between light, moderate, and heavy use of drugs and alcohol.

C. Have a cost similar to drug urinalysis testing.

D. May provide false-indicator results (e.g., positive tests for morphine after consumption of poppy seeds).

E. Have a detection window of about 1–3 days.

CHAPTER 50

Medical Education on Addiction

50.1 Which of the following is a key element of successful change and enhancement to medical school substance abuse curricula?

A. Identify key faculty to champion change.
B. Engage medical students interested in learning.
C. Replace skills-based training with didactic training.
D. Increase curricula hours to incorporate substance abuse training.
E. Implement a single lecture on substance abuse training.

50.2 The Substance Abuse and Mental Health Services Administration's Center for Substance Abuse Treatment (SAMHSA/CSAT) funded medical residency training program cooperative agreements to develop and implement training programs. Which of the following initiatives facilitates sustained practice change in graduating residents?

A. Brief educational half-day programs.
B. Longer clinical rotations in substance abuse treatment.
C. Role-play with supervising clinicians.
D. Feedback provision by simulated patients.
E. Skills-based sessions.

50.3 The U.S. Drug Enforcement Administration approval to prescribe buprenorphine for opiate dependence and withdrawal requires additional training. Psychiatrists who have certification from which of the following boards are exempt from this exam?

A. American Osteopathic Association (AOA).
B. American Society of Addiction Medicine (ASAM).
C. American Board of Addiction Medicine (ABAM).
D. American Board of Pain Medicine (ABPM).
E. American Board of Internal Medicine.

50.4   Identify an effective intervention that targets practicing physicians to improve their substance use practices below.

A. Continuing medical education (CME) programs using didactic sessions.
B. CD-ROM–based CME courses.
C. Online CME courses.
D. Augmentation of brief education training with system-based clinical prompt.
E. Recruitment of physicians to attend substance abuse CME programs.

50.5   Which of the following is an effective educational strategy to optimize substance use curriculum and expansion?

A. Prerecorded interviews.
B. Real patients.
C. Didactic lectures.
D. Virtual reality avatars.
E. Skills-based interactive curricula.

CHAPTER 51

Prevention of Substance Abuse

51.1 In a study of LifeSkills Training (LST), a school-based, curriculum-driven program that uses social influences and social competency, the experimental groups were teachers who received annual provider training with ongoing consultation and teachers who received training via videotape without ongoing consultation, whereas the control arm comprised teachers representing a no-treatment control condition. Students who were exposed to 60% or more lessons were considered "high fidelity" and those receiving less than 60% lessons were considered "low fidelity." After 6 years, which of the following is a key finding?

A. No statistically significant differences in drug use between students whose teachers were personally trained and students whose teachers received training via videotape.
B. Statistically significant differences in drug use between students whose teachers were personally trained and students whose teachers received training via videotape.
C. No statistically significant differences on various measures of drug use between control students and high-fidelity students in the two experimental conditions.
D. Statistically significant differences between experimental students and control students classified as having low fidelity.
E. LST is efficacious for both students with good attendance and those with greater absenteeism.

51.2 Which of the following school-based, curriculum-driven drug prevention programs has the highest level of success in reducing substance abuse?

A. LifeSkills Training (LST).
B. Project ALERT.
C. Take Charge of Your Life (TCYL).
D. Hutchinson Smoking Prevention Program (HSPP).
E. Positive Action (PA).

51.3 The Communities That Care (CTC) community-based and community-placed substance abuse prevention program focuses on "individual-level" changes using a risk-protective factors framework and measures. These risk factors are organized under four concepts: 1) community, 2) family, 3) school, and 4) peer-individual. The outcome variables are substance abuse, delinquency, teen pregnancy, school dropout, violence, depression, and anxiety. Hawkins et al. (2012) found that in communities with CTC, there were lower levels of target risk factors, less initiation of delinquent behavior, lower alcohol and cigarette use, lower prevalence of past-month cigarette use, and lower prevalence of past-year delinquency and violence. Which of the following items is one of the limitations to the CTC intervention?

A. Community-level responses to the CTC survey are used to "prioritize" risk factors to be addressed.
B. Only data from students followed from fifth through tenth grades in 24 small- to medium-sized communities are used to measure change in spite of the fact that each school contains multiple cohorts.
C. Substance use and other problem behaviors targeted by CTC may be expressed by students, who are embedded in "social networks" that are included in the CTC.
D. Students providing data from fifth through tenth grade undergo many changes, and life events are captured in frequent surveys.
E. The CTC survey measures capture dynamic aspects of the lives of the students and the events happening to the adults in their families that affect the students.

51.4   PROSPER, the PROmoting School-community-university Partnerships to Enhance Resilience community-placed coalition, involves a university-community partnership with many teams. It has demonstrated a slower growth in misuse of illicit substances for six and seventh graders who participate in a family- or school-based curriculum-driven program when they enter eleventh and twelfth grade. Which of the following is a limitation of the PROSPER program?

A. The reliance on only two cohorts of students followed longitudinally to assess community-level change.
B. The large number of exposure units for the school-and-family-oriented interventions.
C. The existence of a potential infrastructure for dissemination of prevention.
D. The family and consumer science agricultural extension agents that are an integral component of land-grant universities in the United States.
E. The evaluation was conducted in 28 matched-pair communities, 14 each in Iowa and Pennsylvania.

51.5   Media campaigns have been used as a vector for prevention of substance abuse. Which of the following agency campaigns has demonstrated a dose-response relationship between exposure to media and decline in substance use?

A. National Youth Anti-Drug Media Campaign of the National Drug Control Policy (ONDCP).
B. Partnership for a Drug-Free America.
C. Tobacco industry-sponsored smoking prevention.
D. American Legacy Foundation.

CHAPTER 52

Forensic Addiction Psychiatry

52.1 In which of the following scenarios is the psychiatrist serving as an expert witness, as opposed to a witness of facts?

A. The psychiatrist is subpoenaed to testify about a former patient's diagnoses.
B. The patient asks the psychiatrist to provide copies of treatment records for a disability hearing.
C. The psychiatrist is asked to testify about a current patient's adherence to treatment recommendations.
D. The psychiatrist is asked to provide an independent opinion regarding the role of substance use in a domestic violence dispute.
E. The psychiatrist is accused of medical malpractice and provides testimony regarding treatment rendered to a patient.

52.2 Which of the following diagnoses carries the greatest risk of violence?

A. Schizophrenia.
B. Bipolar disorder.
C. Alcohol use disorder.
D. Co-occurring alcohol and cocaine use disorders.
E. Co-occurring schizophrenia and cocaine intoxication.

52.3 Under which of the following circumstances can intoxication be used as a defense against responsibility for a crime?

A. There was no intent to cause harm.
B. The individual was tricked into using a substance.
C. The crime is nonviolent.
D. The individual's presentation does not meet criteria for a substance use disorder.
E. Laboratory evidence supports the claim of intoxication.

52.4 When asked by a court to make recommendations for a parolee with a substance use disorder, an addiction psychiatrist should recommend treatment for at least what period of time?

A. 1 month.
B. 3 months.
C. 6 months.
D. 1 year.
E. 5 years.

52.5 A psychiatrist is asked to evaluate an individual who was arrested for murder while driving under the influence. The defendant caused a motor vehicle accident which led to the death of the other driver. At the time of the arrest, the individual was acutely intoxicated. In the forensic setting, which of the following requests is appropriate for the psychiatrist to answer?

A. To render an opinion about whether the defendant possessed the intent necessary for a charge of murder.
B. To conduct a complete psychiatric assessment in order to help the court better understand the defendant.
C. To render an opinion regarding the likelihood that the defendant will drive while under the influence in the future.
D. To render an opinion regarding the degree of dangerousness the defendant poses if released while awaiting trial.
E. Estimating the degree of violence possessed by the defendant when under the influence of alcohol.

CHAPTER 53

Substance Abuse and Mental Illness

53.1   Which of the following is most likely to co-occur with a substance use disorder (SUD)?

A. Schizophrenia.
B. Bipolar disorder.
C. Major depressive disorder.
D. Generalized anxiety disorder.
E. Posttraumatic stress disorder.

53.2   A 28-year-old patient is admitted to a psychiatric hospital with acute onset of paranoia, auditory hallucinations, and irritability. The patient admits to recent use of cocaine. Which of the following is most likely to help clarify whether the patient's psychosis is due to a substance-induced disorder or co-occurring schizophrenia and cocaine use disorder?

A. Administering urine toxicology on admission.
B. Making serial assessments of psychiatric symptoms over time.
C. Eliciting a family history of substance use disorders.
D. Using a structured diagnostic interview on admission.
E. Eliciting a history of prescriptions for antipsychotic medication.

53.3   It is prudent to wait several months prior to making a formal diagnosis of a psychotic spectrum disorder when treating a patient with psychotic symptoms and use of which of the following substances?

A. Phencyclidine.
B. Cocaine.
C. Methamphetamine.
D. Marijuana.
E. Inhalants.

53.4   Which of the following medications has the most evidence supporting its effectiveness in treating patients with co-occurring schizophrenia and substance use disorders?

A. Haloperidol.
B. Olanzapine.
C. Fluphenazine.
D. Clozapine.
E. Risperidone.

53.5   In a patient with co-occurring bipolar disorder and alcohol use disorder (AUD), which of the following medications has the most evidence to support its use in addressing both mood symptoms and drinking outcomes?

A. Valproic acid.
B. Lithium.
C. Quetiapine.
D. Aripiprazole.
E. Lamotrigine.

Part II

Answer Guide

CHAPTER 1

Neurobiology of Addiction

1.1　Which of the following neurotransmitter systems plays a shared role in the binge/intoxication stage for all drugs of abuse?

A. γ-Aminobutyric acid (GABA).
B. Opioid.
C. Serotonin.
D. Dopamine.
E. Norepinephrine.

The correct response is option D: Dopamine.

The dopamine system has been implicated in the binge/intoxication stage for all drugs of abuse (option D). The GABA system (option A) has been implicated for alcohol and benzodiazepines. The opioid system has been implicated for opioids, alcohol, and cannabis (option B). The serotonin system has been implicated for alcohol and psychostimulants (option C). The norepinephrine system has not been implicated in binge/intoxication for any drug of abuse, although it does play a role in the withdrawal/negative affect stage (option E). **(Neurobiological Mechanisms in the Addiction Cycle/Binge/Intoxication Stage, p. 6)**

1.2　Which of the following behavioral phenomena is thought to be due to elevated brain reward thresholds during acute drug abstinence?

A. Increased craving.
B. Decreased tolerance.
C. Decreased control over drug seeking.
D. Increased negative motivational/affective state during acute abstinence.
E. Decreased arousal.

The correct response is option D: Increased negative motivational/affective state during acute abstinence.

Elevated brain reward threshold refers to the greater level of stimulation required to elicit dopamine in reward-related regions, such as the nucleus accumbens. Acute abstinence raises this threshold, which causes a negative motivational/affective

117

state that is characterized by dysphoria, anxiety, irritability, and anhedonia (option D). Sensitization of the dopamine system, rather than decreased reward threshold, is associated with increased craving (option A). Tolerance (option B) is mediated by chronic changes at the level of the drug receptor, rather than by changes in the functioning of the dopamine system. Dopamine plays a role in control over drug seeking (option C), but this pathway involves a different form of dopamine release in the prefrontal cortex. Arousal (option E) is mediated to an extent by dopamine, but it is mostly related to noradrenergic system functioning, and mostly within the prefrontal cortex. **(Neurobiological Mechanisms in the Addiction Cycle/Withdrawal/Negative Affect Stage, p. 9)**

1.3   Which of the following brain areas or systems is most directly implicated in emotional dysregulation during the withdrawal/negative affect stage of addictive behavior?

A. Lateral habenula.
B. Mesolimbic dopamine system.
C. Hypothalamic-pituitary-adrenal (HPA) axis.
D. Prefrontal cortex.
E. Insula.

The correct response is option C: Hypothalamic-pituitary-adrenal (HPA) axis.

The "stress" response system, including the HPA axis, has been implicated as playing a central role in the emotional dysregulation that is characteristic of the withdrawal/negative affect stage of addictive behavior (option C). The lateral habenula (option A) signals the absence of expected rewards but does not play a role in drug withdrawal/negative affect. The mesolimbic dopamine system (option B) is implicated in the binge/intoxication stage, not in the withdrawal/negative affect stage. The prefrontal cortex (option D) plays a role in control over drug-seeking behavior during the preoccupation/anticipation stage. The insula (option E) also plays a role in the preoccupation/anticipation stage. **(Neurobiological Mechanisms in the Addiction Cycle/Withdrawal/Negative Affect Stage, p. 9)**

1.4   Which of the following brain areas or systems is most directly involved in executive control over incentive salience/preoccupation?

A. Prefrontal cortex.
B. Basolateral amygdala.
C. Hypothalamic-pituitary-adrenal (HPA) axis.
D. Ventral striatum.
E. Endogenous opioid system.

The correct response is option A: Prefrontal cortex.

The prefrontal cortex, through its projections to the ventral tegmental area, exerts regulatory control over incentive salience and preoccupation (option A). Addiction is associated with deficits in these regulatory functions, leading to loss of control over incentive salience. The basolateral amygdala (option B) is involved in cue-induced reinstatement and relapse. The HPA axis (option C) is involved in withdrawal/negative affect. The ventral striatum (option D) is primarily involved in promoting preoccupation/anticipation. The endogenous opioid system (option E) does not play a role in the incentive salience/preoccupation stage. **(Neurobiological Mechanisms in the Addiction Cycle/Preoccupation/Anticipation Stage, p. 14)**

1.5 Which of the following is the correct sequence of physiological/molecular events leading to the synaptic plasticity that underlies addiction?

  A. Reduction in inhibitory G-protein levels → increased cyclic adenosine monophosphate (cAMP) levels → increased protein kinase A (PKA) activity→ cAMP response element binding protein (CREB) regulation of gene expression → synaptic plasticity.
  B. Increased cAMP levels → CREB regulation of gene expression→ reduction in inhibitory G-protein levels → increased PKA activity → synaptic plasticity.
  C. CREB regulation of gene expression → increased cAMP levels → reduction in inhibitory G-protein levels → increased PKA activity → synaptic plasticity.
  D. Increased PKA activity → increased cAMP levels → CREB regulation of gene expression → reduction in inhibitory G-protein levels → synaptic plasticity.
  E. Increased cAMP levels → reduction in inhibitory G-protein levels → CREB regulation of gene expression → increased PKA activity → synaptic plasticity.

The correct response is option A: Reduction in inhibitory G-protein levels → increased cyclic adenosine monophosphate (cAMP) levels → increased protein kinase A (PKA) activity→ cAMP response element binding protein (CREB) regulation of gene expression → synaptic plasticity.

Chronic exposure to drugs of abuse leads to a reduction in inhibitory G-protein activity, which in turn increases cAMP levels. This increases the activity of cAMP-dependent protein kinases, such as PKA, which activate CREB. CREB is a cAMP-responsive element binding protein that, when activated, binds to DNA regulatory elements and upregulates the transcription of specific genes that promote synaptic plasticity (option A). All other options (B, C, D, E) do not describe this sequence. **(Molecular and Cellular Targets Within the Brain Circuits Associated With Addiction, pp. 16–18)**

CHAPTER 2

Genetics of Addiction

2.1 Which of the following statements best describes the genetic influences on the development of substance use disorders?

A. Substance use disorders follow recessive Mendelian patterns of inheritance.
B. Substance use disorders are inherited via risk alleles that require a gene-by-environment interaction.
C. Twin and adoption studies have demonstrated the heritability of certain substance use disorders.
D. Epidemiologic studies have shown that the development of substance use disorders is dependent on the interaction of risk alleles with socioeconomic status.
E. In determining the risk for developing a substance use disorder, genetic influences are considered roughly equivalent among most individuals.

The correct response is option B: Substance use disorders are inherited via risk alleles that require a gene-by-environment interaction.

Substance use disorders are similar to other complex traits in that they are influenced by both genetic and environmental factors. However, in the case of substance use disorders, there is a necessary component of gene-by-environment interaction. A person cannot become substance dependent without exposure to the substance, regardless of genetic constitution (option B). Substance use disorders do not follow Mendelian genetics, and no specific allele fully determines whether an individual is affected (option A). Although twin, adoption, and family studies can show a range of phenotypes and show that substance use disorders may be familial, they cannot demonstrate direct heritability (option C). In the United States, alcohol dependence, opioid dependence, cocaine dependence, and nicotine dependence pose a significant public health problem that cuts across race, geography, ethnicity, and socioeconomic status (option D). For clinicians and health professionals, it is important to understand that genetic influences on the risk of inheriting a substance use disorder vary among individuals (option E). This means that levels of risk also vary, and the nature of this risk is in part purely biological. **(Introduction, p. 25; Importance of Genes for Risk of Substance Dependence, pp. 26–28)**

2.2   From the evidence to date, which of the following statements about the heritability of alcohol and substance use disorders is most accurate?

A. Twin studies have estimated heritability of alcohol dependence, ranging from 50% to 60%.
B. Twin studies have shown that concordance rates for opioid and stimulant dependence are similar for monozygotic and dizygotic twin pairs.
C. Twin studies have estimated heritability of nicotine dependence, ranging from 80% to 90%.
D. The risk for developing alcohol and opioid use disorders has been correlated in twin studies.
E. Genetic influences for substance abuse in general, but not for specific drugs of abuse, have been demonstrated.

The correct response is option A: Twin studies have estimated heritability of alcohol dependence, ranging from 50% to 60%.

Twin, family, and adoption studies have established that genetic factors are important in the development of alcohol and other substance use disorders. The largest twin studies have yielded heritability estimates for alcohol dependence of 50%–60%, suggesting that more than half of the risk of developing alcohol dependence is genetic (Kendler et al. 1992, 1997; Prescott and Kendler 1999) (option A). Concordance rates for alcohol and for opioid dependence are higher in monozygotic twins relative to dizygotic twins, according to estimates from studies using the Vietnam Era Twin Registry (Tsuang et al. 1996) and the Swedish Twin Registry (Kendler et al. 1997) (option B). Heritability for nicotine dependence has been estimated at >60% (Madden et al. 2000; True et al. 1999), but a meta-analysis of twin studies estimated heritability of smoking persistence to be 0.59 for males and 0.46 for females (Li et al. 2004) (option C). Twin registry studies have also shown the correlations for co-occurring of alcohol and nicotine dependence (Madden et al. 2000), with the correlation estimated at 0.68 in one study (True et al. 1999); however, opioid use disorder has not been directly correlated with alcohol use disorder (option D). On the basis of co-occurrence of different forms of substance abuse using the Vietnam Era Twin Registry, investigators have concluded that genetic factors exist that are both specific to certain drugs of abuse and general to multiple forms of dependence (option E). **(Importance of Genes for Risk of Substance Dependence/ Heritability of Alcohol Dependence, pp. 26–27; Heritability of Drug Dependence, pp. 27–28)**

2.3   Which of the following statements about genetic susceptibility for developing alcohol dependence is most accurate?

A. Decreased metabolism of acetaldehyde increases risk for developing alcohol dependence.
B. Decreased alcohol dehydrogenase function increases risk for developing alcohol dependence.

C. Low level of response to alcohol has been shown to be protective against developing alcohol dependence in a genomewide linkage association study.
D. Increased risk for alcohol dependence has been mapped to an alcohol dehydrogenase gene cluster on chromosome 4q (*ADH4*).
E. *ADH4* codes for a subunit in the alcohol dehydrogenase gene cluster that mainly contributes to enzyme function in the liver and has little bearing on the risk of alcohol dependence.

The correct response is option D: Increased risk for alcohol dependence has been mapped to an alcohol dehydrogenase gene cluster on chromosome 4q (*ADH4*).

Linkage studies by the Collaborative Studies on the Genetics of Alcoholism and the National Institute on Alcohol Abuse and Alcoholism investigating alcohol dependence yielded promising lod (logarithm of odds) scores (a measure of the likelihood that loci mapping to the region is linked to the disorder under study) for a region close to *ADH4*, mapping increased risk for alcohol dependence to this region (Foroud et al. 2000; Long et al. 1998; Reich et al. 1998) (option D). Decreased metabolism of acetaldehyde produces aversive symptoms such as flushing, nausea, lightheadedness, and palpitations, which might decrease drinking behavior and thereby reduce the risk for developing alcohol dependence. A genetic variant that greatly reduces or eliminates acetaldehyde dehydrogenase function and thus decreases acetaldehyde elimination (most commonly occurring in Asian populations) is known to be protective against developing alcohol dependence (option A). Alcohol dehydrogenase variants that increase acetaldehyde function through increased metabolism of alcohol to acetaldehyde may also be protective (Hasin et al. 2002; Konishi et al. 2003; Thomasson et al. 1991) (option B). As with family history of alcohol dependence, low level of response to alcohol has been associated with increased risk for developing alcohol dependence according to findings from genomewide linkage association studies (Schuckit et al. 2006; Wilhelmsen et al. 2003) (option C). *ADH4* codes for the π subunit of the alcohol dehydrogenase enzyme, which mainly contributes to alcohol dehydrogenase activity in the liver and is a disease-influencing locus in the alcohol dehydrogenase cluster on chromosome 4q (Edenberg et al. 1999) (option E). **(Identification of Risk Genes/Genomewide Linkage Studies/Studies of Alcohol Dependence, p. 29; Candidate Gene Studies, p. 31; Alcohol-Metabolizing Enzymes, p. 31)**

2.4   Which of the following statements best describes the role of the *DRD2* locus in susceptibility to drug or alcohol dependence?

A. The *DRD2* locus codes for dopamine D_2 receptors and is a candidate gene for schizophrenia but not for susceptibility to drug or alcohol dependence.
B. Substantial evidence implicates the *DRD2* locus in the heritability of nicotine dependence.
C. Findings implicating the *DRD2* locus in nicotine dependence may be attributable to nearby loci on chromosome 11.

D. *DRD2* has been implicated in increased risk for alcohol dependence.

E. *DRD2* has been implicated in increased risk for opioid dependence.

The correct response is option C: Findings implicating the *DRD2* locus in nicotine dependence may be attributable to nearby loci on chromosome 11.

The *DRD2* locus on chromosome 11 codes for dopamine D_2 receptors and is a candidate gene for substance dependence risk (option A). For nicotine dependence risk, evidence of association is stronger for single nucleotide polymorphisms at loci *TTC12* and *ANKK1*, which are located near the *DRD2* locus on chromosome 11, than for association with the *DRD2* locus itself. Thus, positive findings linking *DRD2* to nicotine dependence may be attributable to variants in these nearby loci (option C). *DRD2* was investigated and shown to have only modest linkage for nicotine dependence (Gelernter et al. 2007) (option B). Additionally, it is this nearby region on chromosome 11 spanning loci *TTC12* and *ANKK1* and not the *DRD2* locus that has been further associated with alcohol dependence risk (Yang et al. 2007) (option D) and heroin dependence risk (Nelson et al. 2013) (option E). **(Identification of Risk Genes/Candidate Gene Studies/*DRD2, ANKK1, TTC12*: Association With Multiple Forms of SD, pp. 34–35)**

2.5   Which of the following statements about susceptibility genes for substance dependence is most accurate?

A. A cluster of nicotinic receptor genes on chromosome 15 has been associated with number of cigarettes smoked per day and with lung cancer, but not with nicotine dependence.

B. Genomewide association studies have mapped susceptibility for nicotine dependence to a cluster of nicotinic receptor genes on chromosome 15.

C. The μ-opioid receptor gene *OPRM1* has been associated with opioid dependence but not with alcohol or other drug dependence.

D. *GABBRA2*, which codes for one of the four subunits of the γ-aminobutyric acid (GABA) receptor, has shown significant associations with large effect sizes on risk of alcohol dependence.

E. 5-HTTLPR, a rare polymorphism in the serotonin transporter gene, has been implicated in drinking and drug-taking behavior among adolescents and college students.

The correct response is option B: Genomewide association studies have mapped susceptibility for nicotine dependence to a cluster of nicotinic receptor genes on chromosome 15.

Genetic markers associated with nicotine dependence were mapped to a cluster of nicotinic receptor genes on chromosome 15 (option B). The nicotinic receptor genes on chromosome 15 were first associated with nicotine dependence (Bierut et al. 2007) and later associated with other smoking traits, such as number of cigarettes smoked per day and lung cancer, in numerous studies (e.g., Thorgeirsson et al. 2010) (option A). The μ-opioid receptor gene has been associated with alcohol and drug dependence in European American and Russian populations (Zhang et al. 2006) (option C). *GABRA2*, which codes for one of the four subunits of the GABA receptor, has shown significant associations with risk for alcohol dependence, but nonreplication of these findings has also been reported. In a meta-analysis of 14 variants including eight studies, significant associations with risk for alcohol dependence were found, but all studies yielded small effects on risk (odds ratio < 1.5 for all four variants) (Zintzaras 2012) (option D). The short allele of 5-HTTLPR is a commonly occurring functional polymorphism in the serotonin transporter protein gene *SLC6A4* that, in one or two copies, has been associated with more depressive symptoms related to stressful life events compared with individuals homozygous for the long allele (Kaufman et al. 2004). A similar gene-by-environment interaction was found among college students, in which this polymorphism together with negative life events was found to moderate drinking and drug use (Covault et al. 2007). The functional polymorphism 5-HTTLPR is common rather than rare (option E). **(Identification of Risk Genes/Candidate Gene Studies/Opioid Receptor Genes, p. 33; *GABRA2*, p. 33; Genomewide Association Studies/Studies of Drug Dependence, p. 36; Next Steps, p. 37)**

References

Bierut LJ, Madden PA, Breslau N, et al: Novel genes identified in a high-density genome wide association study for nicotine dependence. Hum Mol Genet 16:24–35, 2007 17158188

Covault J, Tennen H, Armeli S, et al: Interactive effects of the serotonin transporter 5-HTTLPR polymorphism and stressful life events on college student drinking and drug use. Biol Psychiatry 61:609–616, 2007 16920076

Edenberg HJ, Jerome RE, Li M: Polymorphism of the human alcohol dehydrogenase 4 (ADH4) promoter affects gene expression. Pharmacogenetics 9:25–30, 1999 10208639

Foroud T, Edenberg HJ, Goate A, et al: Alcoholism susceptibility loci: confirmation studies in a replicate sample and further mapping. Alcohol Clin Exp Res 24:933–945, 2000 10923994

Gelernter J, Panhuysen C, Weiss R, et al: Genomewide linkage scan for nicotine dependence: identification of a chromosome 5 risk locus. Biol Psychiatry 61:119–126, 2007 17081504

Hasin D, Aharonovich E, Liu X, et al: Alcohol and ADH2 in Israel: Ashkenazis, Sephardics, and recent Russian immigrants. Am J Psychiatry 159:1432–1434, 2002 12153842

Kaufman J, Yang BZ, Douglas-Palumberi H, et al: Social supports and serotonin transporter gene moderate depression in maltreated children. Proc Natl Acad Sci U S A 101:17316–17321, 2004 15563601

Kendler KS, Heath AC, Neale MC, et al: A population-based twin study of alcoholism in women. JAMA 268:1877–1882, 1992 1404711

Kendler KS, Prescott CA, Neale MC, et al: Temperance board registration for alcohol abuse in a national sample of Swedish male twins, born 1902 to 1949. Arch Gen Psychiatry 54:178–184, 1997 9040286

Konishi T, Smith JL, Lin K, et al: Influence of genetic admixture on polymorphisms of alcohol-metabolizing enzymes: analyses of mutations on the CYP2E1, ADH2, ADH3 and ALDH2 genes in a Mexican-American population living in the Los Angeles area. Alcohol Alcohol 38:93–94, 2003 12554615

Li MD, Ma JZ, Beuten J: Progress in searching for susceptibility loci and genes for smoking-related behaviour. Clin Genet 66:382–392, 2004 15479180

Long JC, Knowler WC, Hanson RL, et al: Evidence for genetic linkage to alcohol dependence on chromosomes 4 and 11 from an autosome-wide scan in an American Indian population. Am J Med Genet 81:216–221, 1998 9603607

Madden PAF, Bucholz KK, Martin NG, et al: Smoking and the genetic contribution to alcohol-dependence risk. Alcohol Res Health 24:209–214, 2000 15986715

Nelson EC, Lynskey MT, Heath AC, et al: ANKK1, TTC12, and NCAM1 polymorphisms and heroin dependence: importance of considering drug exposure. JAMA Psychiatry 70:325–333, 2013 23303482

Prescott CA, Kendler KS: Genetic and environmental contributions to alcohol abuse and dependence in a population-based sample of male twins. Am J Psychiatry 156:34–40, 1999 9892295

Reich T, Edenberg HJ, Goate A, et al: Genome-wide search for genes affecting the risk for alcohol dependence. Am J Med Genet 81:207–215, 1998 9603606

Schuckit M, Smith T, Pierson J, et al: Relationships among the level of response to alcohol and the number of alcoholic relatives in predicting alcohol-related outcomes. Alcohol Clin Exp Res 30:1308–1314, 2006 16899033

Thomasson HR, Edenberg HJ, Crabb DW, et al: Alcohol and aldehyde dehydrogenase genotypes and alcoholism in Chinese men. Am J Hum Genet 48:677–681, 1991 2014795

Thorgeirsson TE, Gudbjartsson DF, Surakka I, et al: Sequence variants at CHRNB3-CHRNA6 and CYP2A6 affect smoking behavior. Nat Genet 42:448–453, 2010 20418888

True WR, Xian H, Scherrer JF, et al: Common genetic vulnerability for nicotine and alcohol dependence in men. Arch Gen Psychiatry 56:655–661, 1999 10401514

Tsuang MT, Lyons MJ, Eisen SA, et al: Genetic influences on DSM-III-R drug abuse and dependence: a study of 3,372 twin pairs. Am J Med Genet 67:473–477, 1996 8886164

Wilhelmsen KC, Schuckit M, Smith TL, et al: The search for genes related to a low level response to alcohol determined by alcohol challenges. Alcohol Clin Exp Res 27:1041–1047, 2003 12878909

Yang BZ, Kranzler HR, Zhao H, et al: Association of haplotypic variants in DRD2, ANKK1, TTC12 and NCAM1 to alcohol dependence in independent case control and family samples. Hum Mol Genet 16:2844–2853, 2007 17761687

Zhang H, Luo X, Kranzler HR, et al: Association between two mu-opioid receptor gene (OPRM1) haplotype blocks and drug or alcohol dependence. Hum Mol Genet 15:807–819, 2006 16476706

Zintzaras E: Gamma-aminobutyric acid A receptor, alpha2 (GABRA2) variants as individual markers for alcoholism: a meta-analysis. Psychiatr Genet 22:189–196, 2012 22555154

CHAPTER 3

Epidemiology of Addiction

3.1   What is the most widely used illicit drug or drug class internationally?

A. Opioids.
B. Cocaine.
C. Alcohol.
D. Cannabis.
E. Stimulants.

The correct response is option D: Cannabis.

Cannabis is the most widely used illicit drug internationally; it is used by an estimated 119–221 million people worldwide (2.6%–5.0% of the population) (option D). The global prevalence of the use of stimulants is estimated to be 0.3%–1.2% (between 14 and 52.5 million users worldwide); opioid use and cocaine use are both estimated to be 0.3%–0.5% of the population (13–21 million users) (options A, B, E). Alcohol is not considered an illicit drug (option C). **(Epidemiology of Substance Use and Related Disorders, pp. 50–55)**

3.2   Globally, epidemiological surveys consistently show that men are much more likely than women to have a substance use disorder. In the United States, use of which substance is associated with being a white female?

A. Cannabis.
B. Stimulant.
C. Alcohol.
D. Cocaine.
E. Nicotine.

The correct response is option B: Stimulant.

Stimulant use is associated with being young, female, and white or Hispanic, with increased use in western and southwestern states of the United States (option B). Cannabis use disorders are associated with being male, Native American, and separated/widowed/divorced; having lower SES; and living in the western states

127

(option A). Globally, being female is associated with greater rates of abstinence from alcohol (option C). In the United States, cocaine dependence is associated with being black and living in urban rather than rural areas (option D). Being young and female is associated with transition from nicotine use to dependence, but when compared with whites, Native Americans, Alaskan Natives, and Native Hawaiians and other Pacific Islanders are more likely to transition to dependence (option E). **(Epidemiology of Substance Use and Related Disorders, pp. 50–55)**

3.3   The revisions introduced in DSM-5 were informed by epidemiological data gathered from large-scale nationally representative surveys. Which of the following statements about DSM-5 and addiction is *not* true?

A. The substance-related legal problems symptom continues to have clinical utility in determining diagnostic thresholds.
B. Abuse and dependence have been combined into a single disorder of graded severity (substance use disorder).
C. Craving is now recognized as a key clinical feature of substance use disorders.
D. Cannabis withdrawal is now a recognized syndrome.
E. Prevalence rates of substance use disorders in the United States may change when DSM-5 criteria are used.

The correct response is option A: The substance-related legal problems symptom continues to have clinical utility in determining diagnostic thresholds.

The substance-related legal problems symptom has been removed from DSM-5 (American Psychiatric Association 2013) because it was of such high severity that it had little clinical utility (option A). The merging of substance abuse and dependence into a single disorder of graded severity has been supported by studies of epidemiological and clinical data (American Psychiatric Association 2010) which suggest that the substance abuse and dependence symptoms represent a single latent dimension rather than two distinct disorders (option B). Clinical and epidemiological research has indicated that craving is a key clinical feature of substance use disorders (option C). Cannabis withdrawal is now a fully recognized syndrome (option D). The epidemiological implications of the DSM-5 revisions are being researched, but early studies suggest modest increases in the prevalence of 12-month substance use disorders in the United States (option E) (Agrawal et al. 2011). **(Effects of DSM-5 Revisions on Epidemiology, p. 55)**

3.4   Large epidemiological surveys suggest that nearly a quarter of alcohol users will become alcohol dependent at some point in their lives. Which of the following is *not* associated with the transition from alcohol use to dependence?

A. Male gender.
B. Being black rather than white.
C. Older age.
D. Family history of substance use disorders.
E. Presence of comorbid disorders.

The correct response is option C: Older age.

The National Epidemiologic Survey on Alcohol and Related Conditions (Lopez-Quintero et al. 2011) indicated that transitions from alcohol use to dependence were associated with being male (option A), young (rather than older in age [option C]), and black rather than white (option B). Comorbid disorders (option E) and a family history of substance use disorders (option D) also increased the risk of transitioning from alcohol use to dependence. **(Epidemiology of Substance Use and Related Disorders/Alcohol, pp. 50–51)**

3.5   Epidemiological surveys are informative about who becomes addicted to substances. In developed countries, having an alcohol use disorder is associated with which of the following?

A. Being male, young, unmarried, and of high socioeconomic status.
B. Being male, older, unmarried, and of low socioeconomic status.
C. Being male, older, married, and of high socioeconomic status.
D. Being male, older, married, and of low socioeconomic status.
E. Being male, young, unmarried, and of low socioeconomic status.

The correct response is option E: Being male, young, unmarried, and of low socioeconomic status.

There is some consistency in the major risk factors for alcohol use disorders internationally (Teesson et al. 2012). In developed countries, having an alcohol use disorder is associated with being male, young, and unmarried as well as being of low socioeconomic status (option E). In the majority of cases, the onset of alcohol abuse and dependence occurs before age 30. **(Epidemiology of Substance Use and Related Disorders/Alcohol, pp. 50–51)**

References

Agrawal A, Heath AC, Lynskey MT: DSM-IV to DSM-5: the impact of proposed revisions on diagnosis of alcohol use disorders. Addiction 106:1935–1943, 2011 21631621

American Psychiatric Association: DSM-5 Development. 2010. Available at: http://www.dsm5.org/Pages/Default.aspx. Accessed January 5, 2014.

American Psychiatric Association: Diagnostic and Statistical Manual of Mental Disorders, 5th Edition. Washington, DC, American Psychiatric Association, 2013

Lopez-Quintero C, Pérez de los Cobos J, Hasin DS, et al: Probability and predictors of transition from first use to dependence on nicotine, alcohol, cannabis, and cocaine: results of the National Epidemiologic Survey on Alcohol and Related Conditions (NESARC). Drug Alcohol Depend 115:120–130, 2011 21145178

Teesson M, Hall W, Proudfoot H, et al: Addictions, 2nd Edition. East Essex, UK, Psychology Press, 2012

CHAPTER 4

Cross-Cultural Aspects of Addiction

4.1   The term *ethnicity* refers to which of the following?

   A. People from diverse cultures who share a common background.
   B. The sum total of a group's life ways.
   C. The comparison of characteristics across culture groups.
   D. Distinct groupings within a culture.
   E. The cumulative social learning process.

   The correct response is option A: People from diverse cultures who share a common background.

   Ethnicity applies to people from diverse cultures who share a common background (option A). *Culture* is the sum total of a group's life ways (option B). *Cross-cultural* refers to the comparison of characteristics across culture groups (option C). *Sub-culture* refers to distinct groupings within a culture (option D). *Acculturation* is the cumulative social learning process in which people assimilate the values of the host culture while retaining the values of the original culture (option E). **(Concepts and Definitions, pp. 59–60)**

4.2   Confounding variables are commonly noted to affect prevalence estimates comparing the impact of addiction between ethnic groups. In which of the following studies would it be important to account for differences in *age distribution*?

   A. A survey of alcohol consumption in Mexican women presenting to a family practice clinic.
   B. A survey of high school students looking at differences in cannabis use between ethnic groups.
   C. A survey comparing alcohol use in Hawaiian residents born in Asia with those born in Hawaii.
   D. A survey examining the prevalence of substance use disorders in Native Americans compared with non–Native Americans.
   E. A survey of drug use in Hispanic persons born in the Unites States versus those born outside the United States.

The correct response is option D: A survey examining the prevalence of substance use disorders in Native Americans compared with non–Native Americans.

Differences in age distribution can affect prevalence rates. A higher proportion of youths, a high-risk group for substance use among Native Americans, could influence the prevalence of substance abuse in that ethnic group (option D). Societal norms can affect prevalence estimates as well; for example, Mexican societal attitudes are more negative toward women's alcohol consumption than men's; therefore, this societal norm is likely to have an impact on the prevalence estimates of women's alcohol consumption (option A). Population sampling is another important variable; school survey results must account for potential ethnic differences in school retention rates (option B). Extent of acculturation is another important variable. Studies have shown that substance use rates can vary between first- and second-generation immigrants (options C, E). **(Risk and Protective Factors Moderating the Impact of Ethnicity, pp. 61–63)**

4.3   Which of the following terms can be applied to a grouping resulting from a specific addiction, such as one might find in a crack house?

A. Culture.
B. Subculture.
C. Background.
D. Ethnicity.
E. Cross-cultural.

The correct response is option B: Subculture.

Subculture refers to distinct groupings within a culture. In the context of addiction, the term can be applied to groupings resulting from specific addictions, such as affiliations with cocktail lounges, gambling outlets, shooting galleries, or crack houses (option B). *Culture* is the sum total of a group's life ways and refers to such things as a shared worldview, social organization, and language (option A). *Background* refers to identity with a national and/or shared language of origin, religious practice, dress, diet, holidays or ceremonial events, traditional family rituals, use of disposable income, and leisure activities (option C). *Ethnicity* applies to people from diverse cultures that share a common background (option D). *Cross-cultural* refers to differences in culture or comparisons across cultural groups (option E). **(Concepts and Definitions, pp. 59–60)**

4.4   The clinical formulation of culture has traditionally been associated with which of the following?

A. Norm conflict.
B. Normative versus deviant behavior.
C. Socially prescribed use.
D. Cultural change.
E. Culture-bound syndromes.

The correct response is option E: Culture-bound syndromes.

Traditionally, diagnostic evocation of culture has been associated with rare culture-bound syndromes (option E) rather than with the much more common clinical presentations found in daily practice, which include the following factors: *Norm conflict* occurs when standards held desirable by a culture conflict with the person's behavior (option A). Any substance use in an abstinence-based group would be considered deviant (option B) but not necessarily pathological from a health perspective. *Socially prescribed use* occurs when use in religious rites is replaced by secular use (option C). *Cultural change* occurs through migration and exposure to new norms (option D). **(Clinical Cultural Formulation, pp. 63–64)**

4.5   Culturally sensitive care can be delivered through all of the following models, and each model has its own challenges. Which model runs the risk of marginalization?

A. Evidence-based manualized interventions.
B. Separate services.
C. Cultural consultation model.
D. Sensitized melting pot approach.
E. Individualized strategy.

The correct response is option B: Separate services.

One of the challenges of *separate services* is fear that separation further marginalizes people who are already marginalized (option B). The challenge of *evidence-based interventions* is striking the balance between adherence to the treatment manual and clinical flexibility (option A). In the *cultural consultation model,* a specialized multidisciplinary team brings together clinical experience with cultural knowledge and linguistic skills (option C). In the *sensitized melting pot approach,* mainstream services are commonly enriched by responding to the needs of all cultural groups, guaranteeing equality of access, and ensuring rights for all individuals (option D). An *individualized strategy* allows for both prescribed medication and ethnically specific interventions such as spiritual therapies (option E). **(Alternative Models of Care, pp. 67–68; Key Points, p. 68)**

CHAPTER 5

Science in the Treatment of Substance Abuse

5.1 By the early 1920s, most of the opioid detoxification clinics were closed. Which of the following was an important factor in this change?

A. Detoxification was not a common treatment for opioid addiction at the beginning of the twentieth century.
B. The clinics were deemed a failure because the patients did not become abstinent.
C. There were numerous treatments other than detoxification available for the treatment of opiate addiction.
D. Physicians could safely prescribe maintenance opioids independently of these clinics.
E. Most state governments discontinued their reimbursement of these clinics.

The correct response is option B: The clinics were deemed a failure because the patients did not become abstinent.

At the beginning of the twentieth century, the treatment for opiate addiction was detoxification (options A, C). However, the relapse was so great that clinics that dispensed morphine (or sometimes heroin) were opened in many U.S. cities. By the early 1920s, the clinics were closed, deemed a failure either because of patient diversion of drugs or because the patients did not become abstinent (option B). Physicians who continued to prescribe maintenance opioids to addicted patients were prosecuted. Between 1925 and 1940, about 25,000 physicians were arrested, and approximately 10% of them went to prison (option D). State funding for detoxification programs was not generally available until the introduction of Medicaid in the 1960s (option E). **(Introduction, pp. 73–75)**

5.2 Many well-known substance abuse treatment programs have historically expressed nonacceptance of medications as treatment options to prevent relapse. Which of the following best accounts for this decision?

A. There are limited medications available for this purpose.
B. Treatment programs are unaware of the potential benefit of these medications.

C. Medication use conflicts with their treatment philosophy.
D. There is insufficient research to support the use of these pharmacological approaches.
E. Medications are not cost-effective for the health care system.

The correct response is option C: Medication use conflicts with their treatment philosophy.

Much research on the treatment of substance use disorders (SUDs) has been conducted over the past 40 years, demonstrating that there are specific behavioral and pharmacological approaches to substance abuse treatment that have been found effective in numerous randomized controlled trials (option D). Unfortunately, only about 1 in 10 individuals with SUDs receives any treatment, and those who do usually do not experience evidence-based treatment techniques. As demonstrated in Dr. Sanjay Gupta's 2009 CNN documentary program *Addiction: Life on the Edge* (Gupta 2009), many treatment programs have expressed the opinion that "we don't *believe* in medications in our program"; thus, patients are deprived of the chance to benefit from medication just because of treatment philosophy (option C). The CNN program clearly shows senior therapists and counselors at well-known programs telling the reporter that they do not believe in the use of medications even though the reporter has just shown them an example of a patient who did extremely well by taking naltrexone (option B). Of course, not all patients will show the remarkable results reported by the patient interviewed in the documentary. If patients do not respond well to naltrexone, other medications that have been found to reduce relapse can be tried (option A). The existing drugs are showing progressively increasing success, not only for preventing relapse in practice but also for saving money for the health care system (option E). **(Introduction, pp. 73–75; Progress in Research, p. 75; Training of Treatment Providers, pp. 75–77; Ethical Considerations, pp. 77–78)**

5.3   Why is detoxification the most common form of treatment for substance use disorders?

A. Detoxification provides long-term benefit for patients with substance use disorders.
B. Detoxification makes the patient more comfortable and therefore more likely to comply with longer-term treatment.
C. Detoxification represents the best use of limited resources.
D. Detoxification alone is a highly effective treatment for substance use disorders.
E. Detoxification is covered by most insurance programs, even state Medicaid programs.

The correct response is option E: Detoxification is covered by most insurance programs, even state Medicaid programs.

The most common form of treatment for substance use disorders is probably *detoxification*, which, in reality, is not treatment at all. Simply reducing withdrawal symptoms by giving a short-term medication may make the patient more comfortable, but there is no long-term benefit (options A, B). However, because detoxification is covered by most insurance programs (that provide any coverage at all for substance abuse), providers tend to detoxify everyone. Even state Medicaid programs for people with low incomes will cover detoxification (option E), which is a waste of precious resources (option C). The data are very clear in showing that detoxification by itself is useless (option D). **(Most Common Treatment, p. 75)**

5.4   Which of the following best describes the position taken by the Central Council of Alcoholics Anonymous (AA) regarding individuals who are taking physician-prescribed treatment medications for substance dependence?

A. Individuals who are taking naltrexone, but not methadone or buprenorphine, are permitted to attend and speak freely at all AA meetings.
B. Use of physician-prescribed treatment medications is permitted.
C. Individuals taking physician-prescribed treatment medications are not permitted to attend any AA meetings.
D. Individuals taking any physician-prescribed treatment medications are permitted to attend and speak freely at all AA meetings.
E. The Central Council of AA has no position on this issue.

The correct response is option B: Use of physician-prescribed treatment medications is permitted.

The position taken by the Central Council of AA permits the use of physician-prescribed treatment medications (option B, not option E). Despite this, many (perhaps most) of the AA and Narcotics Anonymous groups do not permit individuals who are taking methadone or buprenorphine, or at times naltrexone, to speak at meetings. They are invited to stay but cannot speak until they stop taking these medications (options A, C, D). **(Training of Treatment Providers, pp. 75–77)**

5.5   Why have some clinicians denied that naltrexone is effective in patients with alcohol use disorder?

A. Naltrexone does not reliably produce long-term abstinence from alcohol; rather, it reliably produces a reduction in heavy drinking.
B. Studies have shown that naltrexone treatment leads to greater dropout rates from treatment.
C. Opioid receptor antagonists such as naltrexone are not approved in countries outside of the United States.
D. There is no evidence that opioid receptors are relevant in the reward pathway associated with addiction to alcohol.
E. Naltrexone has no effect on drinking patterns in patients with alcohol use disorder.

The correct response is option A: Naltrexone does not reliably produce long-term abstinence from alcohol; rather, it reliably produces a reduction in heavy drinking.

The discovery that reinforcement produced by alcohol significantly involves the endogenous opioid system was a breakthrough in the 1980s, but it still has not been adequately followed up. Many alcohol researchers actively resisted the idea that alcohol had anything in common with heroin. Although evidence from numerous animal models shows clearly that an essential step in the activation of the dopamine reward pathway by alcohol requires μ-opioid receptor activation (option D), no program of research (despite a request for proposals) has been issued by the National Institutes of Health to elucidate the molecular mechanism by which alcohol activates endogenous opioids. Although it has an effect on drinking patterns (option E), some clinicians have denied that naltrexone is effective because it does not reliably produce long-term complete abstinence from alcohol; rather, it reliably produces a reduction in heavy drinking (option A) and therefore is more like antihypertensive medication, which reduces blood pressure only as long as the medication is taken. Recent studies have found that naltrexone treatment leads to alcoholic individuals remaining in treatment longer (option B). In 2013, the European Medicines Agency reviewed the results of three studies using nalmefene, another opioid receptor antagonist, and approved the drug for use by physicians in the European Union for the reduction of heavy alcohol drinking (option C). **(Training of Treatment Providers, pp. 75–77)**

5.6   Which of the following best accounts for why there has been little motivation for pharmaceutical companies to pursue medications to treat substance use disorders?

A. The existing drugs have showed little success in preventing relapse.
B. Medications already available are used so little.
C. Medications to treat substance use disorders do not reduce costs.
D. Medications to treat substance use disorders do not reduce emergency visits.
E. Because of the Affordable Care Act, insurance will not pay for medications for the treatment of substance use disorders.

The correct response is option B: Medications already available are used so little.

Until now there has been little motivation for pharmaceutical companies to pursue medications to treat substance use disorders because already available medications are used so little (option B). Several developments may change this. First, the existing drugs are showing progressively increasing success, not only in preventing relapse in practice but also for saving money for the health care system (option A). Both Kaiser and Aetna systems are showing reduced costs by patients receiving extended-release naltrexone (option C), especially in reduced use of emergency room visits (option D). A second development is implementation of the requirements of the Affordable Care Act by the federal government. The plan is organized to detect substance use disorders early and thereby prevent costly medical and surgical complications later on. The insurance will pay for all U.S. Food and Drug Administration–approved medications for the treatment of substance use disorders (option E). It is expected that this increased coverage will demonstrate the cost-benefit advantage of medications for substance use disorder treatment and also encourage pharmaceutical research aimed at the development of new and more effective medications. **(Training of Treatment Providers, pp. 75–77)**

References

Gupta S: Addiction: life on the edge. CNN, April 2009. Available at: http://transcripts.cnn.com/TRANSCRIPTS/0904/19/cp.01.html. Accessed January 7, 2015.

CHAPTER 6

Assessment of the Patient

6.1   Which of the following interview questions is most likely to make a patient feel comfortable during an initial interview?

A. How long have you been addicted to cocaine?
B. Why do you use cocaine?
C. Is anyone else in your family addicted?
D. What brought you to see me today?
E. Have you ever been to a hospital because of your cocaine use?

The correct response is option D: What brought you to see me today?

Obstacles to obtaining an accurate substance abuse history include the patient's defenses, such as denial, minimization, rationalization, projection, and externalization (Schottenfeld and Pantalon 1999). Asking open-ended questions such as "What brought you to see me today?" (option D) may circumvent these obstacles. Clinicians can also avoid using labels such as "addicted" (options A, C); instead, they can ask patients to describe their pattern of use without labeling it. Maintaining a nonjudgmental stance is helpful to patients who may have feelings of shame or denial. For example, a clinician may ask, "How were you feeling before you used cocaine?" rather than "Why do you use cocaine?" (option B). Option E is not an open-ended question and is likely to make the patient feel defensive. **(Eliciting the Substance Abuse History/Interviewing Style, pp. 81–82)**

6.2   Which of the following substances requires inpatient detoxification?

A. Marijuana.
B. Nicotine.
C. Benzodiazepines.
D. Cocaine.
E. Amphetamines.

The correct response is option C: Benzodiazepines.

Untreated withdrawal from alcohol or from sedatives, hypnotics, or anxiolytics (e.g., benzodiazepines, barbiturates) can result in seizures, delirium tremens, and death (option C). Withdrawal syndromes associated with the use of marijuana or of stimulants such as cocaine and amphetamines do not require inpatient detoxification (options A, D, E) (American Psychiatric Association 2006). Nicotine withdrawal is also managed on an outpatient basis (American Psychiatric Association 2006) (option B). **(Eliciting the Substance Abuse History/Patient Characteristics, pp. 82–84)**

6.3   Which of the following patients has a substance-induced mental disorder?

A. A 16-year-old boy who began drinking to cope with social anxiety.
B. A 31-year-old man who developed auditory hallucinations 2 years after cessation of cocaine use.
C. A 30-year-old woman who complains of depressed mood after 2 years of near-daily marijuana use.
D. A 77-year-old man with a history of daily alcohol use who experiences disorientation and visual hallucinations 3 days after his last drink.
E. A 21-year-old woman who developed depressed mood and suicidal thoughts 1 week after using cocaine for the first time.

The correct response is option E: A 21-year-old woman who developed depressed mood and suicidal thoughts 1 week after using cocaine for the first time.

A diagnosis of a *substance-induced mental disorder* is made when symptoms meeting the full criteria for a mental disorder develop during or within 1 month of intoxication with or withdrawal from a substance that is capable of causing the mental disorder (option E) (American Psychiatric Association 2013). The 2-year time span in option C exceeds the 1-month time noted in the definition. A mental disorder would be considered independent of a substance if the disorder preceded the onset of severe intoxication or withdrawal (option A), or if the mental disorder persisted for a substantial period of time (e.g., at least 1 month) after substance intoxication or substance withdrawal ended (option B). Additionally, the disorder cannot occur exclusively during the course of a delirium (option D), and the disorder must cause clinically significant distress or impairment in important areas of functioning. **(Content of the Interview/Psychiatric History, pp. 88–89)**

6.4   Which of the following medical problems is *least* likely to be related to alcohol dependence?

A. Cerebellar degeneration.
B. Peripheral vascular disease.
C. Cardiomyopathy.
D. Pancreatitis.
E. Aspiration pneumonia.

The correct response is option B: Peripheral vascular disease.

Peripheral vascular disease is most commonly associated with use of nicotine (option B). Cerebellar degeneration (option A), cardiomyopathy (option C), pancreatitis (option D), and aspiration pneumonia (option E) are all associated with alcohol use disorder (Table 6–1). **(Table 6–2, Medical problems associated with substance-related disorders, p. 90)**

TABLE 6–1. **Medical problems associated with substance-related disorders**

Alcohol	Cocaine
Blackouts	Transient ischemic attacks
Hangovers	Cerebral vascular events
Withdrawal tremors	Ischemia of gastrointestinal tract
Withdrawal seizures	Chest pain
Delirium tremens	Myocardial infarction
Aspiration pneumonia	Pneumothorax (intranasal)
Cardiomyopathy	Pneumomediastinum (intranasal)
Cerebellar degeneration	Pulmonary infarction (intranasal)
Gastritis	Dyspnea (intranasal)
Gastroesophageal reflux disease	Cellulitis (intravenous)
Hepatitis	Endocarditis (intravenous)
Pancreatitis	
Wernicke-Korsakoff syndrome	**Opioids**
	Constipation
Nicotine	In overdose:
Chronic obstructive pulmonary disease	Respiratory depression
Emphysema	Coma
Cardiovascular disease	Death
Peripheral vascular disease	
Lung cancer	**Alcohol and illicit drugs**
Oral cancer	Hepatitis B
	Hepatitis C
Sedative-hypnotics	HIV
Withdrawal tremors	Tuberculosis
Withdrawal seizures	
In overdose:	
Respiratory depression	
Coma	
Death	

6.5 Which of the following is true regarding the use of collateral informants when obtaining a substance use history?

    A. Contact with collateral informants should occur only with written permission from the patient.

    B. There is no role for the involvement of collateral informants in treatment planning and recovery.

C. Patients are most likely to maintain abstinence if collateral informants are not involved in treatment.
D. Collateral informant interviews are unlikely to provide helpful information.
E. Collateral informants should not be asked about the patient's substance use, as this violates patient confidentiality.

The correct response is option A: Contact with collateral informants should occur only with written permission from the patient.

Collateral informant interviews may provide helpful information for some patients (option D). A patient's significant others can often serve as collateral informants who can corroborate and provide additional information about the patient's reported substance use history (Carroll 1995). Speaking with the patient's significant others also allows for their early involvement in treatment planning and may help in establishing social networks that can potentially support the patient's recovery and help maintain abstinence (Havassy et al. 1991) (options B, C). Contact with collateral informants should occur only with written permission from the patient (option A, not option E). **(Obtaining Additional Information, p. 94; Key Points, p. 95)**

References

American Psychiatric Association: Practice guideline for the treatment of patients with substance use disorders, 2nd edition, in American Psychiatric Association Practice Guidelines for the Treatment of Psychiatric Disorders: Compendium. Washington, DC, American Psychiatric Association, 2006, pp 291–563
American Psychiatric Association: Diagnostic and Statistical Manual of Mental Disorders, 5th Edition. Washington, DC, American Psychiatric Association, 2013
Carroll KM: Methodological issues and problems in the assessment of substance use. Psychol Assess 3:349–358, 1995
Havassy BE, Hall SM, Wasserman DA: Social support and relapse: commonalities among alcoholics, opiate users, and cigarette smokers. Addict Behav 16:235–246, 1991 1663695
Schottenfeld R, Pantalon M: Assessment of the patient, in The American Psychiatric Press Textbook of Substance Abuse Treatment, 2nd Edition. Edited by Galanter M, Kleber HD. Washington, DC, American Psychiatric Press, 1999, pp 109–120

CHAPTER 7

Screening and Brief Intervention

7.1 For which of the following patients does evidence support the use of screening and brief intervention (SBI)?

A. A patient seeking treatment for moderate alcohol use disorder.
B. A patient seen in an emergency department for chest pain following cocaine use.
C. A patient seen in a primary care clinic for an annual physical.
D. A patient who presents for treatment of a panic attack following cannabis use.
E. A patient who has been arrested for driving under the influence.

The correct response is option C: A patient seen in a primary care clinic for an annual physical.

SBI is simultaneously 1) a preventive intervention aimed at recurring behavioral risks and 2) an initial step in the management of moderate to severe substance use disorders. The best evidence supports preventive intervention—decreasing risk for people who use substances associated with future health harms but who have mild or no substance use disorder (option C). Little evidence supports the second definition, although SBI as a first part of longer-term treatment or as a referral strategy has not been well studied. In addition, little evidence supports the efficacy of SBI for drugs other than alcohol (options B, D). SBI is a clinical preventive service and is not geared primarily to those with symptoms (options A, B, D, E). As such, it is to be implemented in settings in which the main purpose of the health care visit is not attention to substance use (option C). In settings in which patients are seeking help or treatment for substance use and substance use disorders or in which patients have symptoms or diagnoses for which substance use disorders rank high on the differential diagnosis, SBI is not useful (options A, B, D, E). **(Introduction, pp. 99–103)**

7.2 Which of the following screening tools is most useful for brief screening?

A. Alcohol Use Disorders Identification Test (AUDIT-C).
B. Alcohol, Smoking and Substance Involvement Screening Test (ASSIST).

C. CAGE questionnaire.
D. Michigan Alcoholism Screening Test (MAST).
E. Drug Abuse Screening Test (DAST).

The correct response is option A: Alcohol Use Disorders Identification Test (AUDIT-C).

Tools validated as part of controlled trials of screening and brief intervention, such as the AUDIT (Babor et al. 2001), are ideal. The AUDIT-C is a well-validated, short screening version of the AUDIT with three alcohol consumption items (option A).

The ASSIST can have upward of six-dozen items, depending on how many substances the patient reports using, and is unwieldy for screening (option B). The CAGE questionnaire (Mayfield et al. 1974) and the MAST (Selzer 1971) were among the first screening tools developed. However, these tools are no longer recommended for screening because although they can identify alcohol use disorders, they are not sufficiently accurate for identifying the spectrum of unhealthy use (options C, D). The MAST is also too long. DAST (Skinner 1982) has not been found to have better validity than single screening questions in general health care settings (option E). The 10-item version of the DAST is a longer option for screening for drugs; its validity for screening in primary care settings is much lower than that of the AUDIT for alcohol, and the screening results do not provide information on which drug might be a concern. **(Screening/Screening Tools, pp. 100–103)**

7.3   Which of the following problem drinkers is in the *precontemplative* stage of change?

A. A 40-year-old man who recently started drinking after 2 years of abstinence.
B. A 66-year-old woman who has decided to stop drinking.
C. A 42-year-old man who attends Alcoholics Anonymous weekly and has been sober for 3 years.
D. A 27-year-old woman who has experienced blackouts when drinking but denies having a problem with alcohol.
E. A 39-year-old man who has entered a 28-day rehabilitation program.

The correct response is option D: A 27-year-old woman who has experienced blackouts when drinking but denies having a problem with alcohol.

Readiness to change lies on a continuum. In the precontemplative stage, the patient is not considering making a change (option D). In the contemplation stage, the patient is thinking about change. In the determination stage, the patient has decided to change (option B). In the action stage, the patient is making a change (option E). In the maintenance stage, the patient has made a change (option C). In the relapse stage, the patient has returned to unhealthy use (option A). **(Assessment/Assessment of the Patient's Perception and Readiness to Change, pp. 104–105)**

7.4   A patient states that one reason he drinks during the day is because he does not want family and friends to see his hands shake. Which of the following responses exemplifies the technique of reflective listening?

A. "I am concerned that you are putting yourself at risk by drinking during the daytime."
B. "You should tell your family about your drinking."
C. "You are embarrassed about your tremor."
D. "Do you think that other people will notice your tremor?"
E. "Let's set a goal that you will not drink during the daytime."

The correct response is option C: "You are embarrassed about your tremor."

Reflective listening is a key skill of motivational interviewing that is helpful in brief behavior change counseling. Reflective listening involves repeating or paraphrasing what the patient has said in the form of a statement (option C), not a question (option D). When the clinician uses reflective listening, patients feel that the clinician has heard or listened to them; even though what they hear is just a reflection of what they said, it has a powerful impact. Brief intervention, unlike reflective listening, involves feedback about the patient's risks and consequences of substance use (option A), specific advice (option B), and goal setting (option E). **(Brief Counseling Interventions/Performing a Brief Intervention, pp. 105–106)**

7.5 Which of the following is a proven effect of brief intervention (BI) for patients with alcohol use?

A. Reductions in motor vehicle crashes.
B. Reduction in mortality.
C. Reduction in emergency room utilization.
D. Reduction in risky drinking by 10% at 1 year.
E. Reduction in risky drinking by 10 drinks per week.

The correct response is option D: Reduction in risky drinking by 10% at 1 year.

The effect of BI is to decrease risky drinking by about 10%–12% at 1 year (option D) and by about three drinks per week (not 10 drinks per week, option E) (Jonas et al. 2012). Although this is a small effect for an individual, it is significant relative to public health. Although some studies have found benefits for outcomes beyond drinking (e.g., reduction in motor vehicle crashes [option A], less hospital or emergency department utilization [option C], or even lower mortality [option B]), data at present are insufficient to draw firm conclusions about the impact of BI on these outcomes. **(Brief Counseling Interventions/Evidence for Efficacy of Brief Intervention Among Patients Identified by Screening, pp. 106–108)**

7.6 Which of the following patients would be considered a "risky" drinker?

A. A 45-year-old man who consumes 12–14 grams of ethanol 7 times a week.
B. A 35-year-old woman who drinks four 12-ounce beers a day.
C. A 68-year-old man who drinks 2 ounces of 80-proof liquor every other day.
D. A 50-year-old man who drinks 12 ounces of wine over the course of a weekend.
E. A 22-year-old woman who drinks a glass of wine every day.

The correct response is option B: A 35-year-old woman who drinks four 12-ounce beers a day.

The National Institute on Alcohol Abuse and Alcoholism (2007) defines "risky" amounts as more than 14 drinks per week on average or more than 4 drinks in a day for men less than 65 years of age, and more than 7 drinks per week or three in a day for women and for men age 65 or older. A standard drink has 12–14 grams of ethanol, which is the content found in 12 ounces of regular-strength beer, 5 ounces of nonfortified wine, and 1.5 ounces of 80-proof liquor.

A man younger than 65 years who consumes 12–14 grams of ethanol 7 times a week is having one drink daily, for a total of 7 per week; thus, his consumption is below the total needed to qualify his use as risky (option A). A man 65 years or older should not drink more than 10.5 ounces of liquor per week; the man in that age group in this question is drinking a total of 6 ounces of liquor per week (option C). A man who drinks 12 ounces of wine 2 days a week (option D) is drinking approximately 2.5 drinks twice a week; even if he were over 65, he would still not be considered a risky drinker. A 22-year-old woman who drinks one glass of wine daily (option E) remains at the limit for women of 7 drinks weekly. A woman who drinks four 12-ounce beers a day (option B) consumes much more than the limit of 3 drinks daily or 7 drinks weekly for women of all ages. **(Screening/Purpose of Screening, p. 100)**

References

Babor TF, Higgins-Biddle JC, Saunders JB, et al: AUDIT: The Alcohol Use Disorders Identification Test: Guidelines for Use in Primary Health Care (WHO Publ No PSA/92.4). Geneva, Switzerland, World Health Organization, 2001

Jonas DE, Garbutt JC, Amick HR, et al: Behavioral counseling after screening for alcohol misuse in primary care: a systematic review and meta-analysis for the U.S. Preventive Services Task Force. Ann Intern Med 157:645–654, 2012 23007881

Mayfield D, McLeod G, Hall P: The CAGE questionnaire: validation of a new alcoholism screening instrument. Am J Psychiatry 131:1121–1123, 1974 4416585

National Institute on Alcohol Abuse and Alcoholism: Helping Patients Who Drink Too Much: A Clinician's Guide: Updated, 2005 Edition. Bethesda, MD, National Institutes of Health, 2007

Selzer ML: The Michigan Alcoholism Screening Test: the quest for a new diagnostic instrument. Am J Psychiatry 127:1653–1658, 1971 5565851

Skinner H: The Drug Abuse Screening Test. Addict Behav 7:363–371, 1982 7183189

CHAPTER 8

Patient Placement Criteria

8.1   Which of the following is an example of placement matching?

   A. You determine that your patient is suitable for motivational enhancement therapy.
   B. You determine that your patient is not suitable for naltrexone treatment.
   C. You determine that your patient is suitable for family therapy.
   D. You determine that your patient requires intensive outpatient care.
   E. You determine that your patient should be transferred to another provider.

   The correct response is option D: You determine that your patient requires intensive outpatient care.

   To understand patient placement criteria, one must be aware of the distinction between placement matching and modality matching. *Placement matching* refers to patient assignments made to a treatment setting with certain resource intensity rather than to an individual provider (option E). *Modality matching* (options A, B, C) refers to patient assignments made according to the optimal theoretical model or clinical approach that corresponds to a patient's problems (Gastfriend et al. 2000). Placement matching applies to a setting, such as intensive outpatient or residential care (option D), whereas modality matching is focused on the suitability for a particular person of, for example, motivational enhancement therapy (option A), family therapy (option C), or a certain medication (option B). **(Rationale for Patient Placement Criteria, pp. 112–113)**

8.2   As part of the evaluation and treatment of a 47-year-old married real estate agent with alcohol use disorder, you recommend that his spouse and teenage children attend Alanon and Alateen, respectively. This is an example of which of the following American Society of Addiction Medicine (ASAM) Patient Placement Criteria (PPC) assessment dimensions?

   A. Family history of psychiatric illness.
   B. Health insurance status.
   C. Patient demographics.
   D. Recovery environment.
   E. Participation in self-help recovery groups.

The correct response is option D: Recovery environment.

The most widely used and researched patient placement criteria for addiction treatment are the PPC for the Treatment of Substance-Related Disorders of the ASAM (American Society of Addiction Medicine 1996). The revised second edition (ASAM PPC-2R) included criteria for people with co-occurring mental and substance use disorders (Mee-Lee et al. 2001).

To place a patient, the evaluator is required to screen and diagnose the patient, then assess patient characteristics in six dimensions encompassing all pertinent biopsychosocial aspects of addiction that determine the severity of the patient's illness and level of function, as described in Table 8–1. These problem areas (dimensions) have been identified as essential in the formulation of an individual patient's treatment plan and, subsequently, in making patient placement decisions. Recovery environment (option D) involves assessment of need for specific individualized, family, or significant other services and the need for housing, financial, vocational, educational, legal, transportation, or child care services. Options A, B, C, and E, although they may be relevant aspects of an addiction assessment, are not considered formal dimensions of the ASAM PPC. **(Origins and Organization of the ASAM Patient Placement Criteria, pp. 113–118; Table 8–2, American Society of Addiction Medicine criteria assessment dimensions, p. 116)**

8.3   As the treating psychiatrist, you engage a 49-year-old patient with alcohol use disorder in a therapeutic discussion of the pros and cons of his alcohol use. To which American Society of Addiction Medicine (ASAM) Patient Placement Criteria (PPC) assessment dimension does this correspond?

   A. Acute intoxication and/or withdrawal potential.
   B. Biomedical conditions and complications.
   C. Emotional, behavioral, or cognitive conditions and complications.
   D. Readiness to change.
   E. Recovery environment.

The correct response is option D: Readiness to change.

Readiness to change involves assessment of the patient's stage of readiness to change. If the patient is not ready to commit to full recovery, he or she should be engaged with treatment using motivational enhancement strategies (option D). If the patient is ready for recovery, consolidate and expand action for change. While options A, B, C, and E are also ASAM PPC assessment dimensions, they do not involve engaging the patient in readiness to change current patterns of use by discussion of pros or cons of current substance use.

8.4   Which of the following is an American Society of Addiction Medicine (ASAM) Patient Placement Criteria (PPC) basic treatment level?

   A. Early intervention.
   B. Intensive outpatient/partial hospitalization.

TABLE 8–1. American Society of Addiction Medicine criteria assessment dimensions

Dimensions	Assessment and treatment planning focus
1. Acute intoxication and/or withdrawal potential	Assess for intoxication and/or withdrawal management. Manage withdrawal in a variety of levels of care, and make preparations for continued addiction services.
2. Biomedical conditions and complications	Assess and treat co-occurring physical health conditions or complications. Treatment provided within the level of care or through coordination of physical health services.
3. Emotional, behavioral, or cognitive conditions and complications	Assess and treat co-occurring diagnostic or subdiagnostic mental health conditions or complications. Treatment provided within level of care or through coordination of mental health services.
4. Readiness to change	Assess stage of readiness to change. If not ready to commit to full recovery, engage into treatment using motivational enhancement strategies. If ready for recovery, consolidate and expand action for change.
5. Relapse, continued use, or continued problem potential	Assess readiness for relapse prevention services and teach, where appropriate. If still at early stages of change, focus on raising consciousness of consequences of continued use or continued problems as part of motivational enhancement strategies.
6. Recovery environment	Assess need for specific, individualized, family, or significant other services, and the need for housing, financial, vocational, educational, legal, transportation, or child care services.

    C. Student health services.
    D. Emergency room detoxification.
    E. Peer support groups.

The correct response is option B: Intensive outpatient/partial hospitalization.

In the ASAM PPC, one prevention level (Level 0.5) and four basic treatment levels of care exist, within which later editions of the criteria indicate additional sublevels and modalities:

- Level 0.5: Early intervention.
- Level 1: Outpatient services. Level 1 services are provided in regularly scheduled sessions and are designed to help the individual achieve permanent changes in his or her alcohol and drug-using behavior and mental functioning. The services address major lifestyle, attitudinal, and behavioral issues that have the potential to undermine the goals of treatment or inhibit the individual's ability to cope with major life tasks without the nonmedical use of alcohol or other drugs.
- Level 2: Intensive outpatient/partial hospitalization (option B).
- Level 3: Residential/inpatient services.
- Level 4: Medically managed intensive inpatient services.

Option A is an ASAM PPC prevention level. Options C and D are treatment settings but are not part of the ASAM PPC basic treatment levels. Option E is not an ASAM PPC level. **(Origins and Organization of the ASAM Patient Placement Criteria, pp. 113–118)**

8.5   Which of the following tools is used to evaluate the American Society of Addiction Medicine (ASAM) Patient Placement Criteria (PPC) assessment dimension of acute intoxication or withdrawal as part of a multidimensional patient assessment?

   A. CAGE questionnaire.
   B. Alcohol Use Disorders Identification Test-C (AUDIT-C).
   C. Clinical Institute Withdrawal Assessment for Alcohol Scale—Revised (CIWA-Ar).
   D. Drug Abuse Screening Test (DAST).
   E. Michigan Alcoholism Screening Test (MAST).

The correct response is option C: Clinical Institute Withdrawal Assessment for Alcohol Scale—Revised (CIWA-Ar).

Practitioners and others involved in running treatment programs who seek more rigorous and comprehensive multidimensional methods of assessment, especially in research settings, can most effectively evaluate the dimensions through the use of the computer-driven structured interview (Gastfriend et al. 1994). A considerable portion of needed information can be obtained from the most widely used tool in the field, the Addiction Severity Index (McLellan et al. 1992), and also from the CIWA-Ar (Sullivan et al. 1989) and the Clinical Institute Narcotics Assessment (CINA; Fudala et al. 1991). The CIWA-Ar and CINA are standardized scales that can be used to evaluate the first assessment dimension: acute intoxication or withdrawal.

Many screening tools have been validated for their accuracy. The key issues for selecting a tool for practice are brevity, wide applicability to populations, and validity for detecting the full spectrum of unhealthy use. The CAGE questions (Mayfield et al. 1974) and the MAST (Selzer 1971) were among the first screening tools developed. (The acronym CAGE stands for four questions: Have you ever felt you should cut down on your drinking? Have people annoyed you by criticizing your drinking? Have you ever felt bad or guilty about your drinking? Have you ever taken a drink first thing in the morning [eye-opener] to steady your nerves or get rid of a hangover?) However, these tools are no longer recommended for screening because although they can identify alcohol use disorders, they are not sufficiently accurate for identifying the spectrum of unhealthy use; also, the MAST is too long (options A, E).

The AUDIT-C (Babor et al. 2001) is a well-validated, short screening version of the AUDIT with three alcohol consumption items.

The 10-item version of the DAST is a longer option for screening for drugs that may provide additional information useful for discussion during a brief intervention (option D) (Yudko et al. 2007).

The assessment tool most often cited in current alcohol withdrawal literature is the CIWA-Ar (option C). This clinician-rated checklist, a 10-item scale used to monitor the clinical course of withdrawal symptoms, includes assessments of nausea; vomiting; tremor; sweating; anxiety; agitation; tactile, auditory, and visual disturbances; and clouding of sensorium. Higher total scores indicate more severe alcohol withdrawal symptoms and a greater risk of major withdrawal symptoms such as delirium tremens and seizures (Foy et al. 1988). **(Origins and Organization of the ASAM Patient Placement Criteria, pp. 113–118; see also Chapter 7, pp. 100–103)**

References

American Society of Addiction Medicine: Patient Placement Criteria for the Treatment of Substance-Related Disorders: ASAM PPC-2, 2nd Edition. Chevy Chase, MD, American Society of Addiction Medicine, 1996

Babor TF, Higgins-Biddle JC, Saunders JB, et al: AUDIT: The Alcohol Use Disorders Identification Test: Guidelines for Use in Primary Health Care (WHO Publ No PSA/92.4). Geneva, Switzerland, World Health Organization, 2001

Foy A, March S, Drinkwater V: Use of an objective clinical scale in the assessment and management of alcohol withdrawal in a large general hospital. Alcohol Clin Exp Res 12:360–364, 1988 3044163

Fudala PJ, Berkow LC, Fralich JL, et al: Use of naloxone in the assessment of opiate dependence. Life Sci 49:1809–1814, 1991 1943484

Gastfriend DR, Baker SL, Najavits LM, et al: Assessment instruments, in Principles of Addiction Medicine. Edited by Miller N, Doot M. Chevy Chase, MD, American Society of Addiction Medicine, 1994, pp 1–8

Gastfriend DR, Lu SH, Sharon E: Placement matching: challenges and technical progress. Subst Use Misuse 35:2191–2213, 2000 11138721

Mayfield D, McLeod G, Hall P: The CAGE questionnaire: validation of a new alcoholism screening instrument. Am J Psychiatry 131:1121–1123, 1974 4416585

McLellan AT, Kushner H, Metzger DS, et al: The fifth edition of the Addiction Severity Index. J Subst Abuse Treat 9:199–213, 1992

Mee-Lee D, Shulman GD, Fishman M, et al: ASAM Patient Placement Criteria for the Treatment of Substance-Related Disorders, 2nd Edition, Revised (ASAM PPC-2R). Chevy Chase, MD, American Society of Addiction Medicine, 2001

Selzer ML: The Michigan Alcoholism Screening Test: the quest for a new diagnostic instrument. Am J Psychiatry 127:1653–1658, 1971 5565851

Sullivan JT, Sykora K, Schneiderman J, et al: Assessment of alcohol withdrawal: the revised Clinical Institute Withdrawal Assessment for Alcohol Scale (CIWA-Ar). Br J Addict 84:1353–1357, 1989 2597811

Yudko E, Lozhkina O, Fouts A: A comprehensive review of the psychometric properties of the Drug Abuse Screening Test. J Subst Abuse Treat 32:189–198, 2007 17306727

CHAPTER 9

"Recovery" in Chronic Care Disease Management

"Disease Control" in Substance Use Disorders

9.1   Recent federal legislation will promote changes in the way that substance abuse is treated. Which of the following is the most accurate statement about these changes?

   A. The Wellstone and Domenici Mental Health Parity and Affordable Addiction Equity (MHPAE) Act of 2009 requires physicians to report patients who drink and drive, and thus put others at risk, to an appropriate law enforcement agency.
   B. The Patient Protection and Affordable Care (PPAC) Act of 2010 requires all health care plans to offer prevention screening and brief interventions to detect and reduce medically harmful substance abuse.
   C. The MHPAE Act requires that care for substance abuse be administered only by professionals who are trained substance abuse specialists.
   D. The PPAC Act pertains only to patients who self-identify as having substance abuse problems.
   E. Taken together, the MHPAE Act and the PPAC Act will aid in getting substance abuse patients out of primary care and into specialty addiction clinics.

The correct response is option B: The Patient Protection and Affordable Care (PPAC) Act of 2010 requires all health care plans to offer prevention screening and brief interventions to detect and reduce medically harmful substance abuse.

The PPAC Act essentially requires all health plans to offer care for the full spectrum of substance use disorders: prevention, screening, and brief interventions to detect and reduce "medically harmful use" (option B). This will end the long-standing segregation of the substance abuse field from the rest of health care and will likely mean that substance abuse will be treated by the same people and same places that treat other chronic illnesses, namely, in primary care settings (options C and E). The screening and prevention services are thus aimed at a broad range

155

of patients, not just self-identified substance abusers (option D). The MHPAE Act does not deal with reporting requirements (option A). **(The Concept and Measurement of "Recovery," pp. 129–130)**

9.2   Which of the following statements most accurately describes the chronic care management (CCM) model?

    A. The CCM model involves a multidisciplinary team approach focused on tracking disease status with the goal of relapse prevention.

    B. The CCM model prevents the suboptimal outcomes that can derive from patients managing their own care.

    C. Although more effective than traditional episodic-reactive approach, the CCM model is costlier and often resented by patients.

    D. The recovery model is incompatible with the CCM model and will need to be abandoned because the CCM model is implemented more widely.

    E. The CCM model is applicable to type 2 diabetes and rheumatologic disorder because those illnesses involve patient self-management to an important degree.

The correct response is option A: The CCM model involves a multidisciplinary team approach focused on tracking disease status with the goal of relapse prevention.

The CCM model replaces traditional single-clinician care with multidisciplinary team care using new health information technologies to track patient "disease control" and to anticipate and prevent relapses (option A). Care specifically provided by the clinical team is designed to lead to enhanced "patient self-management," not diminish patient participation (Bodenheimer et al. 2002; Wagner et al. 1996) (option B). There is evidence that CCM is more effective than traditional clinical care in the treatment of many chronic medical illnesses (Dobscha et al. 2009) not just a few (option E) and that it is more appreciated by patients (option C) and physicians (Marsteller et al. 2010). In addition, it does not cost more than traditional care (Rosenthal et al. 2010) (option C). The term *recovery* as used in the substance abuse field can be integrated into the language associated with the CCM model (option D). **(The Concept and Measurement of "Recovery"/Chronic Care Management Model, pp. 130–131)**

9.3   Although there are multiple differing definitions of *recovery*, the definitions share some common elements. Which of the following most accurately describes the common elements?

    A. Some definitions use the term *abstinence* and others use the term *sobriety;* however, all definitions agree that the term *recovery* applies only to individuals who have stopped using illicit substances.

    B. Current definitions of *recovery* include adherence to a 12-step approach as a necessary condition.

    C. All definitions recognize that *recovery* describes an outcome of behavior change.

D. Recovery involves a process of behavior change that includes improved health and well-being.
E. Recovery requires abstinence; thus a patient may improve while taking medication, the use of medications, however, precludes being in recovery.

The correct response is option D: Recovery involves a process of behavior change that includes improved health and well-being.

Three widely used definitions of *recovery* cover different aspects but also contain the common notion of a process of change, including improved health and well-being (option D). The three representative definitions are 1) a *process* of change (not an outcome) (option C) through which individuals improve their health and wellness, live a *self-directed life,* and strive to reach their full potential (Substance Abuse and Mental Health Services Administration 2011); 2) a voluntarily maintained *lifestyle* characterized by *sobriety*, *personal health,* and *citizenship* (Betty Ford Institute Consensus Panel 2007); and 3) voluntarily sustained *control over substance use,* which maximizes health and well-being and participation in the rights, roles, and responsibilities of society (U.K. Drug Policy Commission Recovery Consensus Group 2008). Only the Betty Ford Institute definition emphasizes sobriety as a necessary condition for being in recovery (option A). Despite the fact that Alcoholics Anonymous (AA) and other 12-step programs are the most familiar methods presently used to attain recovery, none of the definitions suggests a single approach, method, or formula for achieving recovery (option B). The argument that being "medicated" is inconsistent with being "in recovery" is a relatively recent historical development; even the founders of AA recognized that there were many paths to the same position (Alcoholics Anonymous World Services 2001; Cheever 2004) (option E). **(Defining *Recovery,* pp. 131–133)**

9.4   Which of the following best describes the study by Dawson et al. (2005) examining diagnostic transitions among adults with self-reported alcohol dependence?

A. Abstinence is an effective but not prevalent method of achieving disease control in alcohol-dependent individuals.
B. Only 18% of the total sample of subjects who had prior alcohol dependence were in remission for the past year.
C. Those individuals in the study who were previously treated for alcohol dependence (an indication of a more severe illness) had significantly higher rates of total abstinence than the rest of the total sample.
D. Abstinence is the only method of achieving stable remission from alcohol dependence.
E. Those who had been previously treated were unlikely to still have a diagnosis of alcohol dependence.

The correct response is option A: Abstinence is an effective but not prevalent method of achieving disease control in alcohol-dependent individuals.

The study by Dawson et al. (2005) examined 4,422 adults (age 18 and older) who self-reported alcohol dependence (DSM-IV [American Psychiatric Association 2000] criteria) sometime prior to the past year. These adults were interviewed about their drinking status in the past year and categorized into five levels. Individuals in the first three categories—abstainer, low-risk drinker, and asymptomatic risk drinker—were operationally defined as being "in full remission" because their drinking was below National Institute on Alcohol Abuse and Alcoholism unhealthy limits. However, only individuals in the first two categories were classified as being in recovery. In this regard, it is quite interesting that almost half (48%) of previously addicted drinkers met the operational definition of being in remission for the past year (categories 1–3) (option B). Most surprising is the fact that only 37.5% (18/48) of those who achieved remission did so by maintaining abstinence (option A). In turn, a closer examination of the Dawson et al. (2005) data reveals that among those previously treated for alcohol dependence, roughly one-third were still dependent (option E), one-third were abstinent (option C) and in recovery, and one-third were drinking in a nondependent manner. These findings are somewhat closer to what might be expected from the traditional views about addiction and recovery, but even this more severely affected sample shows a very significant proportion of formerly dependent drinkers maintaining disease control although drinking (option D). **("Disease Control" in Addiction/Recovery From Alcohol Addiction, pp. 134–138)**

9.5   The Look AHEAD (Action for Health in Diabetes) study (Gregg et al. 2012), although focusing on adults with type 2 diabetes, has elements analogous to those in the recovery approach to substance abuse. Which of the following best describes the comparison between these studies?

A. Weight loss was an important outcome variable in the Look AHEAD study, and reduction in alcohol intake also contributes to weight loss.
B. In the Look AHEAD study, the intensive lifestyle intervention (ILI) involved changes in lifestyle supported by individual and group counseling analogous to those supported in a 12-step recovery program.
C. In both the ILI intervention and the recovery approach, individual counseling served to ensure that patients take their prescribed medication.
D. In the ILI intervention, patients only showed improvement if they increased their medication intake over the 4 years of the study.
E. The ILI intervention involved weight loss and exercise, which cannot be compared with the behavior changes required in the recovery approach to substance use.

The correct response is option B: In the Look AHEAD study, the intensive lifestyle intervention (ILI) involved changes in lifestyle supported by individual and group counseling analogous to those supported in a 12-step recovery program.

The Look AHEAD study followed 5,145 obese adults with type 2 diabetes (see Gregg et al. 2012). Its primary objective was to bring about remission of cardiac events and also diabetes, hypertension, and sleep apnea using an intensive lifestyle intervention to change patients' problematic behaviors. The two conditions were 1) diabetes support and education, consisting of usual medical care supplemented by patient education, and 2) ILI, consisting of group and individual counseling sessions to achieve weight loss through planned dieting and increased physical activity (option B). The ILI group lost significantly more weight, showed greater fitness increases, and was significantly more likely to be in partial or complete remission from diabetes than the control participants. The types of lifestyle changes required by ILI are quite in line with the requirements for commitment to "sobriety, personal health, and citizenship" (Betty Ford Institute Consensus Panel 2007), as commonly expected of substance-dependent patients (option E). Indeed, even the methods to attain these personal goals were similar: individual and group counseling sessions and personal case management to support patient self-change (not to focus on medication as a solution) (option C). Interestingly, as in many addiction treatment studies, about one-third of recruited patients showed reduction of diabetes, hypertension, and sleep apnea symptoms to below diagnostic levels, despite elimination of most of their medications (option D). The effect of recovery on weight loss was not discussed in these studies (option A). **("Disease Control" in Addiction/"Recovery" in Type 2 Diabetes, pp. 136–137)**

References

Alcoholics Anonymous World Services: Alcoholics Anonymous: The Story of How Many Thousands of Men and Women Have Recovered From Alcoholism, 4th Edition. New York, Alcoholics Anonymous World Services, 2001

American Psychiatric Association: Diagnostic and Statistical Manual of Mental Disorders, 4th Edition, Text Revision. Washington, DC, American Psychiatric Association, 2000

Betty Ford Institute Consensus Panel: What is recovery? A working definition from the Betty Ford Institute. J Subst Abuse Treat 33:221–228, 2007 17889294

Bodenheimer T, Wagner EH, Grumbach K: Improving primary care for patients with chronic illness: the chronic care model, Part 2. JAMA 288:1909–1914, 2002 12377092

Cheever S: My Name is Bill: Bill Wilson—His Life and the Creation of Alcoholics Anonymous. New York, Simon & Schuster, 2004

Dawson DA, Grant BF, Stinson FS, et al: Recovery from DSM-IV alcohol dependence: United States, 2001–2002. Addiction 100:281–292, 2005 15733237

Dobscha SK, Corson K, Perrin NA, et al: Collaborative care for chronic pain in primary care: a cluster randomized trial. JAMA 301:1242–1252, 2009 19318652

Gregg EW, Chen H, Wagenknecht LE, et al: Association of an intensive lifestyle intervention with remission of type 2 diabetes. JAMA 308:2489–2496, 2012 23288372

Marsteller JA, Hsu YJ, Reider L, et al: Physician satisfaction with chronic care processes: a cluster-randomized trial of guided care. Ann Fam Med 8:308–315, 2010 20644185

Patient Protection and Affordable Care Act, P.L. 111–148, March 23, 2010

Rosenthal MB, Beckman HB, Forrest DD, et al: Will the patient-centered medical home improve efficiency and reduce costs of care? A measurement and research agenda. Med Care Res Rev 67:476–484, 2010 20519426

Substance Abuse and Mental Health Services Administration: SAMHSA announces a working definition of "recovery" from mental disorders and substance use disorders. 2011. Available at: http://www.samhsa.gov/newsroom/advisories/1112223420.aspx. Accessed January 8, 2015.

U.K. Drug Policy Commission Recovery Consensus Group: A vision of recovery: UKPDC recovery consensus group. 2008. Available at: http://www.ukdpc.org.uk/publication/recovery-consensus-group/. Accessed January 8, 2015.

Wagner EH, Austin BT, Von Korff M: Organizing care for patients with chronic illness. Milbank Q 74:511–544, 1996 8941260

Wellstone and Domenici Mental Health Parity and Addiction Equity (MHPAE) Act of 2008 (P.L. 110–343)

CHAPTER 10

Neurobiology of Alcohol Use Disorder

10.1 In which of the following brain regions is neural activity both correlated with cue-induced alcohol craving and reduced by successful treatments?

A. Ventral striatum/nucleus accumbens.
B. Ventral tegmental area.
C. Orbitofrontal cortex.
D. Anterior cingulate cortex.
E. Amygdala.

The correct response is option A: Ventral striatum/nucleus accumbens.

A recent meta-analysis by Schacht et al. (2013) demonstrated that activity in the ventral striatum/nucleus accumbens consistently correlates with cue-induced craving and was reduced by successful treatments, suggesting an important role in the mechanism of treatment effects (option A). The ventral tegmental area (option B) gives rise to dopamine input to the ventral striatum, but activity here has not been shown to be correlated with treatment effects. The orbitofrontal cortex (option C), anterior cingulate cortex (option D), and amygdala (option E) are all activated in functional imaging studies of cue-induced craving, but their activity has not been shown as consistently as the ventral striatum to be related to both self-reported craving and to treatment effects. **(Basic Mechanisms of Action, pp. 146–148)**

10.2 Which of the following acute effects of alcohol is a phenotypic marker of alcoholism risk?

A. High rewarding/euphoric effects.
B. Low neural excitability.
C. Low sedative-ataxic effects.
D. Low behavioral disinhibition.
E. High anxiolytic effects.

The correct response is option C: Low sedative-ataxic effects.

161

Individuals who demonstrate a lower level of acute sedation and ataxia in response to a given dose of alcohol are more likely to develop an alcohol use disorder later on (option C). It is believed that this represents a higher level of tolerance to these specific effects, which allows for consumption of a higher amount of alcohol. Individuals at higher risk, for example, those with an alcoholic parent, also show low sedative-ataxic effects. High rewarding/euphoric effects (option A), low neural excitability (option B), low behavioral disinhibition (option D), and high anxiolytic effects (option E), although all acute effects of alcohol that are plausibly related to increased alcohol intake, have not been shown in prospective studies to predict the development of an alcohol use disorder. (**Complex Actions of Alcohol, pp. 148–149**)

10.3   Which of the following is linked to allelic variation of the *OPRM1* gene?

A. Degree of sedative-ataxic effects of alcohol.
B. Level of alcohol cue-induced neural activity within the ventral striatum/nucleus accumbens.
C. Level of impulsivity caused by alcohol.
D. Level of tolerance to alcohol.
E. Level of alcohol-induced dopamine release within the ventral striatum/nucleus accumbens.

The correct response is option E: Level of alcohol-induced dopamine release within the ventral striatum/nucleus accumbens.

The level of dopamine release induced within the ventral striatum by consuming alcohol has been shown through positron emission tomography studies to be increased in carriers of the 118G allele of the *OPRM1* gene, compared with noncarriers (option E). The *OPRM1* gene is related to the opioid system, which is involved in the rewarding effects of alcohol, through its role in facilitating dopamine release in the ventral striatum. There is no known relationship between *OPRM1* and the degree of sedative-ataxic effects of alcohol (option A); the level of cue-induced neural activity (option B), which is different from neural activity induced by consuming alcohol; the level of impulsivity caused by alcohol (option C); or the level of tolerance to alcohol (option D). (**Individual Variation in Alcohol Reward, pp. 149–150**)

10.4   Which of the following physiological processes is thought to be most directly involved in the acute withdrawal syndrome that occurs upon cessation of heavy drinking?

A. Downregulation of adrenergic neurotransmission.
B. Rebound hyperactivity of glutamatergic neurotransmission.
C. Increased γ-aminobutyric acid (GABA)–ergic tone.
D. Dopamine receptor downregulation in the nucleus accumbens.
E. Hypothalamic-pituitary-adrenal (HPA) downregulation.

The correct response is option B: Rebound hyperactivity of glutamatergic neu-rotransmission.

The acute alcohol withdrawal syndrome upon cessation of heavy alcohol use is driven largely by rebound hyperactivity of glutamatergic neurotransmission (option B). The neuroadrenergic system is hyperactive in withdrawal states (evidenced by tachycardia and hypertension), not downregulated (option A). Similarly, increased GABAergic tone (option C) would lead to reduced neuronal excitability, which is the opposite of what is seen in alcohol withdrawal. The dopamine system (option D) is not known to play a direct role in alcohol withdrawal, although it does play an important role in alcohol reward and craving. HPA axis activity (option E) is increased in acute alcohol withdrawal, not downregulated, followed by a more prolonged blunting of HPA axis function that contributes to negative affect long after acute withdrawal has subsided. **(Alcohol Dependence–Induced Neuro-adaptations, pp. 150–151; Stress Systems and Progression Into Negatively Reinforced Alcohol Use, pp. 151–153)**

10.5   The binding of corticotropin-releasing hormone (CRH) to which of the following brain regions leads to increased behavioral reactivity to stress after cessation of heavy alcohol use?

A. Amygdala complex.
B. Ventral striatum/nucleus accumbens.
C. Anterior pituitary.
D. Lateral hypothalamus.
E. Periaqueductal gray matter.

The correct response is option A: Amygdala complex.

The binding of CRH within the amygdala complex is associated with increased behavioral reactivity to stress after cessation of heavy alcohol use (option A). The ventral striatum/nucleus accumbens (option B) plays a role in signaling the rewarding effects of acute alcohol ingestion, not stress reactivity upon alcohol cessation. The anterior pituitary (option C) mediates the endocrine response to CRH release (e.g., cortisol production), not the behavioral response. The lateral hypothalamus (option D) does not play a role in the stress response, although it does contain dopaminergic fibers projecting from the ventral tegmental area to the nucleus accumbens, which do play a role in signaling alcohol reward. The periaqueductal gray matter (option E) plays a role in visceromotor responses to emotional stimuli but is not known to play a role in stress reactivity after heavy alcohol use. **(Stress Systems and Progression Into Negatively Reinforced Alcohol Use, pp. 151–153)**

References

Schacht JP, Anton RF, Myrick H: Functional neuroimaging studies of alcohol cue reactivity: a quantitative meta-analysis and systematic review. Addict Biol 18:121–133, 2013 22574861

C H A P T E R   1 1

Treatment of Alcohol Intoxication and Alcohol Withdrawal

11.1 Which of the following laboratory assays would be best to utilize during alcohol treatment if your goal is to detect heavy alcohol use and monitor drinking status?

A. Alanine aminotransferase (ALT).
B. γ-Glutamyl transpeptidase (GGT).
C. Aspartate aminotransferase (AST).
D. Carbohydrate-deficient transferrin (CDT).
E. Ethyl glucuronide (EtG).

The correct response is D: Carbohydrate-deficient transferrin (CDT).

CDT is a biological assay that may be a more sensitive and specific indicator of heavy alcohol consumption (Litten et al. 1995). The diagnostic specificity of percentage of CDT (%CDT) for recent heavy drinking is approximately 70% in patients with non-alcohol-induced liver cirrhosis, 88.2% in hepatitis patients, and 93.5% in patients with a nonspecific elevation of GGT, making it a more sensitive and specific indicator of alcohol consumption (Hock et al. 2005). The sensitivity of GGT in detecting alcohol abuse is 40%–60%, with a specificity of about 80% (option B). A limitation of GGT, however, is that it may not be particularly sensitive to relapse. Notably, the combination of GGT and %CDT enhances the detection of problem drinking even further. EtG, a conjugated ethanol metabolite, can be used to confirm or rule out recent drinking (option E). Elevations in ALT and AST are often used to identify alcohol use but are not used to monitor drinking status (options A, C). **(Alcohol Intoxication/General Management, pp. 160–161)**

11.2 A 65-year-old patient with a history or delirium tremens is on your service for management of alcohol withdrawal. If the patient's withdrawal is left untreated, when might you expect to see symptoms of delirium tremens emerge?

A. 0–1 days from last drink of alcohol.
B. 2–4 days from last drink of alcohol.
C. 5–7 days from last drink of alcohol.
D. 6–8 days from last drink of alcohol.
E. 8–10 days from last drink of alcohol.

The correct response is B: 2–4 days from last drink of alcohol.

The most intense and serious syndrome associated with alcohol withdrawal is *delirium tremens*, which is characterized by fluctuating disturbance of consciousness, agitation and tremulousness, autonomic instability, hyperpyrexia, persistent visual and auditory hallucinations, and disorientation. Symptoms usually begin 2–4 days from the last drink. Although the average length of an episode of delirium tremens is less than 1 week, there are reports of cases lasting weeks to months (Hersh et al. 1997). Delirium tremens have been estimated to occur in 5% of patients admitted for alcohol withdrawal and must be considered a medical emergency because the mortality rate can be as high as 20% for those not receiving prompt and adequate treatment for the severe withdrawal (Mayo-Smith et al. 2004). **(Alcohol Withdrawal/Signs and Symptoms, p. 161)**

11.3   You admit a 40-year-old patient with alcohol use disorder to your service. To manage his withdrawal, you would like to use a symptom-triggered approach (versus fixed multiple daily dosing). Which one of the following should you use to assess the severity of alcohol withdrawal symptoms?

A. CAGE questionnaire.
B. Clinical Institute Withdrawal Assessment for Alcohol–Revised (CIWA-Ar).
C. Alcohol Use Disorders Identification Test (AUDIT).
D. Michigan Alcoholism Screening Test (MAST).
E. Addiction Severity Index (ASI).

The correct response is B: Clinical Institute Withdrawal Assessment for Alcohol–Revised (CIWA-Ar).

The CIWA-Ar is the assessment tool most cited in current alcohol withdrawal literature for assessing severity of alcohol withdrawal symptoms (option B) (Sullivan et al. 1991). This clinician-rated checklist, a 10-item scale used to monitor the clinical course of withdrawal symptoms, includes assessments of nausea; vomiting; tremor; sweating; anxiety; agitation; tactile, auditory, and visual disturbances; and clouding of sensorium. Higher total scores indicate more severe alcohol withdrawal symptoms and a greater risk of major withdrawal symptoms such as delirium tremens (Foy et al. 1988). Recent trials have used symptom-triggered treatment with the CIWA-Ar to indicate the need for benzodiazepine (Saitz et al. 1994). The CAGE questions, AUDIT, and MAST are all alcohol screening tools (options A, C, D). The ASI (option E) is a semi-structured interview designed to address seven potential problem areas in substance-abusing patients: medical status, employment and support, drug use, alcohol use, legal status, family/social status, and psychiatric status. It is not designed to assess alcohol withdrawal. **(Alcohol Withdrawal/Measurement of the Withdrawal, p. 162; Medication Management/Benzodiazepines, p. 164)**

11.4 To prevent precipitation of Wernicke's encephalopathy in a patient with alcohol use disorder, thiamine should be administered *before* which of the following?

A. Glucose.
B. Magnesium.
C. Potassium.
D. Phosphate.
E. Folate.

The correct response is A: Glucose.

Individuals with alcohol use disorder often present with electrolyte nutritional abnormalities that should be corrected. Electrolyte deficits include hypomagnesemia, hypophosphatemia, and hypokalemia. Nutritional deficits are secondary to dietary habits as well as alcohol-related changes in the digestive tract. Oral multivitamin preparations containing folic acid should be given for a few weeks. The replacement of thiamine is particularly important given its role in Wernicke's encephalopathy. It is imperative that thiamine be provided prior to glucose administration in order to prevent precipitation of Wernicke's encephalopathy by depletion of thiamine reserves (option A). While deficits in magnesium (option B), potassium (option C), phosphate (option D), and folate (option E) should be corrected, doing so prior to thiamine will not precipitate Wernicke's encephalopathy. **(Alcohol Withdrawal/General Management, p. 162)**

11.5 You are discussing treatment options for alcohol detoxification with a patient who tells you he prefers outpatient detoxification to inpatient. After reviewing his history, you tell him that you do *not* recommend outpatient treatment of alcohol withdrawal. Which of the following in his history *most* led you to recommend inpatient treatment?

A. He was arrested a few years ago for assault and public intoxication.
B. He prefers to drink beer over hard liquor.
C. He has a history of alcohol withdrawal seizures.
D. He smokes one pack of cigarettes per day.
E. He smokes marijuana 3–4 times per week.

The correct response is C: He has a history of alcohol withdrawal seizures.

Over the past two decades, there has been a major shift from the inpatient to the outpatient setting for the treatment of alcohol withdrawal. In a review of the literature on ambulatory detoxification, Abbott et al. (1995) found that less than 10%–20% of patients required admission to an inpatient unit. The completion rates for ambulatory detoxification programs ranged from 35% to 95%, with most having completion rates above 70%. In most studies reviewed, 50% of patients continued in alcohol rehabilitation treatment, including group and individual therapy. Most importantly, this review found no reports of mortality or serious medical complications except for one program reporting a seizure occurring after the start of detoxification.

Despite the lack of specific criteria indicating which patients should be treated on an outpatient basis, there are practical considerations that should be addressed by the treating clinician. These include making sure that the patient has only mild to moderate alcohol withdrawal symptoms, has no concomitant medical or severe psychiatric illnesses that could interfere with the withdrawal process, has no past history of alcohol withdrawal seizures or delirium tremens (option C), and, when possible, has a sober significant other as a reliable support person. Patients should be seen daily to reassess withdrawal symptoms, to watch for the occurrence of medical complications, and to monitor the treatment regimen. (**Alcohol Withdrawal/Inpatient Versus Outpatient Treatment, pp. 162–163**)

References

Abbott PJ, Quinn D, Knox L: Ambulatory medical detoxification for alcohol. Am J Drug Alcohol Abuse 21:549–563, 1995 8561102

Foy A, March S, Drinkwater V: Use of an objective clinical scale in the assessment and management of alcohol withdrawal in a large general hospital. Alcohol Clin Exp Res 12:360–364, 1988 3044163

Hersh D, Kranzler HR, Meyer RE: Persistent delirium following cessation of heavy alcohol consumption: diagnostic and treatment implications. Am J Psychiatry 154:846–851, 1997 9167514

Hock B, Schwarz M, Domke I, et al: Validity of carbohydrate-deficient transferrin (%CDT), gamma-glutamyltransferase (gamma-GT) and mean corpuscular erythrocyte volume (MCV) as biomarkers for chronic alcohol abuse: a study in patients with alcohol dependence and liver disorders of non-alcoholic and alcoholic origin. Addiction 100:1477–1486, 2005 16185209

Litten RZ, Allen JP, Fertig JB: Gammaglutamyltransferase and carbohydrate deficient transferrin: alternative measures of excessive alcohol consumption. Alcohol Clin Exp Res 19:1541–1546, 1995 8749824

Mayo-Smith MF, Beecher LH, Fischer TL, et al: Management of alcohol withdrawal delirium. An evidence-based practice guideline. Arch Intern Med 164:1405–1412, 2004 15249349

Saitz R, Mayo-Smith MF, Roberts MS, et al: Individualized treatment for alcohol withdrawal. A randomized double-blind controlled trial. JAMA 272:519–523, 1994 8046805

Sullivan JT, Swift RM, Lewis DC: Benzodiazepine requirements during alcohol withdrawal syndrome: clinical implications of using a standardized withdrawal scale. J Clin Psychopharmacol 11:291–295, 1991 1684974

CHAPTER 12

Neurobiology of Stimulants

12.1 A 33-year-old woman with a decade-long history of cocaine use tearfully states that she wants nothing more than to reconcile with her ex-husband, have more visits with her children, and get a job. However, she never spends much time on these goals before she prostitutes herself in order to use again. She knows she is making bad decisions, but when faced with a choice between feeling good quickly from cocaine *versus* possibly feeling good later upon achieving a goal, she always chooses the high. What is the term for this decision-making tendency related to chronic stimulant use?

A. Delayed discounting.
B. Tolerance.
C. Cue-induced drug seeking.
D. Dependence.
E. Stimulant-induced drug seeking.

The correct response is option A: Delayed discounting.

Delayed discounting is the tendency to choose immediate rewards over larger, delayed rewards. Both cocaine and methamphetamine abusers show increased delay discounting relative to non–drug users, a pattern of responding associated with decreased recruitment of dorsal brain circuitry including dorsolateral prefrontal cortex and anterior cingulate cortex (option A). Decreased recruitment of this circuitry may reduce the capacity to modulate signaling in ventral regions associated with motivational salience and value of immediate rewards (e.g., ventral striatum. ventromedial prefrontal cortex), leading to immediately gratifying but ultimately disadvantageous choices. *Tolerance* (option B) is the need for larger doses to achieve an effect previously achieved with a smaller dose. Of note, experienced abusers of stimulants do not appear less sensitive to the reinforcing effects of these drugs than do those with less experience, although tolerance to certain stimulant effects, such as those associated with anorexia, does occur. Tolerance is not described in this vignette. *Cue-induced drug seeking* (option C) is drug seeking stimulated by exposure to "people, places, and things" associated with the drug use, whereas *stimulant-induced drug seeking* (option E) is drug seeking stimulated by use of the drug (as even a small amount of stimulant can result in an abstinent drug user returning to preabstinent levels of drug use). The question is not about what stimulates the subject's drug use but is about the subject's tendency to choose a quickly gratifying but very disadvantageous option over one with delayed reward. *Dependence* (option D) is the presence of withdrawal symptoms upon cessation of use. There is no description of withdrawal in this case. **(Consequences of Repeated Stimulant Exposure/Stimulant- and Cue-Induced Drug Seeking, pp. 173–174; Cognitive Control, Impulsivity, and Decision Making, pp. 174–175; Tolerance, pp. 175–176; Dependence, p. 176)**

12.2   Methamphetamine and cocaine have similar properties, but methamphetamine is more neurotoxic because of which feature that cocaine lacks?

A. Interference of dopamine reuptake.
B. Promotion of dopamine release.
C. Short-lasting effect.
D. Faster metabolism.
E. Prolonged increase in dopamine that does not habituate.

The correct response is option B: Promotion of dopamine release.

Methamphetamine blocks reuptake but also promotes dopamine release, which renders this drug more neurotoxic than cocaine (option B). Both cocaine and methamphetamine interfere with dopamine reuptake (option A). Cocaine has a relatively short-lasting effect (option C) and a faster metabolism (option D) than methamphetamine, which has a longer lasting effect. Stimulants, cocaine and methamphetamine included, elicit a prolonged increase in dopamine that does not habituate (option E) and that, by enhancing the signaling in the nucleus accumbens to a greater extent than nondrug reinforcers, may lead to excessive strengthening of the behaviors associated with drug use. **(Acute Stimulant Effects, pp. 169–170; Consequences of Repeated Stimulant Exposure/Toxicity, pp. 176–178)**

12.3   *N*-methyl-D-aspartate (NMDA) antagonists prevent both dopaminergic and serotonergic neurotoxicity, suggesting these medications could decrease methamphetamine toxicity by interference with which NMDA receptor-binding neurotransmitter?

A. Dopamine.
B. Serotonin.
C. Glutamate.
D. Norepinephrine.
E. γ-Aminobutyric acid (GABA).

The correct response is option C: Glutamate.

Glutamate is an excitatory neurotransmitter that binds to NMDA receptors, and toxic doses of methamphetamine increase glutamate efflux in the striatum where neurotoxicity occurs. In several studies, some NMDA antagonists prevented both dopaminergic and serotonergic neurotoxicity, suggesting that these medications could decrease methamphetamine toxicity (option C) (Krasnova and Cadet 2009). The magnitude of dopamine release correlates with the amount of neurotoxicity, and destruction of both serotonin and dopamine neurons can be prevented in laboratory animals if brain dopamine levels are depleted prior to methamphetamine administration (option A) (Krasnova and Cadet 2009). However, dopamine does not bind to the NMDA receptor. Tissue concentration of serotonin (option B) levels is decreased in methamphetamine use, and dysregulation of serotonin is implicated in stimulant withdrawal, but serotonin does not bind to the NMDA receptor. Norepinephrine (option D) seems to mediate the anxiogenic component of cocaine withdrawal but does not bind to the NMDA receptor. GABA (option E) modulates dopamine neurons in the ventral striatum but does not bind to the NMDA receptor. **(Consequences of Repeated Stimulant Exposure/Addiction, pp. 171–173; Dependence, p. 176; Toxicity, pp. 176–178)**

12.4   Which γ-aminobutyric acid (GABA)–modulating medication was found to *decrease* relapse in cocaine users?

A. Gabapentin.
B. Baclofen.
C. Vigabatrin.
D. Tiagabine.
E. Topiramate.

The correct response is E: Topiramate.

Topiramate, which enhances GABA and blocks α-amino-3-hydroxy-5-methyl-4-isoxazolepropionic acid (AMPA) glutamate receptors, decreased the likelihood of relapse to cocaine use (Kampman et al. 2004), suggesting that targeting both glutamate and GABA may be an effective approach (option E). GABA modulates dopamine neurons in the ventral striatum, yet GABA agonists, such as gabapentin (option A), baclofen (option B), vigabatrin (option C), and tiagabine (option D), have not been shown to reduce cocaine use in either the human laboratory studies (Haney et al. 2006; Hart et al. 2004, 2007) or the clinic (Kahn et al. 2009; Winhusen et al. 2007). **(Consequences of Repeated Stimulant Exposure/Addiction, pp. 171–173)**

12.5   What would the expected presentation be for a longtime methamphetamine user who abruptly discontinues use?

A. Diarrhea.
B. Nausea.
C. Depression.
D. Dysautonomia.
E. Pain.

The correct response is option C: Depression.

Abstinence following repeated methamphetamine or cocaine use is primarily characterized by disorders of mood, including depression (option C), fatigue, anxiety, and irritability, but not physical withdrawal symptoms (options A, B, D, E). Unlike with opioids and alcohol, stimulants do not produce neuroadaptations to areas mediating somatic and autonomic function. **(Consequences of Repeated Stimulant Exposure/Dependence, p. 176)**

References

Haney M, Hart CL, Foltin RW: Effects of baclofen on cocaine self-administration: opioid- and non-opioid-dependent volunteers. Neuropsychopharmacology 31:1814–1821, 2006 16407903

Hart CL, Ward AS, Collins ED, et al: Gabapentin maintenance decreases smoked cocaine-related subjective effects, but not self-administration by humans. Drug Alcohol Depend 73:279–287, 2004 15036550

Hart CL, Haney M, Collins ED, et al: Smoked cocaine self-administration by humans is not reduced by large gabapentin maintenance doses. Drug Alcohol Depend 86:274–277, 2007 16879931

Kahn R, Biswas K, Childress AR, et al: Multicenter trial of baclofen for abstinence initiation in severe cocaine-dependent individuals. Drug Alcohol Depend 103:59–64, 2009 19414226

Kampman KM, Pettinati H, Lynch KG, et al: A pilot trial of topiramate for the treatment of cocaine dependence. Drug Alcohol Depend 75:233–240, 2004 15283944

Krasnova IN, Cadet JL: Methamphetamine toxicity and messengers of death. Brain Res Rev 60:379–407, 2009 19328213

Winhusen T, Somoza E, Ciraulo DA, et al: A double-blind, placebo-controlled trial of tiagabine for the treatment of cocaine dependence. Drug Alcohol Depend 91:141–148, 2007 17629631

Clinical Management: Cocaine

13.1 Which of the following agonist approaches to the treatment of cocaine addiction, when combined with contingency management, has been shown to reduce cocaine use more effectively than either treatment alone or placebo?

A. D-Amphetamine.
B. Methylphenidate.
C. Modafinil.
D. Bupropion.
E. Disulfiram.

The correct response is option D: Bupropion.

Bupropion is an antidepressant medication. It is also effective as an aid for smoking cessation. Bupropion is a weak dopamine and norepinephrine reuptake inhibitor, and it enhances extracellular dopamine levels in the nucleus accumbens. In clinical trials, bupropion was not effective in reducing cocaine use. Interestingly, bupropion, when combined with contingency management, reduced cocaine use more effectively than either treatment alone or placebo (Poling et al. 2006) (option D).

Several amphetamines, including D-amphetamine and methylphenidate (options A and B), have been tested for the treatment of addiction. In randomized clinical trials, D-amphetamine reduced drug use in short-term clinical trials in cocaine users (Herin et al. 2010). Another clinical trial reported that a sustained-release formulation of methamphetamine, but not the immediate formulation, reduced cocaine use (Mooney et al. 2009). Methylphenidate, on the other hand, increases synaptic dopamine levels by inhibiting reuptake by monoamine transporters. Methylphenidate has had limited success in reducing cocaine use in cocaine-dependent patients (Levin et al. 2007; Schubiner et al. 2002).

Another agonist approach for cocaine dependence is modafinil, which acts as a weak dopamine transporter inhibitor and increases synaptic dopamine levels (Martinez-Raga et al. 2008). Initial clinical trials with modafinil were promising for cocaine addiction. However, subsequent larger randomized clinical trials have been negative (Dackis et al. 2012) (option C).

Although pharmacologically different from the other agonist-like medications, disulfiram also increases synaptic dopamine levels. Some studies have shown that disulfiram has been promising in reducing cocaine abuse (Sofuoglu and Sewell 2009); however, more recent results have not been as promising (option E). **(Treatment for Cocaine Addiction/Pharmacotherapy/Agonist Approaches, pp. 184, 186)**

13.2   Which of the following medications targeting neuroadaptations to chronic cocaine use, when combined with amphetamine salts, has been shown to reduce cocaine use compared with placebo?

A. *N*-acetyl cysteine (NAC).
B. Vigabatrin.
C. Topiramate.
D. Lofexidine.
E. Doxazosin.

The correct response is option C: Topiramate.

Topiramate, a γ-aminobutyric acid (GABA)–enhancing medication with a primary therapeutic indication for epilepsy, has had promising results for cocaine dependence as well. In a 14-week, double-blind, placebo-controlled outpatient study, subjects assigned to treatment with topiramate had more negative urine cocaine results than those given placebo (option C) (Kampman et al. 2004). In a more recent clinical trial, combination of topiramate with mixed amphetamine salts, compared with placebo, reduced cocaine use (Mariani et al. 2012).

NAC, a medication used for the treatment of acetaminophen overdose, targets brain glutamate. NAC has shown some positive results in small clinical trials for cocaine addiction. Larger studies are under way to test NAC's efficacy for the treatment of cocaine addiction (option A).

Human clinical laboratory studies suggest that lofexidine, an α_2-adrenergic receptor agonist, may attenuate stress-induced relapse in cocaine and opioid users (Sinha et al. 2007) (option D). It has not been studied in combination with amphetamine salts for cocaine dependence. In a pilot randomized clinical trial, doxazosin, an α_1-adrenergic agonist, reduced cocaine use (Shorter et al. 2013) (option E). But doxazosin has also not been tested in combination with amphetamine salts for cocaine dependence.

Medications targeting GABA activity have also been investigated for treating cocaine addiction. Vigabatrin, or γ-vinyl-GABA, is an irreversible inhibitor of GABA transaminase that has been shown to reduce cocaine-induced dopamine release in laboratory animals. In a randomized controlled trial, vigabatrin led to a higher percentage of subjects achieving and maintaining abstinence from cocaine and alcohol (Brodie et al. 2009). However, in a recent multisite clinical trial, vigabatrin was no more effective than placebo in reducing cocaine use (option B) (Somoza et al. 2013) **(Treatment for Cocaine Addiction/Pharmacotherapy/Medications Targeting Neuroadaptations to Cocaine Addiction, pp. 186–187)**

13.3   Chronic cocaine use produces which of the following neurochemical changes?

A. Increased postsynaptic dopamine receptors in cocaine users.
B. Increases in dopamine transporter in acutely abstinent cocaine abusers relative to control subjects.
C. Increases in D_2 dopamine receptor binding in detoxified cocaine users relative to control subjects.
D. Increased cerebral blood flow and cortical perfusion among chronic cocaine users.
E. Deficits in attention without a change in working memory.

The correct response is option B: Increases in dopamine transporter in acutely abstinent cocaine abusers relative to control subjects.

Single-photon emission computed tomography and positron emission tomography studies show increases in dopamine transporter in acutely abstinent cocaine abusers relative to control subjects (Malison et al. 1998) (option B) and *decreased* postsynaptic dopamine receptors in cocaine users (Volkow et al. 2008) (option A). These studies also show *decreases* in dopamine D_2 receptor binding in detoxified cocaine abusers relative to control subjects (option C), and *reduced* cerebral blood flow and cortical perfusion among chronic cocaine abusers (Volkow et al. 2008) (option D). Current evidence indicates that most forms of chronic cocaine use may be associated with significant cognitive impairments, especially in attention, working memory, and response inhibition functions (Sofuoglu et al. 2013) (option E). **(Treatment for Cocaine Addiction/Pharmacotherapy/Medications Targeting Cognitive Deficits, pp. 187–188)**

13.4   For which of the following cognitive enhancers, compared with placebo, have studies demonstrated improvements in sustained attention, reduction in cocaine-positive urine specimens, and fewer self-reports of cocaine use?

A. Varenicline.
B. Modafinil.
C. Amphetamines.
D. Glutamate agonists.
E. Galantamine.

The correct response is option E: Galantamine.

There are many potential cognitive enhancers, including cholinesterase inhibitors, modafinil (option B), amphetamines (option C), partial nicotinic acetylcholine receptor (nAChR) agonists (e.g., varenicline, option A), and metabotropic glutamate agonists (option D). Although these potential cognitive enhancers are all noted by the authors of the textbook chapter on which this study guide is based, there is only one for which the authors present evidence of cognitive enhancement. Among cholinesterase inhibitors, galantamine is one with additional allosteric potentiation at the α_7 and $\alpha_4\beta_2$ nAChR. In a double-blind, placebo-controlled study, galantamine treatment improved sustained attention and working memory functions in abstinent cocaine users (Sofuoglu et al. 2011). In a separate, double-blind study in opioid- and cocaine-dependent individuals, those receiving galantamine submitted fewer cocaine-positive urine specimens and reported less cocaine use than those assigned to receive placebo. Randomized clinical trials are under way to test the efficacy of galantamine for the treatment of cocaine addiction. **(Treatment for Cocaine Addiction/Pharmacotherapy/Medications Targeting Cognitive Deficits, pp. 187–188)**

13.5   Which of the following treatment modalities can be most effectively combined with pharmacotherapies to improve treatment outcomes significantly for individuals with cocaine addiction?

   A. Contingency management.
   B. Standard counseling.
   C. Twelve-step facilitation (TSF).
   D. Cognitive-behavioral therapy (CBT).
   E. Methadone maintenance.

The correct response is option A: Contingency management.

Several behavioral treatments have been used for cocaine addiction, including TSF, CBT, and contingency management. These therapies provide a platform for pharmacological treatment by engaging the patient in the treatment, and they facilitate more long-term changes, including prevention of relapse. A specific behavioral approach using positive contingencies to initiate abstinence and prevent relapse has been quite successful for managing cocaine users. Contingency management (option A) can be readily combined with other forms of psychotherapy or medications. For example, combining contingency management with pharmacotherapies such as bupropion may significantly improve treatment outcomes for individuals with cocaine addiction (Poling et al. 2006).

TSF (option C) is an individual therapy based on spiritual, cognitive, and behavioral principles emphasized by organizations such as Alcoholics Anonymous. Although there are doubts about the efficacy of TSF, a study suggested it has efficacy for cocaine dependence. In a study conducted by Carroll et al. (2012), participants recruited from a methadone maintenance program (option E) were randomly assigned to one of four conditions distinguished by use of disulfiram or placebo and either TSF or standard counseling only. TSF was associated with more self-reported abstinence days and more cocaine-free urine samples than standard counseling only (option B). These findings may support the efficacy of TSF as a component of treatment for cocaine dependence, but they do not suggest that TSF adds to the efficacy of pharmacotherapy for cocaine dependence.

CBT is commonly used for the treatment of cocaine addiction. The goal of CBT is to teach strategies and enhance coping abilities to prevent drug use behavior. The efficacy of CBT for cocaine addiction has been demonstrated in multiple studies (Knapp et al. 2007). However, a number of other studies have failed to show statistically significant advantages for CBT in patients with cocaine addiction (option D). **(Treatment for Cocaine Addiction/Behavioral Therapy, pp. 189–190)**

References

Brodie JD, Case BG, Figueroa E, et al: Randomized, double-blind, placebo-controlled trial of vigabatrin for the treatment of cocaine dependence in Mexican parolees. Am J Psychiatry 166:1269–1277, 2009 19651710

Carroll KM, Nich C, Shi JM, et al: Efficacy of disulfiram and Twelve Step Facilitation in cocaine-dependent individuals maintained on methadone: a randomized placebo-controlled trial. Drug Alcohol Depend 126:224–231, 2012 22695473

Dackis CA, Kampman KM, Lynch KG, et al: A double-blind, placebo-controlled trial of modafinil for cocaine dependence. J Subst Abuse Treat 43:303–312, 2012 22377391

Herin DV, Rush CR, Grabowski J: Agonist-like pharmacotherapy for stimulant dependence: preclinical, human laboratory, and clinical studies. Ann N Y Acad Sci 1187:76–100, 2010 20201847

Kampman KM, Pettinati H, Lynch KG, et al: A pilot trial of topiramate for the treatment of cocaine dependence. Drug Alcohol Depend 75(3):233–240, 2004 15283944

Knapp WP, Soares BG, Farrel M, et al: Psychosocial interventions for cocaine and psychostimulant amphetamines related disorders. Cochrane Database Syst Rev (3):CD003023, 2007 17636713

Levin FR, Evans SM, Brooks DJ, et al: Treatment of cocaine dependent treatment seekers with adult ADHD: double-blind comparison of methylphenidate and placebo. Drug Alcohol Depend 87:20–29, 2007 16930863

Malison RT, Best SE, van Dyck CH, et al: Elevated striatal dopamine transporters during acute cocaine abstinence as measured by [123I] beta-CIT SPECT. Am J Psychiatry 155:832–834, 1998 9619159

Mariani JJ, Pavlicova M, Bisaga A, et al: Extended-release mixed amphetamine salts and topiramate for cocaine dependence: a randomized controlled trial. Biol Psychiatry 72:950–956, 2012 22795453

Martinez-Raga J, Knecht C, Cepeda S: Modafinil: a useful medication for cocaine addiction? Review of the evidence from neuropharmacological, experimental and clinical studies. Curr Drug Abuse Rev 1:213–221, 2008

Mooney ME, Herin DV, Schmitz JM, et al: Effects of oral methamphetamine on cocaine use: a randomized, double-blind, placebo-controlled trial. Drug Alcohol Depend 101:34–41, 2009 19058926

Poling J, Oliveto A, Petry N, et al: Six-month trial of bupropion with contingency management for cocaine dependence in a methadone-maintained population. Arch Gen Psychiatry 63:219–228, 2006

Schubiner H, Saules KK, Arfken CL, et al: Double-blind placebo-controlled trial of methylphenidate in the treatment of adult ADHD patients with comorbid cocaine dependence. Exp Clin Psychopharmacol 10:286–294, 2002 12233989

Shorter D, Lindsay JA, Kosten TR: The alpha-1 adrenergic antagonist doxazosin for treatment of cocaine dependence: a pilot study. Drug Alcohol Depend 131:66–70, 2013

Sinha R, Kimmerling A, Doebrick C, et al: Effects of lofexidine on stress-induced and cue-induced opioid craving and opioid abstinence rates: preliminary findings. Psychopharmacology (Berl) 190:569–574, 2007 17136399

Sofuoglu M, Sewell RA: Norepinephrine and stimulant addiction. Addict Biol 14:119–129, 2009 18811678

Sofuoglu M, Waters AJ, Poling J, et al: Galantamine improves sustained attention in chronic cocaine users. Exp Clin Psychopharmacol 19:11–19, 2011 21341919

Sofuoglu M, DeVito EE, Waters AJ, et al: Cognitive enhancement as a treatment for drug addictions. Neuropharmacology 64:452–463, 2013 22735770

Somoza EC, Winship D, Gorodetzky CW, et al: A multisite, double-blind, placebo-controlled clinical trial to evaluate the safety and efficacy of vigabatrin for treating cocaine dependence. JAMA Psychiatry 70(6):630–637, 2013 23575810

Volkow ND, Fowler JS, Wang GJ, et al: Imaging dopamine's role in drug abuse and addiction. Neuropharmacology 56 (suppl 1):3–8, 2008

CHAPTER 14

Clinical Management: Methamphetamine

14.1 When compared with cocaine, methamphetamine (MA) exhibits which of the following important differences in neuronal effects?

A. MA induces intracellular dopamine-containing vesicles to dock with the cell membrane and leak dopamine into the synaptic cleft.
B. Although cocaine blocks reuptake of dopamine from the synaptic cleft, MA does not.
C. MA has a short half-life and duration of action—barely exceeding 60 minutes.
D. MA exerts its primary action at the dopamine transporter to increase extracellular dopamine.
E. MA decreases the cytoplasmic concentration of dopamine, thus reducing the levels of dopamine oxidation products in the cytoplasm and limiting the neurotoxicity of MA.

The correct response is option A: MA induces intracellular dopamine-containing vesicles to dock with the cell membrane and leak dopamine into the synaptic cleft.

MA is often compared to cocaine, but there are important differences in their mechanisms of action. Cocaine acts primarily by blocking the reuptake of released dopamine in the synaptic clefts of the mesolimbic dopamine neurons. MA also inhibits reuptake of the released dopamine (option B), but MA is carried into the dopaminergic neurons and, unlike cocaine, exerts its primary action intracellularly (option D). MA causes docking of the intracellular dopamine-containing vesicles at the membrane, leading to leakage of dopamine into the synaptic cleft (option A). Additionally, it interferes with dopamine transport into the storage vesicles, thus increasing the cytoplasmic concentration of dopamine, which undergoes oxidation and produces oxidation products that are toxic to the nerve terminals (option E) (Hanson et al. 2004). The neurotoxicity of MA is further accentuated by its prolonged half-life and long duration of action, which exceeds 6 hours (option C). **(How Methamphetamine Works, pp. 196–197)**

14.2   The police bring a 27-year-old man with a history of anxiety and cannabis dependence to the emergency room with new-onset paranoid delusions and acute agitation. A friend provides history that the patient was smoking methamphetamine (MA) for the prior 2 days. To manage the patient's toxicity, including the agitation, which of the following would be the most appropriate intervention?

A. Administer emetics and gastric lavage.
B. Initiate dialysis.
C. Avoid attempting to talk with the patient.
D. Administer haloperidol combined with lorazepam in repeated doses over a 12-hour observation period.
E. Avoid the use of atypical antipsychotics.

The correct response is option D: Administer haloperidol combined with lorazepam in repeated doses over a 12-hour observation period.

The typical syndrome associated with MA intoxication that leads patients to seek or need medical attention is acute agitation, which is often best handled by "talking down" the patients, assuring them that the condition will pass in time, and observing them and ensuring a calm environment (option C). Although little formal research has established the efficacy of any pharmacotherapeutic regimen for severe MA intoxication involving agitation and/or psychosis, the traditional approach has been to provide 5 mg of haloperidol neuroleptic medication, frequently in combination with 1–2 mg of lorazepam, administered orally or parenterally in repeated doses (option D). Other approaches include providing atypical neuroleptics (e.g., quetiapine, olanzapine, risperidone) orally or parenterally, with 1–2 mg of lorazepam orally, administered in several doses over a 12-hour period, with the patient evaluated for 12 hours (option E). Clinicians should observe for and treat possible dehydration and hyperthermia (Brown and Yamamoto 2003). Administration of emetics and/or gastric lavage is only potentially useful to clear the drug from the gastrointestinal tract if it was taken orally (option A). This approach is not useful for toxicity related to smoked (or intravenous) ingestion of MA. Dialysis is not used to clear MA from the blood (option B). In addition, it would likely not be feasible to perform hemodialysis on an agitated patient. **(Clinical Management/ Methamphetamine-Related Syndromes and Therapeutic Approaches/Managing MA Intoxication and Withdrawal, pp. 198–199)**

14.3   Which of the following is a problem uniquely experienced by adult MA-dependent women associated with their methamphetamine (MA) use?

A. Over 70% of adult MA-dependent women report histories of physical and sexual abuse and are more likely than men to present for treatment with greater psychological distress.
B. In one sample of all MA-dependent women, 45% showed serological evidence of hepatitis C infection.
C. Rates of HIV seroprevalence are threefold higher among MA-using women compared with those who do not use MA.

D. Over 63% of women seeking substance abuse treatment reported MA as their primary drug of choice.
E. Women show higher dropout rates and more MA use during treatment than men.

The correct response is option A: Over 70% of adult MA-dependent women report histories of physical and sexual abuse and are more likely than men to present for treatment with greater psychological distress.

Over 70% of MA-dependent women report histories of physical and sexual abuse, and women are more likely than men to present for treatment with greater psychological distress (option A). In a recent sample of MA-dependent users who entered treatment in the Midwest, Hawaii, or California, the rate of hepatitis C infection was 15% (Gonzales et al. 2006). Among the men and women in that study who injected MA, over 45% were infected with hepatitis C (option B). Rates of HIV seroprevalence have been reported to be threefold higher among MA-using MSM (men who have sex with men) than among non-MA-using MSM (option C). One study (Rawson et al. 2005) found that 63.7% of adolescent females seeking treatment reported MA as their primary drug of choice (option D). Injection users, both men and women, also have higher dropout rates and exhibit higher rates of MA use during treatment compared with noninjection users (option E). **(Treatment for Methamphetamine-Related Disorders/Methamphetamine Populations With Unique Clinical Concerns/Women, p. 201)**

14.4 The Matrix Model, a blended treatment approach that has shown efficacy for treatment of methamphetamine (MA) use disorders, incorporates which of the following components?

A. Contingency management, individual psychoeducation, group psychodynamic therapy, and 12-step program participation.
B. Motivational interviewing, contingency management, acceptance and commitment therapy, and 12-step facilitation (TSF).
C. Motivational interviewing, family therapy, TSF, and 12-step program participation.
D. Community reinforcement and family therapy, contingency management, individual psychodynamic psychotherapy, and motivational interviewing.
E. Individual and group cognitive-behavioral therapy (CBT), family education, motivational interviewing, and 12-step program participation.

The correct response is option E: Individual and group cognitive-behavioral therapy (CBT), family education, motivational interviewing, and 12-step program participation.

A CBT-like approach with demonstrated efficacy for MA use disorders is the National Institute on Drug Abuse/Substance Abuse and Mental Health Services Administration–documented Matrix Model, a blended treatment approach that incorporates principles of CBT in individual and group settings, family education, motivational interviewing, and 12-step program participation (option E). Options

A, B, C, and D contain elements that are not part of the Matrix Model. **(Treatment for Methamphetamine-Related Disorders/Behavioral Treatments, p. 203)**

14.5   There are no medications that are approved by the U.S. Food and Drug Administration (FDA) for the treatment of methamphetamine (MA) addiction. Which of the following lists drugs with only positive results from clinical trials in human beings demonstrating reduced stimulant use/prevention of relapse to MA or amphetamine-type stimulants (ATSs)?

A. Citicoline, naloxone, and bupropion.
B. Topiramate, lobeline, and aripiprazole.
C. Mirtazapine, naltrexone, and bupropion.
D. MA vaccine, naloxone, and modafinil.
E. γ-Vinyl-γ-aminobutyric acid (GVG), methylphenidate, aripiprazole.

The correct response is option C: Mirtazapine, naltrexone, and bupropion.

No pharmacotherapy has been submitted for approval to the FDA for treatment of MA-related disorders, although medication trials have examined many compounds, with limited success. The antidepressant/smoking cessation drug bupropion has proven somewhat effective (McCann and Li 2012), and the opioid antagonist naltrexone has also shown effectiveness for preventing relapse among ATS-dependent individuals (Jayaram-Lindström et al. 2008) (option C). Additional work with long-acting depot naltrexone is under way in clinical trials. A small trial found mirtazapine to have promise in preventing relapse to MA use (option C) (Colfax et al. 2011). A Finnish study reported that treatment with methylphenidate reduced MA injection in an early-stage trial (Tiihonen et al. 2007). Lobeline, a nicotinic receptor antagonist, may have neuroprotective properties against the effects of MA (Eyerman and Yamamoto 2005); testing lobeline in humans as a treatment agent is in an early stage of development. On the basis of findings that topiramate reduced cocaine consumption in cocaine-dependent subjects, topiramate has been examined in humans and found safe in Phase I interaction studies with MA administration (Johnson et al. 2007). GVG is an anticonvulsant that can block MA-induced increases in dopamine in the nucleus accumbens and thereby blunt the euphoria and positive-subjective effects of MA; clinical trials of GVG involving MA-using individuals have shown positive findings (Brodie et al. 2005).

Other recently completed trials of medications for MA-related disorders have produced negative findings. For example, aripiprazole did not produce better outcomes than placebo (Coffin et al. 2013) (options B and E), and modafinil was not found to be effective (Anderson et al. 2012) (option D). In a small trial using citicoline, MA-dependent patients with co-occurring bipolar disorder were more likely to remain in treatment than those given placebo, although no reduction in MA use was noted (Brown and Gabrielson 2012) (option A).

Research for a vaccine against MA use continues to move forward in preclinical work. For example, the σ receptor ligand AZ66 showed efficacy in reducing MA effects by antagonizing MA at the σ receptor sites (Seminerio et al. 2012). Also showing promise in animal studies is the use of a protein carrier or an immune-stimulating molecule to create MA antibodies, which block psychoactive effects by binding MA in the bloodstream (Miller et al. 2013; Shen et al. 2013). Clinical trials may commence within the next few years in China, where manufacturers have agreed to produce at least one of the vaccines, which is based on a manipulated meningitis protein developed in research supported by the National Institute on Drug Abuse. (**Treatment for Methamphetamine-Related Disorders/Pharmacotherapy for Methamphetamine-Related Disorders, pp. 203–204**)

References

Anderson AL, Li SH, Biswas K, et al: Modafinil for the treatment of methamphetamine dependence. Drug Alcohol Depend 120:135–141, 2012 21840138

Brodie JD, Figueroa E, Laska EM, et al: Safety and efficacy of gamma-vinyl GABA (GVG) for the treatment of methamphetamine and/or cocaine addiction. Synapse 55:122–125, 2005 15543630

Brown ES, Gabrielson B: A randomized, double-blind, placebo-controlled trial of citicoline for bipolar and unipolar depression and methamphetamine dependence. J Affect Disord 143:257–260, 2012 22974472

Brown JM, Yamamoto BK: Effects of amphetamines on mitochondrial function: role of free radicals and oxidative stress. Pharmacol Ther 99:45–53, 2003 12804698

Coffin P, Santos G, Das M, et al: Aripiprazole for the treatment of methamphetamine dependence: a randomized, double-blind, placebo-controlled trial. Addiction 108:751–761, 2013 23186131

Colfax GN, Santos GM, Das M, et al: Mirtazapine to reduce methamphetamine use: a randomized controlled trial. Arch Gen Psychiatry 68:1168–1175, 2011 22065532

Eyerman DJ, Yamamoto BK: Lobeline attenuates methamphetamine-induced changes in vesicular monoamine transporter 2 immunoreactivity and monoamine depletions in the striatum. J Pharmacol Exp Ther 312:160–169, 2005 15331654

Gonzales R, Marinelli-Casey P, Shoptaw S, et al: Hepatitis C virus infection among methamphetamine-dependent individuals in outpatient treatment. J Subst Abuse Treat 31:195–202, 2006 16919748

Hanson GR, Sandoval V, Riddle E, et al: Psychostimulants and vesicle trafficking: a novel mechanism and therapeutic implications. Ann N Y Acad Sci 1025:146–150, 2004 15542712

Jayaram-Lindström N, Hammarberg A, Beck O, et al: Naltrexone for the treatment of amphetamine dependence: a randomized, placebo-controlled trial. Am J Psychiatry 165:1442–1448, 2008 18765480

Johnson BA, Roache JD, Ait-Daoud N, et al: Effects of acute topiramate dosing on methamphetamine-induced subjective mood. Int J Neuropsychopharmacol 10:85–98, 2007 16448579

McCann DJ, Li SH: A novel, nonbinary evaluation of success and failure reveals bupropion efficacy versus methamphetamine dependence: reanalysis of a multisite trial. CNS Neurosci Ther 18:414–418, 2012 22070720

Miller M, Moreno A, Aarde S, et al: A methamphetamine vaccine attenuates methamphetamine-induced disruptions in thermoregulation and activity in rats. Biol Psychiatry 73:721–728, 2013 23098894

Rawson RA, Gonzales R, Obert JL, et al: Methamphetamine use among treatment-seeking adolescents in Southern California: participant characteristics and treatment response. J Subst Abuse Treat 29:67–74, 2005 16135335

Seminerio MJ, Robson MJ, Abdelazeem AH, et al: Synthesis and pharmacological characterization of a novel sigma receptor ligand with improved metabolic stability and antagonistic effects against methamphetamine. AAPS J 14:43–51, 2012 22183188

Shen XY, Kosten TA, Lopez AY, et al: A vaccine against methamphetamine attenuates its behavioral effects in mice. Drug Alcohol Depend 129:41–48, 2013 23022610

Tiihonen J, Kuoppasalmi K, Föhr J, et al: A comparison of aripiprazole, methylphenidate, and placebo for amphetamine dependence. Am J Psychiatry 164:160–162, 2007 17202560

CHAPTER 15

Hallucinogens and Club Drugs

15.1 A patient would most likely seek acute medical attention for which of the following symptoms after ingesting a classic hallucinogen?

A. Hallucinations.
B. Dysphoria.
C. Panic.
D. Nausea/vomiting.
E. Palpitations.

The correct response is option C: Panic.

The most likely adverse effect for which the user of a classic hallucinogen would seek medical attention is anxiety or panic during the period of acute drug action (option C). Frank visual and auditory hallucinations (option A) are actually quite rare with classic hallucinogen use; perceptual alterations (i.e., illusions) are more common. Dysphoria (option B) is possible during a "bad trip," but this is not as common as anxiety/panic. Nausea and vomiting (option D) would be more expected with serotonin syndrome if a classic hallucinogen is combined with a monoamine oxidase inhibitor (as in ayahuasca brew). Palpitations (option E) could occur related to tachycardia or hypertension but, again, are less common. **(Classic Hallucinogens/Subjective Effects, pp. 211–212; Treatment of Acute Effects, p. 212)**

15.2 Which of the following hallucinogens or club drugs is considered to be a drug of dependence/addiction?

A. Lysergic acid diethylamide (LSD).
B. Psilocybin.
C. Methylenedioxymethamphetamine (MDMA).
D. Ketamine.
E. Mescaline.

The correct response is option D: Ketamine.

Classic hallucinogens (e.g., options A, B, E) are abused (i.e., used in such a way that jeopardizes the safety or well-being of the user or others); however, they are not typically considered drugs of dependence or addiction because they do not engender compulsive drug seeking and are not associated with a known withdrawal syndrome. In contrast to classic hallucinogens, dissociative anesthetics such as phencyclidine (PCP) and ketamine have considerable addiction (e.g., compulsive drug seeking) liability (Lerner and Burns 1978) (option D). Survey studies of frequent ketamine users indicate addictive/dependent behaviors such as using ketamine without stopping and taking steadily increasing doses (Muetzelfeldt et al. 2008). MDMA (option C) is also not noted to have significant addictive potential. **(Classic Hallucinogens/Long-Term Consequences, pp. 212–213; Dissociative Anesthetics/Long-Term Consequences, p. 217)**

15.3   You are performing a psychiatric evaluation on a 31-year-old male who has been using lysergic acid diethylamide (LSD) on a regular basis for several years. Which of the following chief complaints would you be most likely to encounter as a result of his chronic hallucinogen use?

A. Depression.
B. Insomnia.
C. Flashbacks.
D. Memory deficits.
E. Psychosis.

The correct response is option C: Flashbacks.

Classic hallucinogens (of which LSD is a member) possess relatively low physiological toxicity and have not been shown to result in organ damage or neuropsychological deficits (option D). A rare yet *possible* risk of hallucinogens is prolonged adverse psychological reactions, such as psychosis and depression (options A, E). The most commonly associated long-term risk of classic hallucinogen use is hallucinogen persisting perception disorder, frequently referred to as "flashbacks" (option C). A flashback involves unexpectedly reexperiencing the perceptual, emotional, or somatic effects of a previous hallucinogen experience. For the psychiatric diagnostic criteria for hallucinogen persisting perception disorder to be met, perceptual disturbances must last beyond the normal duration of drug effects and must be clinically distressing or impairing. Insomnia (option B) can occur from the use of hallucinogens and club drugs but is not especially common with the use of classic hallucinogens. **(Classic Hallucinogens/Long-Term Consequences, pp. 212–213)**

15.4   A 22-year-old woman presents to the medical emergency department with friends after she complained to them of chest pain at a party. She admits to taking some sort of "pill" around 2 hours prior to presentation. In the emergency department, she tells staff members that she "is in love with them" and wanders into other patients' rooms, trying to hug them. Her pupils are dilated, blood pressure is 180/100, and pulse is 120. Her affect is euphoric, and she exhibits no motor impairment. Which substance did the patient most likely ingest?

A. Phencyclidine (PCP).
B. Dextromethorphan.
C. *Salvia divinorum*.
D. Ketamine.
E. Methylenedioxymethamphetamine (MDMA).

The correct response is option E: Methylenedioxymethamphetamine (MDMA).

MDMA is typically taken orally in tablet or capsule form, with onset of effects about 30–60 minutes after administration and effects lasting around 4–6 hours. MDMA has been labeled an *entactogen* for its ability to promote increases in positive mood, as well as feelings of interpersonal openness, trust, and empathy (Johansen and Krebs 2009; Nichols et al. 1986) (option E). Physiological effects of MDMA include dilated pupils and increases in heart rate and blood pressure. *Salvia divinorum* (option C) is typically smoked or chewed, and its effects are relatively brief (resolving within 10–15 minutes). Thus, it is unlikely that medical professionals would see a patient with acute effects. Unlike classic hallucinogens, dissociative anesthetics (options A, B, D) are associated with strong motor impairment. PCP tends to produce more of a dissociative psychotic-like reaction, including catatonic states and extreme agitation. Dextromethorphan and ketamine have effects that overlap with those of classic hallucinogens, including perceptual distortions, changes in sense of time and space, and alterations in body awareness. **(Salvia Divinorum [Salvinorin A]/Subjective Effects, p. 214; Treatment of Acute Effects, p. 214; MDMA [Ecstasy]/Subjective Effects, p. 215; Dissociative Anesthetics/ Subjective Effects, pp. 216–217)**

15.5 Methylenedioxymethamphetamine (MDMA) has been found to have benefit for which of the following conditions?

A. Major depressive disorder.
B. Posttraumatic stress disorder (PTSD).
C. Chronic pain.
D. Alcohol dependence.
E. Anxiety associated with terminal illness.

The correct response is option B: Posttraumatic stress disorder (PTSD).

Initial clinical trials suggest that MDMA may be a safe and effective treatment for posttraumatic stress disorder, with patients exhibiting clinically significant relief from symptoms for years after initial treatment (Mithoefer et al. 2013) (option B). In clinical trials, ketamine has been shown to promote long-term abstinence in both alcohol- and heroin-dependent populations (Krupitsky and Grinenko 1997) (option D) and to produce rapid antidepressant effects that are clinically robust in patients with treatment-resistant major depression (option A). Classic hallucinogens have also been found to have potential therapeutic applications in the treatment of addiction (Krebs and Johansen 2012) and the treatment of pain, anxiety, and distress associated with terminal illness (options C, E) (Grob et al. 2013). Given its selective κ-opioid agonist activity, there is interest in using *Salvia divinorum* in the treatment of chronic pain (and cocaine drug dependence) (Sheffler and Roth 2003) as well (option C). **(Classic Hallucinogens/Medical and Therapeutic Applications, pp. 213–214; Salvia Divinorum [Salvinorin A]/Medical and Therapeutic Applications, p. 215; MDMA [Ecstasy]/Medical and Therapeutic Applications, p. 216; Dissociative Anesthetics/Medical and Therapeutic Applications, pp. 217–218)**

References

Grob CS, Bossis AP, Griffiths RR: Use of the classic hallucinogen psilocybin for treatment of existential distress associated with cancer, in Psychological Aspects of Cancer. Edited by Carr BI, Steel JL. New York, Springer Science and Business Media, 2013, pp 291–308

Johansen PØ, Krebs TS: How could MDMA (ecstasy) help anxiety disorders? A neurobiological rationale. J Psychopharmacol 23:389–391, 2009 19273493

Krebs TS, Johansen PØ: Lysergic acid diethylamide (LSD) for alcoholism: meta-analysis of randomized controlled trials. J Psychopharmacol 26:994–1002, 2012 22406913

Krupitsky EM, Grinenko AY: Ketamine psychedelic therapy (KPT): a review of the results of ten years of research. J Psychoactive Drugs 29:165–183, 1997 9250944

Lerner SE, Burns RS: Phencyclidine use among youth: history, epidemiology, and acute and chronic intoxication. NIDA Res Monogr (21):66–118, 1978

Mithoefer MC, Wagner MT, Mithoefer AT, et al: Durability of improvement in posttraumatic stress disorder symptoms and absence of harmful effects or drug dependency after 3,4-methylenedioxymethamphetamine-assisted psychotherapy: a prospective long-term follow-up study. J Psychopharmacol 27:28–39, 2013 23172889

Muetzelfeldt L, Kamboj SK, Rees H, et al: Journey through the K-hole: phenomenological aspects of ketamine use. Drug Alcohol Depend 95:219–229, 2008 18355990

Nichols DE, Hoffman AJ, Oberlender RA, et al: Derivatives of 1-(1,3-benzodioxol-5-yl)-2-butanamine: representatives of a novel therapeutic class. J Med Chem 29:2009–2015, 1986 3761319

Sheffler DJ, Roth BL: Salvinorin A: the "magic mint" hallucinogen finds a molecular target in the kappa opioid receptor. Trends Pharmacol Sci 24:107–109, 2003 12628350

CHAPTER 16

Tobacco Use Disorder

16.1 What pharmacological properties make nicotine addictive and promote the maintenance of nicotine dependence?

A. Nicotine-induced symptomatic relief lasts many hours.
B. Nicotine concentrations in the brain decline rapidly.
C. Nicotine is metabolized slowly by the liver.
D. Chronic nicotine exposure increases stress tolerance.
E. Nicotine desensitizes the hypothalamic-pituitary-adrenal (HPA) pathway.

The correct response is option B: Nicotine concentrations in the brain decline rapidly.

Nicotine smoke enters the lungs and is quickly absorbed into the arterial system, and nicotine enters the brain within 7–15 seconds after inhalation. As nicotine is distributed to other bodily tissues, blood concentrations in the brain rapidly begin to decline (option B). With this decrease in nicotine levels, symptoms of cravings may emerge in dependent smokers in as little as 20–30 minutes after smoking a cigarette (option A). Because smoking provides symptomatic relief, a vicious cycle is created, and dependence on nicotine is maintained.

Nicotine is metabolized quickly and has a half-life of about 2 hours (option C). Although nicotine initially stimulates the reward circuitry of the brain, *chronic* nicotine exposure may lower stress tolerance by sensitizing brain structures and pathways involved in stress reactivity—most notably, the HPA pathway and amygdala (options D, E). **(Pharmacokinetics of Nicotine, p. 225; Neurobiology of Nicotine, pp. 225–226)**

16.2 Your patient tells you that she smokes cigarettes. According to the U.S. Preventive Services Task Force recommendations, what should you do next?

A. Assess her level of motivation to quit.
B. Assist her with medication and counseling.
C. Advise her to quit.
D. Assess the severity of her physical dependence.
E. Assess her triggers and social supports.

The correct response is option C: Advise her to quit.

The U.S. Preventive Services Task Force recommends that all health care providers use the five As: Ask, Advise, Assess, Assist, and Arrange follow-up. First, the providers should *ask* all patients about whether they smoke and *advise* them to quit if they do (option C). For all tobacco users, the provider should list nicotine use disorder on the problem list and in the treatment plan and should *assess* for the patient's level of motivation to quit (option A). After assessing whether a patient is ready to quit, the provider should *assist* the patient by encouraging the use of medication and either face-to-face counseling or a telephone quit line (option B). Finally, health care providers should *arrange* to discuss again in a follow-up visit or arrange and refer the patient to treatment.

If time permits, tobacco users should be further screened for the severity of physical dependence, tolerance, and withdrawal symptoms (option D). Craving and wanting to use tobacco are the hallmark symptoms of nicotine use disorder and should be assessed and monitored; the health care provider should also try to understand what triggers the individual's tobacco craving and use (option E). **(Assessment and Treatment Interventions, p. 226/Assessment and Treatment Planning, pp. 226–228)**

16.3   What does motivational interviewing entail?

    A. Asking questions designed to elicit client's own incentives for behavior change.
    B. Providing information about community resources that can help with abstinence.
    C. Educating the client about the consequences of ongoing use.
    D. Informing the client about the benefits of quitting.
    E. Discussing advantages and side effects of different medication options.

The correct response is option A: Asking questions designed to elicit client's own incentives for behavior change.

Rather than directly providing information to promote behavior change (options B, C, D, E), in motivational interviewing, the clinician asks questions that are designed to elicit the client's own motivation for behavior change (i.e., to quit smoking) (option A). In addition to motivational interviewing, education is important in helping motivate smokers to quit. Information on the benefits of quitting and on community resources can be helpful to guide a discussion at the time of literature presentation and at follow-up. Clinicians should provide information on the quitting process, the consequences of ongoing tobacco use, the benefits of quitting, and the advantages and possible side effects of the different medication options. **(Assessment and Treatment Interventions/Brief Psychosocial Interventions for Smokers Not Ready to Quit, pp. 228–229; Psychosocial Interventions for Individuals Ready to Quit, pp. 229–230)**

16.4   Which psychosocial intervention helps individuals quit tobacco by promoting increased awareness of bodily sensations, acceptance of craving symptoms, and uncoupling of cravings and linked positive reinforcements?

A. Motivational interviewing.

B. Learning About Healthy Living.

C. Nicotine Anonymous.

D. Mindfulness.

E. Cognitive-behavioral therapy (CBT).

The correct response is option D: Mindfulness.

Studies support the use of mindfulness in promoting successful quitting (Brewer et al. 2011). Mindfulness skills can promote increased awareness of bodily sensations, acceptance of the craving symptoms, development of mindfulness approaches (meditation, body scan, etc.), and ultimately an uncoupling of cravings and linked positive reinforcements as a way to lessen the reactivity to urges and associated triggers (option D). In motivational interviewing, the clinician asks questions that are designed to elicit the client's own motivation for behavior change (i.e., to quit smoking) rather than directly providing information for this purpose (option A).

Learning About Healthy Living (treatment manual available free online) provides educational resources on wellness and the effects of smoking on health, as well as strategies to help tobacco users who are less motivated, in group or individual treatment, to start to consider setting quit goals (option B). Attending Nicotine Anonymous or other support groups can build confidence and hope (Ziedonis et al. 2006) (option C). CBT focuses on identifying triggers, understanding the triggers and associations, and identifying strategies for coping with or avoiding the triggers (option E). **(Assessment and Treatment Interventions/Brief Psychosocial Interventions for Smokers Not Ready to Quit, pp. 228–229; Psychosocial Interventions for Individuals Ready to Quit, pp. 229–230)**

16.5   Which nicotine replacement therapy (NRT) has the highest abuse liability?

A. Transdermal patch.

B. Gum.

C. Lozenge.

D. Inhaler.

E. Nasal spray.

The correct response is option E: Nasal spray.

NRT medications come in five forms: transdermal patch, gum lozenge, inhaler, and nasal spray. The patch, gum, and lozenge are available over the counter. Compared with tobacco products, NRT medications are relatively safe to use because they contain only nicotine and not the 4,000 additional chemicals, including approximately 70 carcinogens, found in smoking tobacco. In addition, NRT medications have low abuse liability (options A, B, C, D), even the abuse liability of the nicotine nasal spray, which is the highest among NRTs (option E), is still much lower than that of cigarettes and e-cigarettes. **(Assessment and Treatment Interventions/Tobacco Use Disorder Treatment Medications/Nicotine Replacement Therapies, pp. 230–232)**

16.6 You have a patient with schizophrenia and tobacco use disorder, treated with olanzapine and quetiapine. You have recently prescribed varenicline and nicotine replacement therapy (gum), and the patient was able to quit smoking. The patient reports increased sedation, hypersomnia, dizziness, and dry mouth. What would be the best course of action to take with this patient?

A. Increase the nicotine replacement therapy dose because these symptoms are consistent with nicotine withdrawal.
B. Discontinue nicotine replacement therapy because it is increasing olanzapine and quetiapine levels.
C. Discontinue varenicline because these symptoms are side effects of varenicline.
D. Decrease quetiapine dose because discontinuation of tobacco increased quetiapine levels.
E. Decrease olanzapine dose because discontinuation of tobacco increased olanzapine levels.

The correct response is option E: Decrease olanzapine dose because discontinuation of tobacco increased olanzapine levels.

The tar and non-nicotine polycyclic aromatic hydrocarbons from tobacco smoke alter the metabolism of many psychiatric medications by increasing the rate of metabolic clearance of the medications, and they can lower blood concentrations of the medications by up to 40% (Desai et al. 2001). Medications metabolized by the cytochrome P450 system's CYP1A2 isoenzyme are affected. Olanzapine has a faster (by 98%) medication clearance (option E). Nicotine is metabolized through CYP2D6 isoenzyme and does not alter the psychiatric medication blood levels; therefore, NRT medications do not change blood level of psychiatric medications (option B). Nicotine withdrawal includes symptoms of cravings, difficulty sleeping, irritability, moodiness/anxiety, restlessness, decreased heart rate, and difficulty concentrating (option A). Nausea is the most common side effect of varenicline; however, there are also risks of other gastrointestinal symptoms (constipation, flatulence, vomiting) and sleep disturbances (insomnia, abnormal dreams) (option C). Quetiapine has no known effect on serum levels of psychiatric medications (option D) **(Assessment and Treatment Interventions/Assessment and Treatment Planning, pp. 226–228; Tobacco Use Disorder Treatment Medications, pp. 230–233; Tobacco Use and Psychiatric Comorbidity/Tobacco Smoke's Effect on Psychiatric Medication Metabolism, p. 234; Table 16–3, Effect of smoking on serum levels of psychiatric medications, p. 235)**

References

Brewer JA, Mallik S, Babuscio TA, et al: Mindfulness training for smoking cessation: results from a randomized controlled trial. Drug Alcohol Depend 119:72–80, 2011 21723049
Desai HD, Seabolt J, Jann MW: Smoking in patients receiving psychotropic medications: a pharmacokinetic perspective. CNS Drugs 15:469–494, 2001 11524025
Ziedonis DM, Williams JM, Steinberg M, et al: Addressing tobacco addiction in office-based management of psychiatric disorders: practical considerations. Primary Psychiatry 13:51–63, 2006

CHAPTER 17

Benzodiazepines and Other Sedatives and Hypnotics

17.1   The weight of evidence suggests that all sedative-hypnotics as well as alcohol interact with which receptor?

A. β_1-Adrenergic.
B. Histamine$_1$ (H$_1$).
C. Serotonin 1A (5-HT$_{1A}$).
D. γ-Aminobutyric acid type A (GABA$_A$).
E. Serotonin 2A (5-HT$_{2A}$).

The correct response is option D: γ-Aminobutyric acid type A (GABA$_A$).

There is considerable evidence that all sedative-hypnotics and alcohol interact with the GABA$_A$ receptor (option D). Other non–sedative-hypnotic agents with reported anxiolytic effects interact with other receptors, and their lack of affinity for the GABA complex likely explains why they have little tendency to cause physiological dependence, for example, propranolol (β_1-adrenergic), hydroxyzine (H$_1$) buspirone (5-HT$_{1A}$), or mirtazapine (5-HT$_{2A}$) (options A, B, C, E). **(Behavioral Pharmacology/GABA$_A$ Receptors, p. 240)**

17.2   For benzodiazepines, which of the following adverse effects is most likely to persist even after several years of daily administration?

A. Lethargy.
B. Memory impairment.
C. Weakness.
D. Dizziness and falls.
E. Ataxia.

The correct response is option B: Memory impairment.

Most adverse effects induced by benzodiazepines are dose dependent and related to excessive sedation and intoxication produced by these drugs. These effects in-

193

clude sleepiness and lethargy (option A), weakness (option C), dizziness and falls (option D), ataxia (option E), confusion, and disorientation. Benzodiazepines may also contribute to the risk of falls among elderly patients. Individuals receiving maintenance therapy of stable doses of benzodiazepines usually develop tolerance to their sedative effects. However, there is no comparable development of tolerance for the memory-impairing effects of these medications, which can persist even after several years of daily administration (option B). **(Behavioral Pharmacology/Behavioral Effects/Other Adverse Effects, pp. 244–245)**

17.3   Physiological dependence to benzodiazepines occurs in approximately half of patients who have received daily medication for which length of time?

A. 1 week.
B. 2 weeks.
C. >1 month.
D. >2 months.
E. >4 months.

The correct response is option E: >4 months.

Regardless of the pharmacokinetics of the particular benzodiazepine used, physiological dependence is almost never seen in patients treated with them for less than 2 weeks (options A, B), and it occurs in approximately 50% of patients treated daily for more than 4 months (option E). Some patients treated for shorter intervals may still be at risk, although the risk is less (options C, D). All patients prescribed benzodiazepines for 4 months or longer should be warned of this possibility and instructed not to discontinue the medications abruptly, because withdrawal symptoms, seizures, or delirium may occur. **(Neurobiology of Sedative-Hypnotic Use Disorder/Physiological Dependence, p. 245)**

17.4   A 36-year-old woman with generalized anxiety disorder is being treated with lorazepam, 0.5 mg twice daily. She has no other medical or psychiatric history and is taking no other medications. She initially experiences a good effect, but on a 6-month follow-up visit, she tells her physician that she recently had to take extra tablets beyond what is prescribed to achieve symptom relief. Her doctor's investigation at this point should first focus on which of the following possible explanations for her complaint?

A. Nonadherence.
B. Drug diversion.
C. Misdiagnosis.
D. Substance use disorder.
E. Pseudoaddiction.

The correct response is option E: Pseudoaddiction.

Many individuals who are chronically prescribed benzodiazepines for the treatment of anxiety disorders will develop physiological dependence. This is often seen as a serious adverse effect that warrants discontinuation of medication, because otherwise it will lead to the development of iatrogenic addiction, with detrimental medical and behavioral consequences for the patient and possibly legal implications for the prescriber. Trepidation among physicians was based on the general lack of awareness that physiological dependence may occur even with therapeutic doses and their confusion in differentiating physiological dependence from addiction. As a result, benzodiazepines are often prescribed in subtherapeutic dosages and for an inadequate period. However, considerable data accumulated since the late 1980s do not support the validity of such concerns, and substance use disorders in patients with no predisposing history are uncommon and by no means the inevitable result of physiological dependence (option D). Inadequate treatment of patients with anxiety disorder can lead to a "pseudoaddiction" presentation (option E), in which inadequately treated patients (e.g., low dosages, long interdose intervals) request more medication and are wrongly presumed to be developing a substance use disorder (option C). In the vignette, it is unlikely that the patient's complaints can be attributed to a misdiagnosis given the initial good response to treatment (option C). Misuse of the medication, such as seen with drug diversion, is possible, although less common (option B). Some patients, out of their own fear of addiction, will take less medication than prescribed; however, such patients are usually willing to discuss their concerns and are unlikely to request even more medication (option A). **(Treatment/Prevention/ Managing Physiological Dependence, pp. 250, 252)**

17.5   A 52-year-old man with a history of sedative-hypnotic use disorder and comorbid panic disorder presents to a hospital seeking detoxification from alprazolam. He has been taking the drug daily for the past year at dosages as high as 12 mg/day. He has no other medical problems and is physically healthy on examination. He appears motivated for detoxification albeit fearful of side effects and admits that in the past he has left detoxification facilities prematurely because of a worsening of his anxiety symptoms. Which of the following first steps would be most helpful to successfully detoxify this patient?

A. Begin a rapid taper of alprazolam.
B. Rapidly cross-taper the patient to clonazepam.
C. Very slowly taper the alprazolam.
D. Slowly infuse flumazenil.
E. Discontinue alprazolam and begin oxazepam.

The correct response is option B: Rapidly cross-taper the patient to clonazepam.

In patients with comorbid psychiatric disorders, discontinuation of a short-acting agent, such as alprazolam, is usually more problematic than discontinuation of a long-acting agent because the former results in a faster onset of withdrawal symptoms and greater likelihood of the emergence of rebound anxiety. Therefore, the first stage of detoxification may involve transitioning to and stabilizing on a medication with more favorable pharmacokinetics (slower onset and longer duration of action), such as clonazepam (option B) or chlordiazepoxide (note that oxazepam [option E] would be less preferred given its shorter duration of action). Most benzodiazepines have comparable profiles of receptor activity, but their tolerability may be related to pharmacokinetic properties. Therefore, change to an equivalent dose of another benzodiazepine may result in better tolerability without change in efficacy. This can usually be accomplished by a fairly rapid cross-taper (over 1–2 weeks) to equivalent doses of a new agent and stabilization on a new medication (options B, C). The use of a slow infusion of the benzodiazepine antagonist flumazenil (option D) has been shown to be feasible and may target the purported changes in the GABA$_A$ receptor associated with physiological dependence; *however, it carries a high risk of seizures in this patient* (Hood et al. 2009). **(Treatment/Cessation of Use/Patients With Primary Psychiatric Comorbidity and Sedative-Hypnotic Use Disorders, pp. 252–255)**

17.6   Which of the following best describes the evidence supporting the use of long-acting benzodiazepines for maintenance treatment of patients with sedative, hypnotic, or anxiolytic use disorder who have been unsuccessful at remaining abstinent?

A. No peer-reviewed literature exists to support or refute benzodiazepine maintenance treatment.
B. Maintenance treatment is not an effective way to treat most substance use disorders.
C. Treatment with maintenance benzodiazepines usually leads to a worsening of substance use disorders.
D. Outside of uncontrolled trials, there is little empirical evidence to support this approach.
E. Clonazepam maintenance has comparable efficacy to methadone treatment for opioid use disorder.

The correct response is option D: Outside of uncontrolled trials, there is little empirical evidence to support this approach.

Maintenance treatment with benzodiazepines has been suggested, particularly for patients with substantial psychiatric comorbidity who are usually doing poorly during and following complete discontinuation of sedative-hypnotics (Joughin et al. 1991). This approach may involve transitioning to and maintenance treatment with a long-acting agent, such as clonazepam, with close monitoring of effectiveness and safety. Maintenance treatment as a general course is supported by extensive successful experience with the treatment of opioid dependence using methadone or buprenorphine (option B). However, experimental evidence to support clonazepam's safety and efficacy in the treatment of sedative-hypnotic dependence, although in existence (option A), is scarce. What literature exists suggests that clonazepam may have some use (option C); however, the effect is not comparable to that for methadone (option E) and relies mostly on uncontrolled trials and anecdotal reports (Weizman et al. 2003) (option D). **(Treatment/Cessation of Use/Patients With Coexisting Psychiatric Disorders, pp. 257–258)**

17.7   A 26-year-old patient has successfully detoxified from diazepam after 5 years of daily use. The patient currently denies withdrawal symptoms but reports continued craving for the drug. Outside of the substance use disorder, the patient has no other medical or psychiatric diagnoses. Which of the following is a first-line treatment for helping this patient maintain the gains achieved during detoxification and attain sustained, long-term abstinence?

A. Carbamazepine.
B. Behavioral therapy.
C. Flumazenil.
D. Oxazepam.
E. Imipramine.

The correct response is option B: Behavioral therapy.

Until more is known about the neurobiology of relapse and more medications become available, psychosocial approaches will remain a mainstay of relapse prevention treatment. Numerous approaches are available, and implementation of behavioral therapy following discontinuation of medication taper can be very effective in preventing relapse (option B). Abstinence rates have been maintained in over 75% of patients with panic disorder who discontinued alprazolam pharmacotherapy (Bruce et al. 1999). Medications currently have an adjunctive role in this setting (options A, C, E). Among medication choices, preliminary clinical evidence supports the use of indirect GABAergic agonists, such as carbamazepine or valproate, in early abstinence. Another approach that remains under investigation at this stage involves treatment with the benzodiazepine antagonist flumazenil (Hood et al. 2014). Patients who received flumazenil infusions during detoxification had significantly lower relapse rates during the first month after detoxification than did patients who were treated with oxazepam or placebo (Gerra et al. 2002). The safety of this approach requires further studies, given that flumazenil may precipitate withdrawal and induce seizures in physically dependent patients (Lugoboni et al. 2011). Imipramine may also help alleviate symptoms of withdrawal during the detoxification phase. **(Treatment/Relapse Prevention, pp. 258–259)**

References

Bruce TJ, Spiegel DA, Hegel MT: Cognitive-behavioral therapy helps prevent relapse and recurrence of panic disorder following alprazolam discontinuation: a long-term follow-up of the Peoria and Dartmouth studies. J Consult Clin Psychol 67:151–156, 1999 10028220

Gerra G, Zaimovic A, Giusti F, et al: Intravenous flumazenil versus oxazepam tapering in the treatment of benzodiazepine withdrawal: a randomized, placebo-controlled study. Addict Biol 7:385–395, 2002 14578014

Hood S, O'Neil G, Hulse G: The role of flumazenil in the treatment of benzodiazepine dependence: physiological and psychological profiles. J Psychopharmacol 23:401–409, 2009 19164495

Hood SD, Norman A, Hince DA, et al: Benzodiazepine dependence and its treatment with low dose flumazenil. Br J Clin Pharmacol 77(2):285–294, 2014 23126253

Joughin N, Tata P, Collins M, et al: In-patient withdrawal from long-term benzodiazepine use. Br J Addict 86:449–455, 1991 1675899

Lugoboni F, Faccini M, Quaglio GL, et al: Intravenous flumazenil infusion to treat benzodiazepine dependence should be performed in the inpatient clinical setting for high risk of seizure. J Psychopharmacol 25:848–849, 2011 21262854

Weizman T, Gelkopf M, Melamed Y, et al: Treatment of benzodiazepine dependence in methadone maintenance treatment patients: a comparison of two therapeutic modalities and the role of psychiatric comorbidity. Aust N Z J Psychiatry 37:458–463, 2003 12873331

CHAPTER 18

Treatment of Anabolic-Androgenic Steroid–Related Disorders

18.1 Which drug is often combined with anabolic-androgenic steroids (AASs) to reduce undesirable side effects?

A. Furosemide.
B. Probenecid.
C. Human growth hormone.
D. Tamoxifen.
E. Thyroid hormone.

The correct response is option D: Tamoxifen.

Users often combine other drugs (e.g., tamoxifen, letrozole, anastrozole) with AASs to reduce undesirable side effects such as gynecomastia (option D). Diuretics such as furosemide (option A) and probenecid (option B) are used as masking agents for urine testing. Human growth hormone and thyroid hormone (options C, E) augment performance- and image-enhancing effects of AASs. **(Identification and Assessment/History, pp. 265–266)**

18.2 Which of the following is the most likely physical exam finding associated with anabolic-androgenic steroid (AAS) use in men?

A. Male-pattern baldness.
B. Prostatic hypertrophy.
C. Testicular atrophy.
D. Hepatomegaly.
E. Hypertension.

The correct response is option C: Testicular atrophy.

The testicles become atrophic as they shut down testosterone production when exogenous AASs are administered in high doses (option C); this may lead to azoospermia and sterility (de Souza and Hallak 2011; Kanayama et al. 2010). Male-pattern bald-ness (option A), hirsutism, hypertension (option E), hepatomegaly (option D), ten-derness of the right-upper quadrant of the abdomen, jaundice, and prostatic hyper-trophy (option B) are also possible but are not reliably associated with AAS use. **(Identification and Assessment/Physical Examination, p. 266)**

18.3   Which of the following psychotropic medications is most appropriate for treating muscle dysmorphia, a form of body dysmorphic disorder seen in users of anabol-ic-androgenic steroids (AASs)?

A. Fluoxetine.
B. Bupropion.
C. Lithium.
D. Amphetamine.
E. Haloperidol.

The correct response is option A: Fluoxetine.

Muscle dysmorphia is a form of body dysmorphic disorder in which the individual perceives himself to be small and frail, even though he is actually large and mus-cular (Rohman 2009). Although systematic studies of the treatment of muscle dys-morphia are not known, it is recommended to follow the general treatment principles for other forms of body dysmorphic disorder, using cognitive-behavioral therapy and selective serotonin reuptake inhibitors (SSRIs) (option A). Bupropion (option B) is an antidepressant but not an SSRI. Lithium (option C) and haloperidol (option E) would be indicated to treat mania or psychosis resulting from AAS use. Amphet-amines (option D) may be abused along with AASs and is not a standard treatment for body dysmorphia. **(AAS Issues That May Garner Clinician Attention/Body Im-age Disorders Associated With AAS Use, p. 272)**

18.4.   Which of the following laboratory abnormalities is most reliably found in men using anabolic-androgenic steroids (AASs)?

A. Elevated high-density lipoprotein (HDL) cholesterol.
B. Elevated luteinizing hormone (LH).
C. Elevated testosterone level.
D. Decreased testosterone level.
E. Increased red blood cell (RBC) count.

The correct response is option E: Increased red blood cell (RBC) count.

AASs stimulate production of RBCs, although the magnitude of this effect varies substantially across individuals (option E). This can place patients at risk of throm-botic or hemorrhagic complications. HDL cholesterol (option A) is typically *decreased* during AAS use, particularly when individuals use orally active, 17α-alkylated AASs such as methandienone, oxymetholone, or stanozolol. Blood testosterone concentrations may be grossly elevated (option C) in patients who are administering exogenous testosterone, with serum concentrations typically several times the upper limit of normal (Kanayama et al. 2013). Conversely, testosterone concentrations may be grossly depressed (option D) in patients who are administering other types of AASs and hence inhibiting their own endogenous testosterone production. Hence testosterone may be either elevated or decreased with AAS use. The level of luteinizing hormone (option B) is typically *depressed*, not elevated. See Table 18–1 for a summary of laboratory abnormalities in AAS users. **(Identification and Assessment/Laboratory Examination, p. 267)**

TABLE 18–1. Laboratory abnormalities in anabolic-androgenic steroid users

Laboratory tests	Abnormalities
Blood work	
Muscle enzymes	↑ ALT, AST, LDH, and CK
Liver function tests	↑ ALT, AST, LDH, GGT, and total bilirubin (caution: ↑ ALT, AST, and LDH are often muscular in origin and do not indicate liver disease)
Cholesterol levels	↓ HDL-C, ↑ LDL-C, ↑ or no change in total cholesterol and triglycerides
Hormonal levels	↑ Testosterone and estradiol (with use of testosterone esters), ↓ testosterone (without use of testosterone esters or during withdrawal), or ↓ LH and FSH
Complete blood count	↑ RBC count, hemoglobin, and hematocrit
Urine testing	
Anabolic-androgenic steroids	Positive
Other drugs of abuse	May be positive
Cardiac testing	
Electrocardiogram	Left ventricular hypertrophy (seen also in intensive weight trainers)
Echocardiogram	Decreased ventricular ejection fraction, impaired diastolic function
Semen analysis	↓ Sperm count and motility, abnormal morphology

Note.   ALT=alanine aminotransferase; AST=aspartate aminotransferase; CK=creatine kinase; FSH=follicle-stimulating hormone; GGT=γ-glutamyltransferase; HDL-C=high-density lipoprotein cholesterol; LDH=lactate dehydrogenase; LDL-C=low-density lipoprotein cholesterol; LH=luteinizing hormone; RBC=red blood cell.

18.5 A 42-year-old man comes to your office reporting new onset of anhedonia, low mood, poor concentration, decreased sex drive, and fatigue. He admits that 1 week ago, he abruptly stopped using anabolic-androgenic steroids (AASs). What would the best treatment strategy be for you and your endocrinologist colleague to address the patient's complaints?

A. Start fluoxetine, and reevaluate symptoms in 4–6 weeks.

B. Start testosterone, then in 1 month discontinue the testosterone and start clomiphene.

C. Start naltrexone to reduce hedonic effects in the event of relapse.

D. Start clomiphene and human chorionic gonadotropin (HCG), with the addition of testosterone depending on level.

E. Start testosterone, then in 1 month discontinue the testosterone and start HCG.

The correct response is option D: Start clomiphene and human chorionic gonadotropin (HCG), with the addition of testosterone depending on level.

Use of exogenous AASs leads to suppression of the hypothalamic-pituitary-gonadal (HPG) axis (de Souza and Hallak 2011; Tan and Scally 2009). Thus, when a man discontinues an AAS course, especially if that course has been prolonged, he will likely experience hypogonadism. Hypogonadism may be associated with loss of sex drive, fatigue, and occasionally serious depression, the symptoms described in this patient. For individuals displaying AAS-withdrawal hypogonadism and expressing a desire not to resume AAS use, it is desirable to institute aggressive endocrinological treatment to stimulate the HPG axis to "jump-start" natural endogenous testosterone production and thus reduce the individual's desire to resume illicit exogenous AAS use (Tan and Scally 2009). Such treatment may include clomiphene to stimulate pituitary secretion of luteinizing hormone and follicle-stimulating hormone, together with HCG to stimulate testicular production of testosterone and spermatozoa. Initially, the patient may also require temporary exogenous testosterone administration to maintain adequate testosterone levels while waiting for clomiphene and/or HCG to stimulate resumption of endogenous function (option D). Although fluoxetine and other selective serotonin reuptake inhibitors (option A) can treat depression and address muscle dysmorphia that contributes to AAS dependence, they would not address the hypogonadism of this patient. Naltrexone (option C) could help block the hedonic effects of AAS that contribute to dependence, but it does not have widespread clinical use in humans and, again, would not address the hypogonadism issues in this patient. Starting testosterone, then later stopping it and starting clomiphene (option B) or HCG (option E) is incorrect because the clomiphene and HCG need to be started right away to stimulate endogenous function of the pituitary and testicles. Starting testosterone first, then stopping it and adding the stimulating agents will likely result in recurrent hypogonadism when the testosterone is stopped. **(AAS Issues That May Garner Clinician Attention/AAS Dependence, pp. 267–270)**

References

de Souza GL, Hallak J: Anabolic steroids and male infertility: a comprehensive review. BJU Int 108:1860–1865, 2011 21682835

Kanayama G, Brower KJ, Wood RI, et al: Treatment of anabolic-androgenic steroid dependence: emerging evidence and its implications. Drug Alcohol Depend 109:6–13, 2010 20188494

Kanayama G, Kean J, Hudson JI, et al: Cognitive deficits in long-term anabolicandrogenic steroid users. Drug Alcohol Depend 130:208–214, 2013

Rohman L: The relationship between anabolic androgenic steroids and muscle dysmorphia: a review. Eat Disord 17:187–199, 2009 19391018

Tan RS, Scally MC: Anabolic steroid-induced hypogonadism—towards a unified hypothesis of anabolic steroid action. Med Hypotheses 72:723–728, 2009 19231088

CHAPTER 19

Neurobiology of Opiates and Opioids

19.1 A cancer patient with painful bony lesions has been getting prescriptions for oxycodone from her oncologist for the pain. She reports to her oncologist that for 2 months her 8/10 pain would go down to 3/10 with the prescribed dose, but recently, she found she was getting less and less relief with that same dose. She tried an increased dose, and the pain went down to 3/10. She now worries about running out of medication too quickly. Which best describes the phenomenon?

A. Withdrawal.
B. Abuse.
C. Dependence.
D. Addiction.
E. Tolerance.

The correct response is option E: Tolerance.

Tolerance is defined as the need for increasing amounts of compound to achieve a specific physiological or pharmacological effect caused by that compound when acting at a specific site, such as a receptor. Thus, tolerance to a μ-opioid receptor (MOPR) agonist is defined as the need for increasing amounts of agonist to be administered to achieve a given effect. In this case, there is no description of withdrawal, nor has the patient been abstinent from the medication for withdrawal to occur (option A). The patient is using the medication for its prescribed purpose (option B). There are no withdrawal symptoms, which would indicate dependence (option C), and the description of requiring more medication for the same therapeutic effect fits the definition of tolerance (option E). However, it is probable that this patient is dependent after prolonged use of the opioid. Note that one can be tolerant and not necessarily dependent. Although dose escalation is a hallmark of addiction, this patient's dose escalation occurs without the context of compulsive drug seeking, drug craving, and negative consequences to self and others (option D). **(Neurobiology of Tolerance, Dependence, and Addiction, pp. 280–284/ Tolerance, pp. 281–282; Dependence, pp. 282–284)**

19.2   How long can a newly abstinent, seriously heroin-dependent person expect to experience the most intense signs and symptoms of withdrawal?

A. 6–12 hours.
B. 48–96 hours.
C. Weeks to months.
D. More than 1 year.
E. The signs and symptoms can be expected to persist even while receiving maintenance treatment.

The correct response is option B: 48–96 hours.

When withdrawal is precipitated by abrupt cessation of heroin or other short-acting opioid administration, there is rapid onset of withdrawal symptoms, which then crescendo and may be followed by a deep, or so-called "yen," sleep, lasting for 1 hour or more. Upon awakening, the dependent person in withdrawal suffers a recrudescence of withdrawal symptoms, which then gradually abate over the ensuing 48–96 hours (option B). The onset of signs and symptoms of μ-opioid receptor (MOPR) agonist dependence in humans occurs within *6–12 hours* (option A) after the last dose of short-acting drug such as heroin. Some signs and symptoms of abstinence persist long after the initial 48- to 96-hour period of intense withdrawal, potentially lasting for *weeks or months* (option C) (particularly signs of hypothalamic-pituitary-adrenal [HPA] axis hyperresponsivity). There is a reduction in dopaminergic tone during chronic MOPR agonist exposure, coupled with decreased binding capacity of dopamine D_2 receptors (Bart et al. 2003; Wang et al. 1997). There are also a few studies suggesting that recovery of this system is slow. Laboratory results have also documented persistent changes in the HPA stress-responsive system, which remains abnormal for very protracted periods of time (*more than 1 year*) (option D) following termination of exposure to MOPR agonists (either illicit use or part of chronic pharmacotherapy) (Kreek et al. 1984). Some HPA axis abnormalities persist during stabilized methadone treatment (Schluger et al. 2003) (option E). **(Neurobiology of Tolerance, Dependence, and Addiction/Dependence, pp. 282–284)**

19.3   What kind of neuron tonically inhibits dopaminergic neurons in the ventral tegmental area (VTA) and is of main importance in opioid addiction?

A. Dopaminergic.
B. γ-Aminobutyric acid (GABA)–ergic.
C. Cholinergic.
D. Noradrenergic.
E. Serotonergic.

The correct response is option B: γ-Aminobutyric acid (GABA)–ergic.

By inhibiting release of GABA (by way of direct inhibition of that neurotransmitter release of the intracellular presynaptic vesicles), neuronal activation or excitatory actions may ensue. Of main importance to addiction to μ-opioid receptor (MOPR) agonists is the inhibition of GABAergic neurons (option B) in the VTA and thus inhibition of GABAergic release. GABA normally tonically inhibits the dopaminergic neurons in the VTA. Thus, MOPR agonist-induced inhibition of GABA results in greater activation of mesolimbic-mesocortical dopaminergic fields. Simply put, MOPR agonists inhibit GABAergic neurons leading to activation of areas involved in reward and reinforcement. Dopaminergic neurons (option A) discussed above are influenced by GABAergic neurons, which can be inhibited by MOPR agonists. Cholinergic neurons (option C) and noradrenergic neurons (option D) are not directly involved in this mechanism. However, the use of clonidine to ameliorate some of the acute signs and symptoms of abstinence indicate that many signs and symptoms are a part of a cascade of overactive sympathetic and noradrenergic systems. Brain centers that mediate these effects include the locus coeruleus and the periaqueductal gray region. Serotonergic neurons (option E) are not directly involved in this mechanism. **(The Endogenous Opioid System/Opioid Peptides and Receptors, pp. 278–279; Signal Transduction Mechanisms, pp. 279–280)**

19.4   Which medication or category of medication is made from the opium poppy?

   A. Opiate.
   B. Opioid.
   C. Methadone.
   D. Fentanyl.
   E. β-Endorphin.

The correct response is option A: Opiate.

The word *opiate* (option A) is correctly used only to refer to a subset of the opioids, namely, natural products of the opium poppy (especially thebaine and morphine) and compounds directly derived therefrom (most notably heroin, a semisynthetic diacetylated derivative of morphine). The term *opioid* (option B) is used to refer to the entire class of compounds, including peptides, natural alkaloids, and synthetic chemicals, that bind to one or more types of opioid receptors. *Methadone* (option C) and *fentanyl* (option D) are synthetic opioids and are not derived from the opium poppy. β-Endorphin (option E) is an endogenous opioid and is not derived from the opium poppy. **(The Endogenous Opioid System/Opioid Peptides and Receptors, pp. 278–279)**

19.5   The stress-responsive hypothalamic-pituitary-adrenal (HPA) axis is profoundly disrupted by heroin addiction and normalized by maintenance treatment with which substance?

   A. Naltrexone.
   B. Naloxone.
   C. Metyrapone.
   D. Methadone.
   E. Adrenocorticotropic hormone (ACTH).

The correct response is option D: Methadone.

Whereas profound disruption of the stress-responsive HPA axis occurs during cycles of heroin addiction, normalization occurs during methadone (option D) maintenance treatment (Cushman and Kreek 1974; Kreek 1973; Kreek et al. 1984). Response to negative-feedback control by glucocorticoids normalizes during methadone maintenance treatment. There is a profound disruption of β-endorphin, ACTH, and cortisol levels during daily chronic naltrexone (option A) maintenance treatment for opiate addiction (Culpepper-Morgan and Kreek 1997; Schluger et al. 1998). Very small doses of the opioid antagonist naloxone (option B) can result in modest elevation of ACTH and cortisol levels, which precedes the signs and symptoms of withdrawal. When metyrapone (option C), a compound that temporarily blocks the last step of cortisol synthesis, was given to well-stabilized, non-drug-abusing, long-term methadone maintenance patients, signs and symptoms of opiate withdrawal would ensue transiently. Emergence of signs and symptoms of opioid withdrawal after administration of metyrapone led to the hypothesis that surges of ACTH (option E) may signal, in former heroin addicts, the onset of abstinence syndrome (Kennedy et al. 1990), and, as noted above, onset of signs and symptoms of withdrawal was preceded by modest elevation of ACTH following naloxone administration. **(Endogenous and Exogenous Opioid Role in Stress Responsivity: Recent Molecular Genetics Findings/Stress Responsivity and the Addictions, pp. 287–288)**

References

Bart G, Borg L, Schluger JH, et al: Suppressed prolactin response to dynorphin A1–13 in methadone-maintained versus control subjects. J Pharmacol Exp Ther 306:581–587, 2003 12730354

Culpepper-Morgan JA, Kreek MJ: Hypothalamic-pituitary-adrenal axis hypersensitivity to naloxone in opioid dependence: a case of naloxone-induced withdrawal. Metabolism 46:130–134, 1997 9030816

Cushman P Jr, Kreek MJ: Methadone-maintained patients. Effect of methadone on plasma testosterone, FSH, LH, and prolactin. N Y State J Med 74:1970–1973, 1974 4528642

Kennedy JA, Hartman N, Sbriglio R, et al: Metyrapone-induced withdrawal symptoms: symptoms in methadone-maintained patients. NIDA Res Monogr 105:416, 1990 1876057

Kreek MJ: Medical safety and side effects of methadone in tolerant individuals. JAMA 223:665–668, 1973 4739193

Kreek MJ, Ragunath J, Plevy S, et al: ACTH, cortisol and beta-endorphin response to metyrapone testing during chronic methadone maintenance treatment in humans. Neuropeptides 5:277–278, 1984 6099512

Schluger JH, Ho A, Borg L, et al: Nalmefene causes greater hypothalamic-pituitaryadrenal axis activation than naloxone in normal volunteers: implications for the treatment of alcoholism. Alcohol Clin Exp Res 22:1430–1436, 1998 9802524

Schluger JH, Bart G, Green M, et al: Corticotropin-releasing factor testing reveals a dose-dependent difference in methadone maintained vs control subjects. Neuropsychopharmacology 28:985–994, 2003 12700714

Wang GJ, Volkow ND, Fowler JS, et al: Dopamine D2 receptor availability in opiate-dependent subjects before and after naloxone-precipitated withdrawal. Neuropsychopharmacology 16:174–182, 1997 9015800

CHAPTER 20

Opioid Detoxification

20.1 Which one of the following objective signs is consistent with opioid intoxication rather than opioid withdrawal?

A. Constricted pupils.
B. Dilated pupils.
C. Diarrhea.
D. Lacrimation.
E. Rhinorrhea.

The correct response is option A: Constricted pupils.

Withdrawal symptoms are usually opposite the acute effects of the drug. For example, opioids acutely constrict pupils (option A) and slow peristalsis; in withdrawal, pupils are dilated (option B) and diarrhea occurs (option C). Symptoms of withdrawal can be separated into two categories for clinical utility: objective (what the clinician sees) and subjective (what the patient reports). The subjective symptoms typically cause the greatest discomfort and can be present in the absence of objective signs.

Withdrawal symptoms begin with intense craving and anxiety and possibly also with profound dysphoria and agitation. Symptoms then progress to perspiration, yawning, lacrimation (option D), rhinorrhea (option E), akathisia, and insomnia and later to piloerection, hot and cold flashes, bone aches, myalgias, muscle spasms, nausea/vomiting/diarrhea, abdominal cramps, mydriasis, weight loss, exquisite tactile sensitivity, and low-grade fever (Table 20–1). **(Clinical Characteristics of the Opioid [μ-Agonist] Withdrawal Syndrome/Signs and Symptoms of Opioid Withdrawal, pp. 297–298)**

20.2 You admit a 25-year-old patient for opioid detoxification. He tells you he is using five bags of heroin intravenously per day. Approximately how many hours after his last heroin use would you expect withdrawal to begin?

A. 3–5 hours.
B. 4–6 hours.
C. 8–12 hours.

TABLE 20–1. Signs and symptoms of opioid withdrawal

Early to moderate	Moderate to advanced
Anorexia	Abdominal cramps
Anxiety	Broken sleep/insomnia
Craving/drug-seeking behavior	Hot or cold flashes
Dysphoria	Hypertension (mild/moderate)
Fatigue	Low-grade fever
Fear of withdrawal (anticipatory anxiety)	Myalgia and bone pain
Headache	Muscle spasm ("kicking the habit")
Irritability	Mydriasis (with dilated fixed pupils at the peak)
Lacrimation	Nausea and vomiting
Mydriasis (mild)	Tachycardia (mild/moderate)
Oscitation (yawning)	
Perspiration	
Piloerection (gooseflesh, or "cold turkey")	
Restlessness	
Rhinorrhea	
Tachypnea (mild/moderate)	

    D. 13–17 hours.
    E. 36–72 hours.

The correct response is option C: 8–12 hours.

Withdrawal symptoms vary, depending on the opioid. With heroin (a short-acting opioid), symptoms manifest 8–12 hours after last use (option C), beginning with intense craving and anxiety, but possibly also with profound dysphoria and agitation. Symptoms then progress to perspiration, yawning, lacrimation, rhinorrhea, akathisia, and insomnia, and later to piloerection, hot and cold flashes, bone aches, myalgias, muscle spasms, nausea/vomiting/diarrhea, abdominal cramps, mydriasis, weight loss, exquisite tactile sensitivity, and low-grade fever. These symptoms peak 2–3 days after the last dose and should resolve by day 5. Appearance of withdrawal from intravenous fentanyl occurs 3–5 hours after last dose (option A), and meperidine withdrawal begins 4–6 hours after last dose (option B). In contrast, withdrawal from methadone, a long-acting agent, presents 36–72 hours after last dose (option E) (Table 20–2). The 13- to 17-hour time frame does not have any opioid withdrawal correlate (option D). **(Clinical Characteristics of the Opioid [μ-Agonist] Withdrawal Syndrome/Signs and Symptoms of Opioid Withdrawal, pp. 297–298, 299)**

20.3   You are teaching a medical student about buprenorphine. The medical student asks you why there are two forms of buprenorphine (buprenorphine alone and buprenorphine combined with naloxone). What do you tell her about the purpose of the naloxone in the combination formulation?

TABLE 20–2. Duration of effects and first appearance of withdrawal

Drug	Effects wear off (hours[a])	Appearance of nonpurposive withdrawal symptoms (hours)	Peak withdrawal effects (hours)	Majority of symptoms over
Fentanyl[b]	1	3–5[c]	8–12	4–5 days
Meperidine	2–3	4–6	8–12	4–5 days
Oxycodone[d]	3–6	8–12	36–72	Approximately 7–10 days
Hydromorphone	4–5	4–5	36–72	Approximately 7–10 days
Heroin	4[e]	8–12	36–72	7–10 days
Morphine	4–5	8–12	36–72	7–10 days
Codeine	4	8–12	36–72	Approximately 7–10 days
Hydrocodone	4–8	8–12	36–72	Approximately 7–10 days
Methadone	8–12	36–72	96–144	14–21 days

[a]Duration may vary with chronic dosing
[b]Intravenous formulation described.
[c]Because of continued skin absorption after the patch is removed, withdrawal symptoms can take 16–24 hours to occur with use of transdermal fentanyl.
[d]The long-acting oral form of oxycodone may last up to 12 hours unless crushed, at which time it reverts back to being short acting.
[e]Usually taken two to four times per day.

A. To allow one to check blood levels.
B. To deter intravenous abuse.
C. To make it more safe in overdose.
D. To enhance the oral bioavailability.
E. To increase the half-life.

The correct response is option B: To deter intravenous abuse.

Buprenorphine comes in two forms: combined with naloxone (Suboxone), as individually wrapped sublingual strips, or alone (Subutex), as tablets. Naloxone has limited oral bioavailability (option D), so it is added to buprenorphine to deter intravenous abuse by putatively inducing withdrawal if injected (option B). Intravenous Suboxone elicits less positive subjective effects and has a lower abuse potential than heroin or the generic tablet form of buprenorphine (Subutex), especially at higher doses (24 mg vs. 2 mg) (Comer et al. 2010). Blood levels for buprenorphine or the combination of buprenorphine and naloxone are not monitored in clinical practice (option A). Buprenorphine is safer than methadone in overdose; however, naloxone has no bearing on its overdose potential, as it has limited oral bioavailability (option C). Buprenorphine has a much longer half-life than naloxone; thus, naloxone is not added to buprenorphine to increase the half-life (option E). **(Detoxification Options/Opioid Agonist Substitution and Taper/Buprenorphine, pp. 300–301)**

20.4   A 35-year-old woman presents to the emergency room in opioid withdrawal. What is the largest *initial* dose of methadone that you can safely give to her?

A. 10 mg.
B. 20 mg.
C. 30 mg.
D. 40 mg.
E. 50 mg.

The correct response is option C: 30 mg.

Initial doses of methadone should not exceed 30 mg (option C), and the 24-hour total should not exceed 40 mg (option D) in the first few days. A safe initial dose in a nontolerant individual can become dangerous if continued beyond 1 or 2 days, because methadone accumulates. When withdrawal is not initially present (e.g., when methadone is used as a prophylactic treatment for a previously dependent patient to prevent relapse), the patient should be observed for drowsiness or depressed respiration. Overdose manifests with drowsiness, motor impairment, miosis, nausea, mild hyperthermia, and QT prolongation, for which methadone carries a black box warning. (QT intervals should be checked regularly, especially if the patient is taking drugs that may synergistically increase the QT interval [e.g., antipsychotics].) Regardless of the setting, medical personnel should be present to manage problems. Overmedication is treated with 0.4–0.8 mg of naloxone, and repeated doses may be required because of methadone's long half-life (Chhabra and Bull 2008). **(Detoxification Options/Opioid Agonist Substitution and Taper/Methadone, pp. 301–302)**

20.5   What is one potential advantage of a clonidine-naltrexone opioid detoxification compared with either methadone taper or clonidine detoxification?

A. Reduction in time to detoxification.
B. Higher patient acceptance.
C. Less need for medical monitoring.
D. Fewer staff required.
E. Less precipitated withdrawal.

The correct response is option A: Reduction in time to detoxification.

The opioid antagonist naltrexone can hasten opioid withdrawal and detoxification, speeding the patient's move to the next phase of treatment. Naltrexone displaces opioids from the receptors and causes a shorter, more severe withdrawal (option E) that is mitigated with early, aggressive use of clonidine and benzodiazepines (Riordan and Kleber 1980). Although the more severe withdrawal requires greater medical oversight, clonidine-naltrexone detoxification and antagonist induction techniques appear to be safe, effective, and economical alternatives to either methadone taper or clonidine detoxification. In trained hands, advantages of the techniques include a dramatic reduction in the time necessary to detoxify (option

A), high completion rates (e.g., 55%–95%), and the ability to move rapidly to the next stage of rehabilitation with fewer withdrawal symptoms. Disadvantages include generally poorer patient acceptance relative to other therapies (option B), the need for intensive medical monitoring (option C), and the need for facilities and staff to accommodate potentially very sick patients (option D). **(Detoxification Options/Clonidine-Naltrexone Detoxification and Antagonist Induction, pp. 304–305)**

References

Chhabra S, Bull J: Methadone. Am J Hosp Palliat Care 25:146–150, 2008 18445864

Comer SD, Sullivan MA, Vosburg SK, et al: Abuse liability of intravenous buprenorphine/naloxone and buprenorphine alone in buprenorphine-maintained intravenous heroin abusers. Addiction 105:709–718, 2010 20403021

Riordan CE, Kleber HD: Rapid opiate detoxification with clonidine and naloxone. Lancet 1:1079–1080, 1980 6103408

CHAPTER 21

Methadone and Buprenorphine Maintenance

21.1 What distinguishes methadone from prior treatments for opioid dependence?

A. Strong *N*-methyl-D-aspartate (NMDA) antagonism.
B. Efficacy.
C. Lack of respiratory depression.
D. Predictable half-life.
E. Mostly renal excretion.

The correct response is option B: Efficacy.

Although methadone was not the first medication used to treat addictive disorder, methadone's dramatic efficacy for what has been a significant problem that has been unresponsive to other treatments made it a life-saving intervention for countless opioid-dependent persons (option B). The half-life of methadone is somewhat complicated, because it can vary considerably between indications as a function of factors such as genetic differences in enzymatic activity, the duration of treatment, and the pH of the urine (option D). Methadone is metabolized in the liver, and a small percentage (about 10%) is excreted unchanged in the urine (option E). Methadone's primary therapeutic effect is mediated by its action as a μ-agonist opioid. However, it also has activity at the NMDA receptor, where it acts as a weak antagonist (option A). Methadone can also function as a respiratory depressant, reflecting its μ-agonist function (option C). **(Methadone Treatment, pp. 311–315)**

21.2 In treatment of opioid addiction, methadone exerts its therapeutic effect via which pharmacological mechanism?

A. Withdrawal suppression.
B. *N*-methyl-D-aspartate (NMDA) agonism.
C. μ-Receptor antagonism.
D. Decreased cross-blockade.
E. Long-lasting analgesia.

The correct response is option A: Withdrawal suppression.

Even at low doses, methadone can effectively suppress spontaneous withdrawal in an opioid-dependent person who stops his or her usual dose of opioid (option A). In a person who takes methadone daily (i.e., is tolerant to its effects), an adequate dose of methadone produces cross-blockade to the other effects of a μ-agonist opioid (i.e., the person who takes an opioid while taking an adequate dose of methadone will not experience a "high" effect from that opioid) (options C, D). Withdrawal suppression and cross-blockade are two of the critical pharmacological effects of methadone that help to exert its therapeutic effect (option A). Methadone's primary therapeutic effect is mediated by its action as a μ-agonist opioid. However, methadone also has activity at the NMDA receptor, where it acts as a weak antagonist (option B). The duration of methadone's analgesic effects is shorter than its pharmacokinetic half-life would suggest, necessitating dosing two or three times per day when used for pain control (option E). **(Pharmacology of Methadone, pp. 311–312)**

21.3   In the United States, methadone treatment for opioid dependence is usually provided in which type of setting?

   A. Substance abuse psychiatrists' offices.
   B. Pain management clinics.
   C. Inpatient substance abuse rehabilitation units.
   D. Outpatient substance abuse rehabilitation units.
   E. Opioid treatment programs.

The correct response is option E: Opioid treatment programs.

Methadone treatment for opioid dependence in the United States is usually provided at a special clinic devoted to this modality of care (often referred to as an *opioid treatment program,* or OTP) (option E). These clinics are health care sites that provide methadone medication as well as other services, such as counseling, urine testing, and vocational assistance. Only opioid treatment programs specifically licensed and approved to dispense methadone for opioid dependence can do so. Psychiatrists' offices and inpatient and outpatient substance abuse rehabilitation units do not fall under this category and do not usually provide methadone treatment (options A, C, and D). Pain management clinics provide methadone for pain management but not for opioid dependence (option B). **(Treatment of Opioid Dependence With Methadone, pp. 312–313)**

21.4   Which of the following correlates with better outcomes in methadone treatment for opioid dependence?

   A. Gradual methadone dose reduction over time.
   B. Lower daily maintenance dosing.
   C. Higher methadone blood levels.

D. Nonpharmacological treatment.

E. Decreased availability of methadone take-home doses.

The correct response is option D: Nonpharmacological treatment.

Whereas methadone *medication* can be very useful for suppressing withdrawal and blocking effects of other opioids, methadone *treatment* provides a context in which a number of other prosocial activities and other health issues can be addressed. Greater amounts of nonpharmacological treatment in the context of methadone are associated with better outcomes (option D). Slower and more gradual withdrawals are more effective than shorter ones, although outcomes from opioid withdrawal are often poor, as demonstrated by a high rate of relapse (option A). Methadone maintenance treatment, on the other hand, consists of an induction period, followed by stable dosing of daily methadone; patients in maintenance treatment may continue taking methadone for many years. Outcomes with methadone medication are dose related; lower doses (20–40 mg/day) are effective at suppressing opioid withdrawal but may not suffice in decreasing craving or blocking effects of other opioids (option B). The blood level of methadone does not correspond well to dose, and the effective dose varies considerably across patients (option C). Contingency management is particularly useful in the context of methadone treatment. The availability of methadone take-home doses can serve as a very useful and powerful reward for behavior change (e.g., stopping problematic drug or alcohol use or improving adherence to counseling sessions) (option E). **(Methadone Treatment/Treatment of Opioid Dependence With Methadone, pp. 312–313; Efficacy and Safety of Methadone, pp. 314–315)**

21.5   What is one of the most common adverse effects of methadone maintenance therapy?

A. QTc prolongation.

B. Constipation.

C. Decreased sweating.

D. Cognitive impairment.

E. Poor psychomotor performance.

The correct response is option B: Constipation.

Methadone maintenance is a safe treatment (Center for Substance Abuse Treatment 2005; Kreek 1973). Despite the potential side effects associated with methadone (e.g., *increased* sweating [option C], constipation [option B]), persons maintained on a steady dose of methadone do not appear to have problems with psychomotor performance or clinically significant cognitive impairment (options D, E). There has been some controversy as to whether methadone can produce prolongation of the QTc interval, but studies to date have been quite variable in their electrocardiogram findings on this matter (option A). **(Methadone Treatment/Efficacy and Safety of Methadone, pp. 314–315)**

21.6 What is the mechanism of action of buprenorphine?

A. Short-acting opioid antagonism.
B. Long-acting opioid agonism.
C. Mixed opioid agonism-antagonism.
D. Long-acting γ-aminobutyric acid (GABA) agonism.
E. Positive allosteric modulation of GABA.

The correct response is option C: Mixed opioid agonism-antagonism.

Buprenorphine is one of a number of analgesic medications that have been classified as mixed agonist-antagonist opioids. Naloxone is a short-acting opioid antagonist (option A). Many opioid agonists have long-acting formulations, such as fentanyl extended-release transdermal system, morphine sulfate extended-release, and oxycodone hydrochloride controlled-release, among others. Buprenorphine is not one of them (option B). Benzodiazepines bind the GABA receptors and increase the activity of the GABA receptor protein, enhancing the effect of GABA at the GABA receptor. Thus, they are positive allosteric modulators and not GABA agonists. Buprenorphine does not act at the GABA receptor (options D and E). **(Pharmacology of Buprenorphine, pp. 316–317)**

21.7 Who can prescribe buprenorphine for opioid dependence in the United States?

A. Opioid treatment programs only.
B. General psychiatrists anywhere in the world.
C. Physicians with special training and a special Drug Enforcement Administration number.
D. Physicians who are board certified in addiction psychiatry with a regular Drug Enforcement Administration number.
E. Physicians who have treated at least 30 patients with buprenorphine under supervision.

The correct response is option C: Physicians with special training and a special Drug Enforcement Administration number.

In the United States, buprenorphine can be prescribed for the treatment of opioid dependence by a physician in an office-based setting (in contrast to methadone, which is essentially available only through opioid treatment programs) (option A). Before prescribing buprenorphine, a physician must complete a special 8-hour training course (or achieve qualification through some other mechanism, such as being board certified in addiction psychiatry) and then must apply for a special Drug Enforcement Administration number (often called an "X number" because the first letter of the number is the letter X) (options C, D). The Drug Addiction Treatment Act of 2000 (Public Law 106-310; referred to as DATA 2000) limits the number of patients a physician can concurrently treat with buprenorphine (30 in the first year, and then up to 100 in subsequent years after requesting this increase) (option E). At this time, in the United States, only physicians can prescribe buprenorphine for opioid dependence (option B). **(Buprenorphine Treatment/ Treatment of Opioid Dependence With Buprenorphine, pp. 317–318)**

21.8   You start a patient on buprenorphine and the patient complains of anxiety, insomnia, nausea, and diaphoresis. What would be the best course of action to take?

    A. Do not do anything differently because these symptoms are unlikely to be related to the medication.

    B. Stop buprenorphine because these symptoms are the side effects of the medication and will not improve.

    C. Increase the dose of buprenorphine to increase the opioid agonism and improve the symptoms.

    D. Wait a few days or decrease the starting dose to minimize opioid withdrawal.

    E. Add a benzodiazepine for anxiety and insomnia.

The correct response is option D: Wait a few days or decrease the starting dose to minimize opioid withdrawal.

A partial agonist can occupy a receptor but produce less activation of that receptor than does a full agonist opioid. This means that a dose of buprenorphine administered to a person who is physically dependent on a full agonist opioid such as heroin could produce a net decrease of receptor effect, resulting in opioid withdrawal. Indeed, this effect has been shown to occur in opioid-dependent persons under laboratory conditions (Rosado et al. 2007; Strain et al. 1995) and has been reported anecdotally by some clinicians. To minimize the risk of buprenorphine-precipitated withdrawal, it is best to have the first dose be low (e.g., 2–4 mg), to give it well after the last dose of opioid agonist (ideally having the patient in early opioid withdrawal), and to be careful if the person has a higher level of opioid physical dependence. Anxiety, insomnia, nausea, and diaphoresis are consistent with opioid withdrawal and are likely related to the medication (option A). The symptoms should improve with decreased starting dose and with time (option B). Increasing the buprenorphine dose may worsen withdrawal symptoms, since buprenorphine will occupy the receptors and produce less activation of the receptors than a full agonist (option C). It is not advisable to add a potentially addictive medication, such as benzodiazepine, to the patient's regimen, given that the patient presumably already has an addiction to opioids (option E). **(Pharmacology of Buprenorphine, pp. 316–317)**

References

Center for Substance Abuse Treatment: Medication-Assisted Treatment for Opioid Addiction in Opioid Treatment Programs. Treatment Improvement Protocol (TIP) Series 43 (HHS Publ No SMA-12-4214). Rockville, MD, Substance Abuse and Mental Health Services Administration, 2005

Kreek MJ: Medical safety and side effects of methadone in tolerant individuals. JAMA 223:665–668, 1973 4739193

Rosado J, Walsh SL, Bigelow GE, et al: Sublingual buprenorphine/naloxone precipitated withdrawal in subjects maintained on 100 mg of daily methadone. Drug Alcohol Depend 90:261–269, 2007 17517480

Strain EC, Preston KL, Liebson IA, et al: Buprenorphine effects in methadone-maintained volunteers: effects at two hours after methadone. J Pharmacol Exp Ther 272:628–638, 1995 7853176

CHAPTER 22

Opioid Antagonists

22.1 What medication acts exclusively as a nonselective opioid antagonist, with no opioid agonist properties?

A. Methadone.
B. Naloxone.
C. Naltrexone.
D. Buprenorphine.
E. Clonidine.

The correct response is option B: Naloxone.

Naloxone (*N*-allylnoroxymorphone), a semisynthetic opiate derivative, is a nonselective opioid antagonist with high lipid solubility that rapidly crosses the blood-brain barrier and competitively binds to μ-opiate receptors but has no intrinsic opioid agonist activity (it binds with lower affinity to κ- and δ-opioid receptors) (option B) (Peng et al. 2007). Naltrexone (option C) is also an antagonist of opioid receptors, but it is also a partial, low-efficacy agonist at the κ-opioid receptor. Methadone (option A) is an opioid agonist, and buprenorphine (option D) is a partial opioid agonist. Clonidine (option E) is an α_1 agonist and is used for symptom relief in opioid detoxification. **(Clinical Pharmacology, pp. 323–325; Use in Opiate Detoxification and Naltrexone Induction, pp. 327–328)**

22.2 Naltrexone's effect on hypothalamic-pituitary-adrenal (HPA) and hypothalamic-pituitary-gonadal (HPG) activity may account for what adverse response in some patients upon treatment initiation?

A. Nausea.
B. Insomnia.
C. Anxiety.
D. Headache.
E. Appetite disturbances.

The correct response is option C: Anxiety.

A small proportion of patients experience severe anxiety reactions, panic, or dysphoria following the first dose of naltrexone or early in treatment, and this may lead to medication discontinuation (option C). The anxiogenic effects of opioid antagonists may be mediated by effects at δ or κ receptors or antagonism of μ receptors. Opioid antagonists increase HPA activity and alter HPG functioning by blocking the tonic, inhibitory effects of β-endorphins on the hypothalamus. Increased HPA activity or stress reactivity may also contribute to the anxiogenic effects of naltrexone experienced by some patients (Vuong et al. 2010). Although nausea, insomnia, headache, and appetite disturbances (options A, B, D, E) are common side effects, these answers are incorrect as they are not primarily due to HPA- and HPG-mediated effects. **(Adverse Effects, pp. 325–326)**

22.3 What accounts for approximately half of the deaths of heroin users in the United States?

A. Liver failure.
B. Malnutrition.
C. Cardiac arrhythmia.
D. Overdose.
E. Stroke.

The correct response is option D: Overdose.

Approximately half of all deaths of heroin users in the United States are attributed to overdose, and there has also been a substantial increase in overdose deaths in the general population associated with the recent rapid increase in opioid analgesic prescriptions and use (option D). Tolerance develops more slowly to the respiratory depressant effects of opioids than to the analgesic or euphoric effects, leading to an increased risk of overdose following opioid dose escalations to maintain analgesic or euphoric effects. Heroin users are at risk for liver failure (option A) from diseases such as hepatitis C (transmitted by shared needles), malnutrition (option B), and other medical problems (options C, E), but these are not the primary causes of death in this patient population. **(Use for Acute, Emergency Treatment of Opioid Overdose, pp. 326–327)**

22.4 In addition to supportive care, what is the treatment of choice in acute opioid overdose?

A. Naloxone.
B. Naltrexone.
C. Clonidine.
D. General anesthesia.
E. Benzodiazepines.

The correct response is option A: Naloxone.

Management of opioid overdose includes maintenance of adequate ventilation, administration of naloxone (administered intravenously, intramuscularly, or intranasally, depending on the setting and availability), and evaluation and treatment of commonly associated problems (option A). Naloxone is favored over naltrexone (option B) for the treatment of overdose because its onset of effects is more rapid, the dose can be titrated more easily to reverse respiratory depression without precipitating severe withdrawal, and precipitated withdrawal, if it occurs, is of shorter duration. Clonidine and benzodiazepines (options C, E) may be used for symptom relief during the first few days of withdrawal from opioids but not in the management of overdose. In certain situations, general anesthesia or conscious sedation (option D) can be used for ultrarapid detoxification from opioids but should not be used to manage acute, life-threatening overdose. **(Use for Acute, Emergency Treatment of Opioid Overdose, pp. 326–327)**

22.5   Compared with those who discontinue opioid agonist treatment, individuals who discontinue opioid antagonist treatment are at much greater risk for what outcome, cited by experts as a reason that antagonist treatment is "unacceptable"?

A. Relapse and overdose.
B. Depression and suicide.
C. Cognitive impairment.
D. Social stigmatization.
E. Panic attacks.

The correct response is option A: Relapse and overdose.

The risk of resumption of opioid use and opioid overdose increases rapidly following discontinuation of oral naltrexone, and high mortality rates have been found following discontinuation of oral naltrexone maintenance treatment (option A). In a pooled analysis of studies in Australia, the rate of heroin overdose for patients after leaving naltrexone treatment was six times higher than the rate during naltrexone treatment and eight times higher than the rate among patients who left opioid agonist maintenance treatment (Digiusto et al. 2004). Options B, C, D, and E are incorrect because they are not the major reason cited to support the superiority of agonist-to-antagonist treatment. **(Mortality Following Naltrexone Discontinuation, pp. 330–331)**

References

Digiusto E, Shakeshaft A, Ritter A, et al: Serious adverse events in the Australian National Evaluation of Pharmacotherapies for Opioid Dependence (NEPOD). Addiction 99:450–460, 2004 15049745

Peng X, Knapp BI, Bidlack JM, et al: Pharmacological properties of bivalent ligands containing butorphan linked to nalbuphine, naltrexone, and naloxone at mu, delta, and kappa opioid receptors. J Med Chem 50:2254–2258, 2007 17407276

Vuong C, Van Uum SH, O'Dell LE, et al: The effects of opioids and opioid analogs on animal and human endocrine systems. Endocr Rev 31:98–132, 2010 19903933

CHAPTER 23

Neurobiology of Marijuana

23.1 After consumption of marijuana, which of the following symptoms is most likely to persist?

A. Impairment in motor coordination.
B. Appetite stimulation.
C. Increase in sociability.
D. Altered perception of time.
E. Heightened sensitivity of stimuli.

The correct response is option A: Impairment in motor coordination.

The consumption of marijuana causes a unique combination of calmness and euphoria, referred to as a *high*. During this state of acute intoxication, the user's sociability and sensitivity to certain stimuli (e.g., colors) are heightened, perception of time is altered, and appetite for sweet and fatty foods is stimulated (options B, C, D, E). These pleasant changes are often associated with, and outlasted by, substantial impairments in cognition, judgment, and motor coordination (option A). **(Clinical Features, pp. 336–337)**

23.2 Which of the following acute symptoms is a person most likely to experience when smoking hash oil compared with marijuana?

A. Increased craving for marijuana.
B. Sensitivity to colors.
C. Decreased appetite.
D. Paranoid thoughts.
E. Altered perception of time.

The correct response is option D: Paranoid thoughts.

Three preparations of different potencies currently dominate the marijuana market: a rough mixture of flowers, leaves, stems, and seeds, known as *bhang* or *grass*, with an average Δ^9-tetrahydrocannabinol (Δ^9-THC) content of 1%–3%; a more refined selection of unfertilized female lowers, called *ganja* or *sinsemilla*, with a Δ^9-THC content of 3%–8%; and a collection of resin glands ("trichomes") obtained from the sterile buds of the plant, called *charas* or *hashish*, with a Δ^9-THC content of 10%–15% (Iversen 2000; Russo 2007). Extraction of *Cannabis* preparations with an organic solvent yields a product (variedly named *hash oil*, *dabs*, or *shatter*) that contains up to 30%–35% Δ^9-THC (Mehmedic et al. 2010). During the state of acute intoxication with the consumption of marijuana, the user's sociability and sensitivity to certain stimuli (e.g., colors) are heightened, perception of time is altered, and appetite for sweet and fatty foods is stimulated (Options B, C, E). When high blood levels of Δ^9-THC are attained with the smoking of hashish oil, the person may experience panic, paranoid thoughts (option D), and hallucinations. Increased craving (option A) is a diagnostic criterion for cannabis use disorder and is not associated with acute symptoms of different potencies of Δ^9-THC potencies achieved. **(Marijuana Preparations, pp. 335–336; Cannabis Use Disorder, p. 337)**

23.3   Which of the following is a DSM-5 criterion for marijuana withdrawal?

A. Apathy.
B. Increased appetite.
C. Craving.
D. Sleep difficulty.
E. Tachycardia.

The correct response is option D: Sleep difficulty.

DSM-5 (American Psychiatric Association 2013) introduces diagnostic criteria for *marijuana withdrawal*, which it defines as the concurrence of at least three of the following symptoms: irritability, anger, or aggression; nervousness or anxiety (option A); sleep difficulty (option D); decreased appetite or weight loss (option B); restlessness; depressed mood; or one or more physical symptoms causing significant discomfort (e.g., stomach pain, headache, sweating, shakiness) (option E). **(Cannabis Use Disorder, p. 337)**

23.4   Which of the following is a rationale for the illicit use of JWH-018 as an alternative to marijuana?

A. Ability to activate both CB_1 and CB_2 cannabinoid receptors.
B. Psychotropic effects.
C. Low potency.
D. Numerous therapeutic utilities.
E. Chemical structures that are almost identical.

The correct response is option B: Psychotropic effects.

In addition to nabilone, a number of other synthetic cannabinoid agonists have been described in the scientific literature and widely tested on experimental animals to investigate the consequences of cannabinoid receptor activation (e.g., CP-55940,

Win-55212-2, and JWH-018; see Figure 23–1 (Iversen 2000; Pertwee 2012) (option E). The therapeutic utility of these highly potent ligands is limited (options C, D) by their CB_1-mediated psychotropic side effects (option A), which presumably provide the rationale for the illicit use of some of them as alternatives to marijuana (option B) (Wells and Ott 2011). Internet-marketed products such as Spice, K2, and Eclipse are blends of various types of plant material (typically herbs and spices) that have been sprayed with a synthetic cannabinoid (e.g., JWH-018). Their effects are assumed to be similar to those of marijuana, but preclinical and clinical data in support of this claim are still very limited. **(Cannabinoid Receptor Agonists and Antagonists, pp. 339–341)**

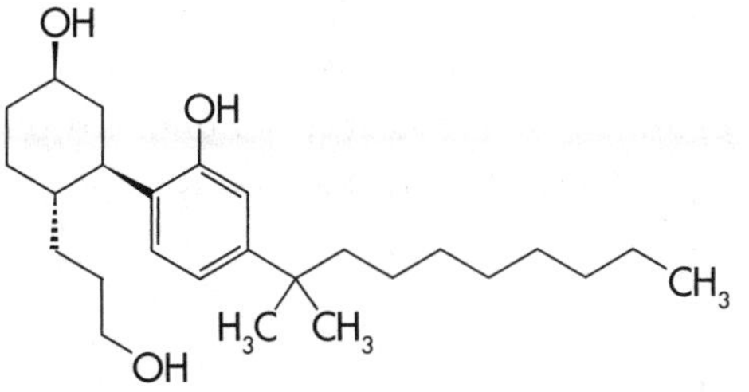

CP-55940

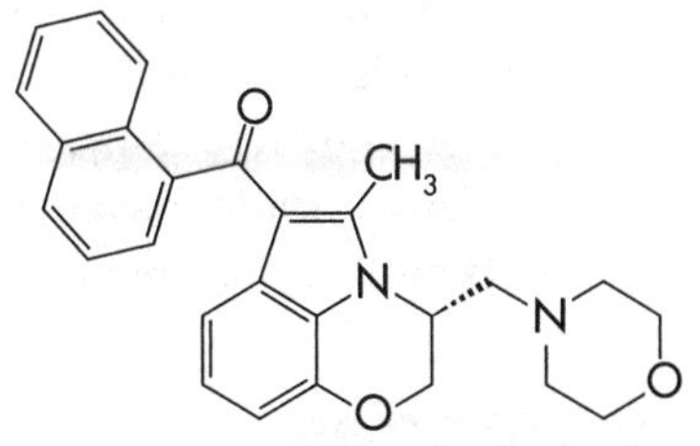

Win-55212-2

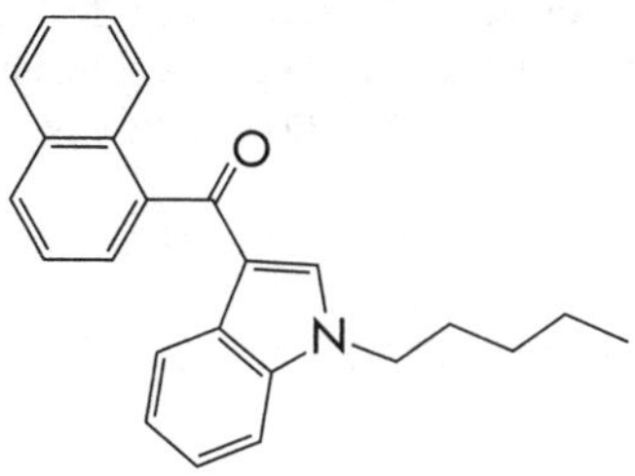

JWH-018

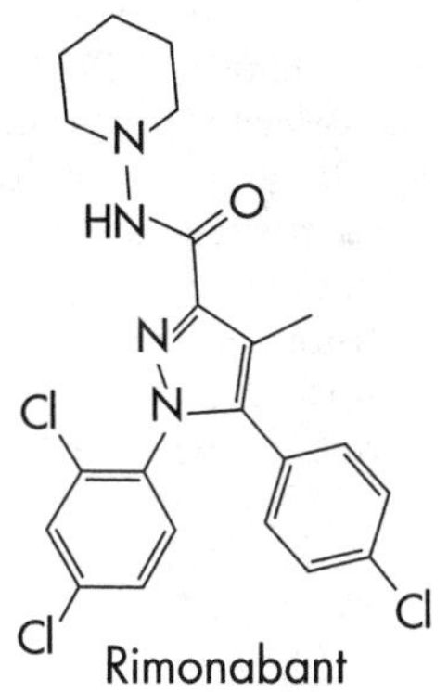

Rimonabant (SR141716A)

FIGURE 23–1. Chemical structures of synthetic CB_1 cannabinoid receptor agonists and antagonists.

CP-55940 and Win-55212-2 (developed by pharmaceutical companies Pfizer and Winthrop, respectively) and JWH-018 (originally synthesized by medicinal chemist J.W. Huffman) are cannabinoid receptor agonists. CP-55940 and Win-55212-2 are widely used experimentally, whereas JWH-018 is a component of Spice and other street drugs. Rimonabant or SR141716A (developed by Sanofi) is a CB_1 receptor inverse agonist.

23.5   Why was the clinical development of rimonabant stopped?

    A. CB_1-antagonist effects in human subjects.
    B. Similarity to nabilone.
    C. Propensity to produce CB_1-agonist psychotropic side effects.
    D. Propensity to worsen lipid profiles and insulin resistance in humans.
    E. Weight gain.

The correct response is option A: CB_1-antagonist effects in human subjects.

Rimonabant is a CB_1 antagonist. Indeed, CB_1 receptor blockade produces in human subjects a series of psychiatric adverse events (including anxiety, depression, and suicidal thoughts), which stopped the clinical development of rimonabant and other CB_1 antagonists as antiobesity medications (options A, C, E) (Engeli 2012). Nabilone is a synthetic analog of Δ^9-tetrahydrocannabinol (option B). Rimonabant has been shown to improve lipid profiles and insulin resistance in humans (option D). **(Cannabinoid-Based Medications, pp. 338–339; Cannabinoid Receptor Agonists and Antagonists, pp. 339–341)**

References

American Psychiatric Association: Diagnostic and Statistical Manual of Mental Disorders, 5th Edition. Washington, DC, American Psychiatric Association, 2013

Engeli S: Central and peripheral cannabinoid receptors as therapeutic targets in the control of food intake and body weight. Handb Exp Pharmacol (209):357–381 2012

Iversen LL: The Science of Marijuana. New York, Oxford University Press, 2000

Mehmedic Z, Chandra S, Slade D, et al: Potency trends of ?9-THC and other cannabinoids in confiscated cannabis preparations from 1993 to 2008. J Forensic Sci 55:1209–1217, 2010 20487147

Pertwee RG: Targeting the endocannabinoid system with cannabinoid receptor agonists: pharmacological strategies and therapeutic possibilities. Philos Trans R Soc Lond B Biol Sci 367:3353–3363, 2012 23108552

Russo EB: History of cannabis and its preparations in saga, science, and sobriquet. Chem Biodivers 4:1614–1648, 2007 17712811

Wells DL, Ott CA: The "new" marijuana. Ann Pharmacother 45:414–417, 2011 21325097

C H A P T E R   2 4

Treatment of
Cannabis Use Disorder

24.1   The synthetic cannabinoids such as K2 and Spice generally have which of the following characteristics?

A. They are partial agonists at CB_1 and CB_2 cannabinoid receptors and are less potent than Δ^9-tetrahydrocannabinol (Δ^9-THC).
B. They are full agonists at CB_1 and CB_2 receptors but are less potent than Δ^9-THC.
C. They are partial agonists at CB_1 and CB_2 receptors with similar potency to Δ^9-THC but have a greater risk of adverse effects.
D. They are full agonists at CB_1 and CB_2 receptors and are more potent than Δ^9-THC, with a greater risk of adverse effects.
E. They are full agonists at CB_1 and CB_2 receptors and have few adverse effects.

The correct response is option D: They are full agonists at CB_1 and CB_2 receptors and are more potent than Δ^9-THC with greater risk of adverse effects.

Synthetic cannabinoids are a large family of unrelated molecules that act on cannabinoid receptors. Common synthetic cannabinoids are known as Spice and K2 and are sold as herbal incense marked "not for human consumption," although they are often ingested for their purported euphorigenic effects. Other similar products are JWH-018, JWS-073, JWH-398, JWH-250, HU-210, and CP-47,497. These synthetic cannabinoids are generally full agonists (options A, C) and far more potent than Δ^9-THC, a partial agonist (options D, B). As a result, they have a potential for more adverse effects, behaviorally and otherwise (options D, E). **(Pharmacology, pp. 351–353)**

24.2   The reinforcing effects of cannabis are attributable to which of the following neurochemical properties?

A. Decreased activity of dopamine neurons in the ventral tegmental area.
B. Decreased extracellular dopamine in the nucleus accumbens.
C. Dopamine release in the ventral striatum.
D. Serotonin release in the ventral striatum.
E. Enhanced synaptic plasticity in the nucleus accumbens.

The correct response is option C: Dopamine release in the ventral striatum.

Cannabis use corresponds to *dopamine* release in the ventral striatum (option C, not option D), *increased* extracellular dopamine in the nucleus accumbens (option B), and *increased* activity of dopamine neurons in the ventral tegmental area (option A). Δ^9-Tetrahydrocannabinol (Δ^9-THC) also *blocks* synaptic plasticity in the nucleus accumbens (Bossong et al. 2009; Chen et al. 1990; Hoffman et al. 2003) (option E). Thus, Δ^9-THC appears to share in common with other drugs of abuse a similar mechanism of generating reinforcing effects via the dopaminergic system that increases the potential for addiction. **(Pharmacology/Neurochemical Actions Mediating Reward for Cannabis Use, pp. 352–353)**

24.3   Which of the following statements about cannabis withdrawal is most accurate?

A. Cannabis withdrawal may include increased appetite and weight gain.
B. Cannabis withdrawal may include hypersomnia.
C. Cannabis withdrawal is driven by a compensatory upregulation of the endo-cannabinoid system.
D. Cannabis withdrawal does not affect any neurotransmitter systems other than the endocannabinoid system.
E. Cannabis withdrawal is alleviated by marijuana use or dronabinol administration.

The correct response is option E: Cannabis withdrawal is alleviated by marijuana use or dronabinol administration.

Cannabis has a withdrawal syndrome, characterized by increased anger and aggression, anxiety, depressed mood, irritability, restlessness, sleep difficulty (option B), and strange dreams, *decreased* appetite and weight *loss* (option A), that is common in regular cannabis users and is alleviated by marijuana use or dronabinol administration (Budney et al. 2007; option E). Chronic Δ^9-tetrahydrocannabinol (Δ^9-THC) administration in rats results in downregulation and desensitization of CB_1 receptors (Breivogel et al. 2003), suggesting that the withdrawal syndrome is driven by a compensatory *downregulation* of the endocannabinoid system (option C). Furthermore, Δ^9-THC decreases sensitivity to opioids as well as cannabinoids at γ-aminobutyric acid–ergic and glutamatergic synapses (Hoffman et al. 2003), and CB_1 receptors are coexpressed with serotonin and dopamine receptors such that a compensatory *downregulation* of the endocannabinoid system with chronic cannabis use would interact with other neurotransmitter systems (option D) (Best and Regehr 2008; Melis et al. 2004). **(Pharmacology/Neurobiological Effects of Chronic Cannabis Use, p. 353)**

24.4   Psychotherapeutic interventions for the treatment of cannabis use disorder have been shown to have which of the following effects?

A. Cognitive-behavioral therapy (CBT) and motivational enhancement therapy (MET) may be potentiated when combined with contingency management (CM) strategies.

B. Longer treatments reduce marijuana use more than brief treatments.

C. For adolescents, more resource-intensive family treatments are superior to other psychotherapeutic interventions in reducing use.

D. Twelve-step facilitation (TSF) is likely to improve treatment efficacy.

E. Long-term abstinence rates achieved by individuals participating in CM alone are higher than those achieved by individuals receiving other psychotherapy treatments.

The correct response is option A: Cognitive-behavioral therapy (CBT) and motivational enhancement therapy (MET) may be potentiated when combined with contingency management (CM) strategies.

Several different psychotherapies have been studied as potential treatments for cannabis dependence. The most commonly used therapies are TSF counseling, motivational interviewing, CBT, and CM. At present, there are no known efficacy trials for TSF counseling for marijuana dependence (option D). CBT and MET may be potentiated when combined with CM strategies, especially in promoting initial abstinence (option A).

In two randomized controlled studies, CM was superior to other psychotherapeutic approaches and to the combination of psychotherapy and CM in maintaining abstinence during the trial period. However, at later follow-ups, the combined treatment groups in both studies—either CBT+CM (Budney et al. 2006) or MET+CBT+CM (Kadden et al. 2007)—had the highest percentages of individuals abstinent (option E).

For adolescents, skills-based treatments and CM have similar clinical efficacy, and the benefits of more resource-intensive family therapy have not been shown (option C). There is growing support for brief interventions for treating cannabis use disorder in both adults and adolescents. Trials comparing brief versus longer treatments have found that treatment groups reduced their marijuana use more than control groups, but no difference was found between the brief and long treatment groups (Dennis et al. 2004; Stephens et al. 2000) (option B). **(Treatment of Cannabis Use Disorder/Psychotherapeutic Approaches, pp. 354–355)**

24.5 Which of the following is a finding of randomized controlled trials (RCTs) studying medications for the treatment of cannabis use disorder?

A. *N*-Acetylcysteine (NAC) and gabapentin have been shown to reduce marijuana use.

B. Dronabinol has been shown to reduce marijuana use.

C. Bupropion has been shown to minimize marijuana withdrawal symptoms.

D. Divalproex sodium has been shown to reduce marijuana use.

E. Nefazodone has been shown to reduce marijuana use, but not marijuana withdrawal symptoms.

The correct response is option A: *N*-Acetylcysteine (NAC) and gabapentin have been shown to reduce marijuana use.

Psychopharmacological interventions for cannabis use disorder are less well studied and less utilized than psychotherapeutic interventions, and to date no pharmacotherapies have been approved by the U.S. Food and Drug Administration for this indication. Promising preliminary findings with NAC and gabapentin have recently emerged, but these medications require further study. NAC, an antioxidant that has modulatory effects on glutamatergic transmission, was evaluated in an RCT with adolescent marijuana users and was more effective than placebo in reducing marijuana use in this group (option A) (Gray et al. 2012). Gabapentin has also shown promise in treating marijuana dependence in an RCT (Mason et al. 2012) (option A).

Agonist therapy fared no better than placebo in reducing marijuana use in an RCT of dronabinol (Levin et al. 2011) (option B). Similarly, an RCT comparing nefazodone (300 mg bid), bupropion SR [sustained release] (150 mg bid), and placebo showed no effects of either medication on reducing marijuana use or minimizing withdrawal symptoms (Carpenter et al. 2009) (options C, E).

Divalproex sodium was tested in the RCT of pharmacological treatment for marijuana dependence. It was found to be no more effective than placebo in reducing marijuana use, but patients in both arms reported reduced irritability (Levin et al. 2004) (option D). **(Treatment of Cannabis Use Disorder/Pharmacotherapy, pp. 355–357)**

References

Best AR, Regehr WG: Serotonin evokes endocannabinoid release and retrogradely suppresses excitatory synapses. J Neurosci 28:6508–6515, 2008 18562622

Bossong MG, van Berckel BN, Boellaard R, et al: Delta 9-tetrahydrocannabinol induces dopamine release in the human striatum. Neuropsychopharmacology 34:759–766, 2009 18754005

Breivogel CS, Scates SM, Beletskaya IO, et al: The effects of delta9-tetrahydrocannabinol physical dependence on brain cannabinoid receptors. Eur J Pharmacol 459:139–150, 2003 12524139

Budney AJ, Moore BA, Rocha HL, et al: Clinical trial of abstinence-based vouchers and cognitive-behavioral therapy for cannabis dependence. J Consult Clin Psychol 74:307–316, 2006 16649875

Budney AJ, Vandrey RG, Hughes JR, et al: Oral delta-9-tetrahydrocannabinol suppresses cannabis withdrawal symptoms. Drug Alcohol Depend 86:22–29, 2007 16769180 Breivogel et al. 2003

Carpenter KM, McDowell D, Brooks DJ, et al: A preliminary trial: double-blind comparison of nefazodone, bupropion-SR, and placebo in the treatment of cannabis dependence. Am J Addict 18:53–64, 2009 19219666

Chen JP, Paredes W, Li J, et al: Delta 9-tetrahydrocannabinol produces naloxone-blockable enhancement of presynaptic basal dopamine efflux in nucleus accumbens of conscious, freely moving rats as measured by intracerebral microdialysis. Psychopharmacology (Berl) 102:156–162, 1990 2177204

Dennis M, Godley SH, Diamond G, et al: The Cannabis Youth Treatment (CYT) Study: main findings from two randomized trials. J Subst Abuse Treat 27:197–213, 2004 15501373

Gray KM, Carpenter MJ, Baker NL, et al: A double-blind randomized controlled trial of N-acetylcysteine in cannabisdependent adolescents. Am J Psychiatry 169:805–812, 2012 22706327

Hoffman AF, Oz M, Caulder T, et al: Functional tolerance and blockade of long-term depression at synapses in the nucleus accumbens after chronic cannabinoid exposure. J Neurosci 23:4815–4820, 2003 12832502

Kadden RM, Litt MD, Kabela-Cormier E, et al: Abstinence rates following behavioral treatments for marijuana dependence. Addict Behav 32:1220–1236, 2007 16996224

Levin FR, McDowell D, Evans SM, et al: Pharmacotherapy for marijuana dependence: a double-blind, placebo-controlled pilot study of divalproex sodium. Am J Addict 13:21–32, 2004 14766435

Levin FR, Mariani JJ, Brooks DJ, et al: Dronabinol for the treatment of cannabis dependence: a randomized, double-blind, placebo-controlled trial. Drug Alcohol Depend 116:142–150, 2011 21310551

Mason BJ, Crean R, Goodell V, et al: A proof of-concept randomized controlled study of gabapentin: effects on cannabis use, withdrawal and executive function deficits in cannabis-dependent adults. Neuropsychopharmacology 37:1689–1698, 2012 22373942

Melis M, Pistis M, Perra S, et al: Endocannabinoids mediate presynaptic inhibition of glutamatergic transmission in rat ventral tegmental area dopamine neurons through activation of CB1 receptors. J Neurosci 24:53–62, 2004 14715937

Stephens RS, Roffman RA, Curtin L: Comparison of extended versus brief treatments for marijuana use. J Consult Clin Psychol 68:898–908, 2000 11068976

CHAPTER 25

Psychodynamic Psychotherapy

25.1   The clinician considering implementation of psychodynamic and psychoanalytic theory in the treatment of addiction would do so based on which of the following?

A. Universal support among theorists for a major role for psychodynamic and psychoanalytic theory in addiction treatment.
B. Awareness that psychodynamic treatment of addiction is not efficacious for patients with comorbid borderline personality disorder and alcohol use disorders.
C. Awareness that psychodynamic treatment of addiction is not efficacious for patients with comorbid major depression and alcohol use disorders.
D. Awareness that psychodynamic theory cannot be of use to individuals in 12-step programs.
E. Awareness that psychodynamic theory can be of use in individual and group rehabilitation settings.

The correct response is option E: Awareness that psychodynamic theory can be of use in individual and group rehabilitation settings.

The use of psychoanalytic and psychodynamic theory in addiction treatment has significant, but not universal, theoretical support. Although many investigators have argued for the benefit of integrating psychodynamic and psychoanalytic practice in treating substance use disorders, Vaillant (1995) has maintained that such interventions have only a minor role in addiction treatment (option A). Dynamic psychotherapy may be particularly efficacious in the treatment of comorbid conditions such as major depressive disorder and alcohol dependence (Gibbons et al. 2008) or borderline personality disorder and alcohol use disorder (Gregory et al. 2009) (options B, C). Other researchers have shown how psychodynamic understanding can add depth to work with individuals and groups and further the rehabilitation process (option E), and increase the usefulness of 12-step programs (option D) (Frances et al. 1989; Khantzian 2012). **(Introduction, pp. 365–366)**

25.2   The self-medication hypothesis of substance use is based on which of the following?

   A. Freud's early psychoanalytic observations of cocaine-using patients.
   B. Observations over the past 30 years of dual-diagnosis patients' specific substance choice.
   C. The use of cocaine to counter patients' feelings of rage and aggression.
   D. The use of opioids to counter patients' feelings of depressive anergic restlessness.
   E. The use of alcohol to prevent the tolerance of loving or aggressive feelings.

The correct response is option B: Observations over the past 30 years of dual diagnosis patients' specific substance choice.

The self-medication hypothesis has evolved over the past three decades and is based on observations of patients with dual diagnoses (option B) and was not described by Freud (option A). Theorists such as Wieder and Kaplan (1969), Milkman and Frosch (1973), and Khantzian (2012) have investigated the importance of the specific effects of particular drugs on patients' affects. Khantzian (2012) highlighted this self-medication hypothesis in describing the use of opioids to assuage feelings of rage and aggression and the use of cocaine to counter feelings of depressive anergic restlessness or to augment grandiosity (options C, D). Alcohol has been related to deep-seated fears of closeness, dependence, and intimacy, with the effects of alcohol promoting the tolerance of loving or aggressive feelings (option E). (**Modern Psychoanalysis and Psychodynamics, p. 366**)

25.3   The application of psychodynamic theory to the treatment of substance abuse includes which of the following?

   A. Modification of the traditional psychoanalytic approach to avoid patient regression.
   B. Postponement of 12-step group participation until the psychodynamic treatment is completed.
   C. Focus on childhood history to the exclusion of the patient's current conflicts.
   D. The requirement that one psychodynamic theory be used exclusively with any single patient.
   E. Avoidance of discussion of the therapist-patient relationship.

The correct response is option A: Modification of the traditional psychoanalytic approach to avoid patient regression.

Applied psychodynamic theory must be distinguished from psychoanalysis. Psychodynamic principles can be used to inform individual and group therapies, rehabilitation, and other aspects of addiction treatment, but psychoanalysis in not appropriate for most recovering addicted patients, until recovery has lasted several years. Psychodynamic psychotherapy for addicted patients is a modified form of psychoanalysis: individual sessions usually occur one or two times per week, possibly in addition to other modalities, such as 12-step groups (option B), with the patient sitting up and facing the therapist. (Use of the couch is generally avoided because it may facilitate regression [option A].) Psychodynamic approaches with patients with addiction focus on current conflicts as they relate to the past rather than dwelling on childhood experiences, not exclusively on childhood history as noted in option C. The therapist-patient relationship is discussed openly to work through resistances of different kinds (option E). An eclectic approach, rather than one limited to one particular psychoanalytic theory (option D), may be the most beneficial for patients with addiction (Potik et al. 2007). **(Application of Psychodynamic Theory to Treatment, pp. 366–367)**

25.4 Which one of the following is a clear indication for individual psychodynamic psychotherapy for a patient with addiction?

A. Active use of substances.
B. Severe organicity.
C. Psychosis.
D. Antisocial personality.
E. Social phobia associated with avoidance of groups.

The correct response is option E: Social phobia associated with avoidance of groups.

The indication for individual psychotherapy for patients with addiction may be based on positive factors such as patients' psychological mindedness or wish to understand or find meaning in behavior, or on negative factors such as social phobia, avoidance, and fears (option E), which make attendance at Alcoholics Anonymous or Narcotics Anonymous meetings difficult. Relative contraindications for psychodynamic psychotherapy include active use of substances, severe organicity, psychosis, and antisocial personality disorder (options A, B, C D). **(Indications and Rationale for Individual Psychodynamic Psychotherapy, pp. 367–370; Contraindications for Individual Psychodynamic Psychotherapy, p. 370)**

25.5 Which of the following is true about the use of group treatment for patients in addiction treatment?

A. Group therapies, including Alcoholics Anonymous or Narcotics Anonymous, are not indicated for patients in individual psychotherapy.
B. Group treatments can help defuse powerful negative transferences that can develop in individual psychotherapy.
C. Only exploratory, not supportive, psychotherapy groups are of use to patients in addiction treatment.
D. Patients seeking abstinence should attend substance abuse groups only.
E. The 12-step groups should be avoided when a patient's primary therapist is not available.

The correct response is option B: Group treatments can help defuse powerful negative transferences that can develop in individual psychotherapy.

The addition of group psychotherapy, Alcoholics Anonymous, or Narcotics Anonymous can be of use when individual psychotherapy alone is not enough to help a patient maintain abstinence (option A). Group treatments can help defuse the powerful negative transference that can emerge in the early stages of an individual psychotherapy (option B). Supportive groups focusing on self-care, self-esteem, and affect regulation are of use to addiction patients in their treatment (Khantzian 2012) as well as exploratory groups (option C). Groups targeted to specific additional diagnoses, such as anxiety disorders, can help patients with substance use disorder (option D). The 12-step groups can be particularly helpful during periods of relapse and during periods when the primary therapist may be unavailable because either the therapist or the patient is away (option E). **(Applications of Psychodynamics to Groups and Self-Help, pp. 375–376)**

25.6   Exploration of defenses commonly seen in patients with addictions supports which of the following?

   A. Higher-level defenses are always encountered initially in the treatment of patients with addiction.
   B. Higher-level defenses often emerge with time and treatment in recovery from addiction.
   C. The alcoholic patient ignoring the effects of liver damage is using intellectualization as a defense.
   D. The alcoholic patient curious about the effects of liver damage is using splitting as a defense.
   E. Higher-level defenses such as reaction formation preclude noncompliance in the treatment of patients with addiction.

The correct response is option B: Higher-level defenses often emerge with time and treatment in recovery from addiction.

The defenses initially encountered in treatment of addiction are usually the most primitive and include denial, rationalization, splitting, projection, and projective identification (option A). With time and treatment, higher-level defenses such as intellectualization, reaction formation, repression, and sublimation will emerge (option B). The patient ignoring alcohol's harmful effects on the liver, reflecting the use of the more primitive defense of denial (option C), may be replaced with curiosity about how liver damage occurs, reflecting the defense of intellectualization, not splitting (option D). Use of reaction formation can lead to noncompliance with psychiatric and other prescribed medications, with the rationale that they could have unknown negative effects on liver and other organ functions (option E). **(An Ego Psychological Model of Rehabilitation, pp. 374–375)**

25.7   Treatment outcome research for patients with addiction supports which of the following?

   A. Standardized treatment for all addiction patients.
   B. Postponement of treatment for comorbid conditions until substance use disorders are in full remission.

C. Mandatory participation in 12-step programs and individual psychotherapy.

D. Avoidance of Alcoholics Anonymous participation because of a possible association with higher substance-related health care costs.

E. Significant health care cost savings resulting from investment in substance abuse treatment.

The correct response is option E: Significant health care costs savings resulting from investment in substance abuse treatment.

The American Psychiatric Association's (2006) practice guideline for treating patients with substance use disorders recommends individualizing treatment planning and including treatment of comorbid conditions (options A, B). Outcome research in addiction treatment provides useful information but not definitive instructions to clinicians. Although many clinicians agree on certain points, the value of 12-step programs and psychodynamic psychotherapy has not been strongly proved in controlled studies although these interventions are in wide use and are supported by a commonsense rationale (option C). Studies of cost-effectiveness and outcomes are increasingly important in substance use treatment. Research has shown that participation in Alcoholics Anonymous has reduced substance-related health care costs for veterans (Humphreys and Moos 1996) (option D). In addition, studies have supported significant cost savings in the long run when substance abuse treatment is available (O'Brien 1997) (option E). **(Treatment Outcome Research, pp. 378–379)**

25.8 Neurobiology studies informing the role of psychotherapy in the treatment of addiction have suggested which of the following?

A. Psychotherapy can be understood as a controlled form of learning in the context of the therapeutic relationship.

B. Environmental signals, including those from psychotherapy, have no effect on the plasticity of the brain.

C. Neuroimaging studies have shown that psychotherapy has no influence on biological activity in the brain.

D. Psychotherapy is not indicated with addiction patients, as the acute and chronic reinforcing effects of drug addiction lead to enhancement of voluntary control.

E. Cognitive-behavioral psychotherapy for patients with addiction discounts the functional characteristics of the individual patient's brain.

The correct response is option A: Psychotherapy can be understood as a controlled form of learning in the context of the therapeutic relationship.

Psychodynamics integrated with neurobiological models of addiction provide a deeper understanding of the patient and the factors that may help a particular patient to change. From a neurobiological perspective, psychotherapy can be understood as a controlled form of learning that occurs in the context of a therapeutic relationship (Etkin et al. 2005) (option A). Research into the plasticity of the brain has shown that once genes are activated by cellular developmental processes, the rate at which those genes are expressed is highly regulated by environmental signals, such as those from psychotherapy (Gabbard 2000) (option B). There is a growing body of evidence, particularly as demonstrated by neuroimaging studies, that psychotherapy influences biological activity in the brain (option C). Studies of the acute and chronic reinforcing effects of drug addiction (Volkow and Li 2004) have been shown to lead to long-lasting neurobiological changes in the brain that undermine, not enhance (option D), voluntary control. Greater understanding of the process and psychology of addiction is achieved through psychodynamic psychotherapy. This understanding may add to the development of treatment methods, such a cognitive-behavioral techniques (Beck et al. 2004), that take into account not only complex human motivating factors in the treatment of addiction but also the functional characteristics of an individual's brain (option E). **(Neurobiology, pp. 379–380)**

25.9   Which of the following is true regarding the treatment of patients with comorbid personality disorders?

A. Alcoholism and drug abuse are rare in patients with personality disorders.
B. Treatments targeting alcohol abuse only were more effective than treatments targeting maladaptive behavioral and interpersonal patterns.
C. An acute substance-induced personality change is easily distinguished from personality disorder symptoms.
D. Addiction patients with narcissistic traits or personality disorder are not treatable.
E. Psychotherapy with patients with borderline personality disorder and addiction requires an emphasis on structure and limit setting.

The correct response is option E: Psychotherapy with patients with borderline personality disorder and addiction requires an emphasis on structure and limit setting.

The application of psychodynamic theory to the treatment of patients with comorbid psychiatric problems such as personality disorders is important especially because alcoholism and drug abuse are overrepresented, not rare (option A), in these patients. Treatments targeting chromic maladaptive behavior and interpersonal patterns were more effective than treatments solely targeting alcohol use disorders in patients with comorbid borderline personality disorder and alcohol use disorders (Gianoli et al. 2012) (option B). It may be especially hard to identify the boundaries of temperament, acute substance-induced personality change, and personality disorders (option C). Many addicted patients have narcissistic traits or personality disorder; for these patients, successful rehabilitation often involves acceptance of vulnerability and of being ordinary and similar to others with the same problem. Such rehabilitation may be achieved through 12-step programs and application of Beck's cognitive therapy (Beck et al. 2004), and psychodynamic exploration of the narcissistic vulnerability (option D). Exploratory psychotherapy with patients with borderline personality disorder and a history of addiction requires an emphasis on structure and limit setting (option E). **(Indications and Rationale for Individual Psychodynamic Psychotherapy, pp. 367–370)**

25.10 The course of addiction recovery for patients treated with psychodynamic psychotherapy will include which of the following?

A. An immediate acceptance of an addiction diagnosis at the outset of individual psychotherapy.
B. A high level of motivation for addiction treatment maintained throughout the treatment process.
C. No need for 12-step program participation or additional psychotherapy after achieving abstinence.
D. Relapse prevention, which can include laboratory tests or family meetings.
E. Less emphasis on patient confidentiality if the patient is forced into treatment by an employer or probation office.

The correct response is option D: Relapse prevention, which can include laboratory tests or family meetings.

Research on the treatment of addictions supports a model in which patients develop awareness of their addiction problems in stages (Prochaska et al. 1992), not immediately at the onset of psychotherapy (option A). A focus on the motivational aspect of treatment and confronting denial are essential elements in initiating treatment because addiction patients may have variable levels of motivation for treatment and may not have a high level of motivation throughout the treatment process (option B). It is unlikely that a patient treated with psychodynamic psychotherapy will never need additional help through a 12-step program or additional psychotherapy (option C). Relapse prevention can include laboratory tests, meetings with family, or other sources of collateral information (option D). When a patient is forced into a consultation for an addiction disorder by an employer, probation office, family member, or physician, the therapist may be required to make a considerable effort to develop trust and a working alliance. The therapist's integrity and adherence to confidentiality can contribute to the establishment of trust, suggesting that more, not less (option E), emphasis on patient confidentiality is indicated. **(Treatment Overview, pp. 370–374)**

References

American Psychiatric Association: Practice Guideline for the Treatment of Patients With Substance Use Disorders, 2nd Edition. Arlington, VA, American Psychiatric Association, 2006

Beck JS, Liese BS, Najavits LM: Cognitive therapy, in Clinical Textbook of Addictive Disorders, 3rd Edition. Edited by Frances RJ, Miller SI, Mack AH. New York, Guilford, 2004, pp 474–501

Etkin A, Pittenger C, Polan HJ, et al: Toward a neurobiology of psychotherapy: basic science and clinical applications. J Neuropsychiatry Clin Neurosci 17:145–158, 2005 15939967

Frances RJ, Khantzian EJ, Tamerin JS: Psychodynamic psychotherapy, in Treatments of Psychiatric Disorders: A Task Force Report of the American Psychiatric Association, Vol 2. Washington, DC, American Psychiatric Association, 1989, pp 1103–1111

Gabbard GO: A neurobiologically informed perspective on psychotherapy. Br J Psychiatry 177:117–122, 2000 11026950

Gianoli MO, Jane JS, O'Brien E, et al: Treatment for comorbid borderline personality disorder and alcohol use disorders: a review of the evidence and future recommendations. Exp Clin Psychopharmacol 20:333–344, 2012 22686496

Gibbons MB, Crits-Christoph P, Hearon B: The empirical status of psychodynamic therapies. Annu Rev Clin Psychol 4:93– 108, 2008 17716035

Gregory RJ, Remen AL, Soderberg M, et al: A controlled trial of psychodynamic psychotherapy for co-occurring borderline personality disorder and alcohol use disorder: six-month outcome. J Am Psychoanal Assoc 57:199–205, 2009 19270255 Gibbons et al. 2008

Humphreys K, Moos RH: Reduced substance abuse-related health care costs among voluntary participants in Alcoholics Anonymous. Psychiatr Serv 47:709–713, 1996 8807683

Khantzian EJ: Reflections on treating addictive disorders: a psychodynamic perspective. Am J Addict 21:274–279, 2012

Milkman H, Frosch WA: On the preferential abuse of heroin and amphetamine. J Nerv Ment Dis 156:242–248, 1973

O'Brien CP: A range of research-based pharmacotherapies for addiction. Science 278:66–70, 1997 9311929

Potik D, Adelson M, Schreiber S: Drug addiction from a psychodynamic perspective: methadone maintenance treatment (MMT) as transitional phenomena. Psychol Psychother 80:311–325, 2007 17535602

Prochaska JO, DiClemente CC, Norcross JC: In search of how people change. Applications to addictive behaviors. Am Psychol 47:1102–1114, 1992 1329589

Vaillant GE: The Natural History of Alcoholism Revisited. Cambridge, MA, Harvard University Press, 1995, pp 362–373

Volkow ND, Li TK: Drug addiction: the neurobiology of behaviour gone awry. Nat Rev Neurosci 5:963–970, 2004 15550951

Wieder H, Kaplan EH: Drug use in adolescents. Psychodynamic meaning and pharmacogenic effect. Psychoanal Study Child 24:399–431, 1969

CHAPTER 26

Cognitive-Behavioral Therapies

26.1 Cognitive-behavioral therapy (CBT) treatments have a number of theoretical sources and empirical roots in the psychological literature. Which of the following is the most accurate statement about these sources and roots?

A. Drug use behaviors are learned through their association with the positively reinforcing (reward) properties of the substances themselves, and thus operant conditioning is important in creating a therapy to counter these behaviors.
B. As reinforcement learning is the basis of substance abuse according to the CBT approach, other risk factors such as family history or personality traits are incidental and not relevant to the treatment.
C. CBT must incorporate an understanding of unconscious conflicts, as described in the psychoanalytic literature, if it is to be effective in eliminating root causes of substance use.
D. Albert Ellis and Aaron Beck emphasized a purely behavioral approach to therapy that was later challenged for its narrow focus.
E. Drug related cues or stimuli are related to drug craving only in those individuals who have a genetic vulnerability, and thus are not relevant to CBT for substance use.

The correct response is option A: Drug use behaviors are learned through their association with the positively reinforcing (reward) properties of the substances themselves, and thus operant conditioning is important in creating a therapy to counter these behaviors.

Cognitive-behavioral treatments have their roots in classical behavioral theory and the pioneering work of Ivan Pavlov, John Watson, B.F. Skinner, and Albert Bandura (for review, see Craighead et al. 1995). Pavlov's work on classical conditioning is the basis of several behavioral approaches to substance use treatment, particularly cue exposure approaches, which are active in all subjects (option E). Skinner's work on operant conditioning demonstrated that behaviors that are positively reinforced are likely to be exhibited more frequently. The field of behavioral pharmacology, which has convincingly demonstrated the reinforcing properties of abused substances in both humans and animals, is grounded in operant conditioning theory and principles (option A). CBT conceives substance use disorders as complex, multidetermined problems (Marlatt and Donovan 2005) with influences that include family history and genetic factors; the presence of comorbid psychopathology; personality traits such as sensation seeking or impulsivity; and a host of environmental factors, all of which are taken into consideration in CBT (option B). Cognitive-behavioral treatments also reflect the pioneering work of Albert Ellis and Aaron Beck, which emphasized the importance of the person's thoughts and feelings as determinants of behavior (option D), but CBT does not incorporate theories of unconscious conflicts (option C). **(Theoretical Basis, pp. 385–386)**

26.2   Which of the following is the most accurate description of the "sleeper effect" phenomenon described by Carroll et al. (1994)?

A. Individuals receiving desipramine reported less insomnia, and this was seen to be a mediator of overall improvement.
B. After a clinical treatment trial for substance abuse ended, individuals receiving cognitive-behavioral therapy (CBT) continued to further reduce their frequency of substance abuse.
C. Individuals receiving CBT maintained their clinical improvement over the following year, as measured by frequency of cocaine use.
D. CBT combined with lifestyle changes, including exercise and improved sleep hygiene, showed a better response rate than CBT alone.
E. Baseline circadian abnormalities, especially with day-night reversal, predicted poorer outcome.

The correct response is option B: After a clinical treatment trial for substance abuse ended, individuals receiving cognitive-behavioral therapy (CBT) continued to further reduce their frequency of substance abuse.

The Carroll et al. (1994) study used a 2×2 factorial design, in which desipramine was compared with placebo, and CBT was compared with supportive clinical management, a supportive psychotherapy control condition. Desipramine had no reported effect on sleep (option A). However, this study was the first to describe the "sleeper effect" phenomenon: after the treatments were terminated, those individuals who had been assigned to receive CBT continued to reduce the frequency of their cocaine use even further (not sustain the frequency [option C]) throughout the 1-year follow-up (option B). Baseline circadian rhythms and lifestyle changes were not part of any of these studies by Carroll (options D, E). **(Empirical Support, pp. 386–389)**

26.3   Multiple clinical trials conducted by Carroll and her team at Yale over a 20-year period focused on cognitive-behavioral therapy (CBT) treatment for substance abuse. Which of the following is the most accurate statement about these studies?

A. The series of studies was marked by a progressively larger effect size for CBT over comparison or control conditions.
B. In these studies, when CBT was conducted to rigorous standards of adherence, subjects showed an equivalent improvement independent of the subject's baseline substance use.
C. Although CBT was more effective than supportive clinical management, all subjects who demonstrated skill acquisition achieved equivalent improvement.
D. Those receiving CBT did better than those receiving interpersonal therapy (IPT), but disulfiram was no better than placebo.
E. Although skill acquisition was strongly associated with long-term reduction in cocaine use, subjects' compliance with homework exercises did not significantly correlate with improved outcomes.

The correct response is option A: The series of studies was marked by a progressively larger effect size for CBT over comparison or control conditions.

The series of studies by Carroll et al. has been marked by progressively larger effect sizes for CBT over the comparison or control conditions (option A). In the team's first randomized trial (Carroll et al. 1991), CBT was not found to have a main effect over IPT, but was found to be significantly more effective among the more severely dependent cocaine abusers (option B). This in turn led to increasing interest in mechanisms that might underlie the effect of CBT, with skills training and behavioral practice through homework assignments as prime candidates. The results indicated that coping skills increased significantly after CBT and that greater acquisition of CBT-specific behavioral and cognitive coping skills was associated with less cocaine use over the 1-year follow-up (option C) (Carroll et al. 2000). In a subsequent study (Carroll et al. 2004), patients assigned to receive CBT reduced their cocaine use significantly more than those assigned to receive IPT, and patients assigned to receive disulfiram reduced their cocaine use significantly more than those assigned to receive placebo (option D). The team also found that participants who complete homework consistently stay in treatment significantly longer, have more consecutive days of cocaine abstinence, and have fewer cocaine-positive urine tests during treatment (option E) (Carroll et al. 2005). **(Empirical Support, pp. 386–389)**

26.4   Cognitive-behavioral therapy (CBT) has been shown to be an effective treatment for substance abuse. Which of the following is the most accurate description of the therapeutic approach used in CBT?

A. Framing the role of the therapist as the expert on substance-related disorders and in charge of the therapy aids patients in developing confidence that the therapist can help them reduce their substance use.
B. Patients are helped to identify the large issues in their lives and avoiding focusing on smaller decisions.

C. The key defining features of CBT are functional analysis of drug use and an emphasis on skill training.

D. Patients receive training to improve their relationships by focusing on the needs of others in their lives and reducing their own assertiveness.

E. CBT is most effective when the patient defines the focus of sessions depending on patient's emotions in the "here and now."

The correct response is option C: The key defining features of CBT are functional analysis of drug use and an emphasis on skill training.

Two key defining features of most cognitive-behavioral approaches for substance use disorders are 1) an emphasis on functional analysis of drug use (i.e., understanding drug use with respect to its antecedents and consequences) and 2) an emphasis on skills training (option C) (Carroll 1998; Monti et al. 1989). Cognitive-behavioral approaches include increasing awareness of the consequences of even small decisions (e.g., which route to take home from work) and the identification of "seemingly irrelevant" decisions that can culminate in high-risk situations (option B). Developing skills for assertively refusing offers of drugs can be transferred to more effective and assertive responses in a number of situations in which assertiveness, rather than a focus on the needs of others, may be the skill that is needed (option D). In comparison with many other behavioral approaches, CBT is typically highly structured. That is, CBT is generally brief (12–24 weeks) and organized closely around well-specified treatment goals. An articulated agenda usually exists for each session, and the clinical discussion remains focused on issues directly related to substance use (option E). The therapeutic relationship is seen as principally collaborative. Thus, the role of the therapist is one of consultant, educator, and guide who can lead the patient through the desired behavior changes (option A). **(Cognitive-Behavioral Techniques and Strategies, pp. 389–390)**

26.5   A trial evaluating training methods for CBT demonstrated which of the following training methods in cognitive-behavioral therapy (CBT) to be the most efficacious for clinicians?

A. Review of the National Institute on Drug Abuse (NIDA) CBT manual only.

B. Review of the NIDA CBT manual plus access to a Web-based training site.

C. Participation in a didactic seminar plus review of the NIDA CBT manual.

D. Participation in a didactic seminar plus supervision from a CBT trainer.

E. Access to CBT manual plus completion of three CBT cases.

The correct response is option D: Participation in a didactic seminar plus supervision from a CBT trainer.

In a trial evaluating training methods for CBT (Sholomskas et al. 2005), 78 clinicians were assigned to one of three training conditions: 1) review of the National Institute on Drug Abuse (NIDA) CBT manual only; 2) access to a Web-based training site (which included additional frequently asked questions, role-plays, and practice exercises) plus the NIDA CBT manual; or 3) a 3-day didactic seminar plus up to three sessions of supervision from a CBT expert trainer based on actual session tapes submitted by the participants. Outcomes focused on clinician behavior and included 1) between-group comparisons of the clinicians' ability to demonstrate key CBT techniques based on structured role-plays administered before and after training and 2) scores on a CBT knowledge quiz. The videotaped role-plays were scored by independent raters who were blind to the participants' training condition as well as time (e.g., pretraining vs. posttraining) and based on adherence and competence ratings of specific CBT techniques from the Yale Adherence and Competence Scale.

Although the conditions described in options A, B, and D all resulted in improved adherence and competence scores, the only training condition that reached levels of skill consistent with those required of clinicians participating in the CBT efficacy trials was the didactic seminar plus supervision condition (option D), with intermediate ratings for the Web condition. Participation in a didactic seminar plus review of the NIDA CBT manual (option C) and CBT manual review plus completion of CBT cases (option E) were not evaluated. Importantly, studies on training clinicians in CBT demonstrated that the availability of manuals alone does not tend to have an enduring effect on clinicians' ability to incorporate new treatments. **(Training and Competence in CBT, pp. 390–391)**

References

Carroll KM: A Cognitive-Behavioral Approach: Treating Cocaine Addiction (NIH Publ No 98-4308). Rockville, MD, National Institute on Drug Abuse, 1998

Carroll KM, Rounsaville BJ, Gawin FH: A comparative trial of psychotherapies for ambulatory cocaine abusers: relapse prevention and interpersonal psychotherapy. Am J Drug Alcohol Abuse 17:229–247, 1991 1928019

Carroll KM, Rounsaville BJ, Gordon LT, et al: Psychotherapy and pharmacotherapy for ambulatory cocaine abusers. Arch Gen Psychiatry 51:177–187, 1994 8122955

Carroll KM, Nich C, Ball SA, et al: One-year follow-up of disulfiram and psychotherapy for cocaine-alcohol users: sustained effects of treatment. Addiction 95:1335– 1349, 2000 11048353

Carroll KM, Fenton LR, Ball SA, et al: Efficacy of disulfiram and cognitive behavior therapy in cocaine-dependent outpatients: a randomized placebo-controlled trial. Arch Gen Psychiatry 61:264–272, 2004 14993114

Carroll KM, Nich C, Ball SA: Practice makes progress? Homework assignments and outcome in treatment of cocaine dependence. J Consult Clin Psychol 73:749– 755, 2005 16173864

Craighead WE, Craighead LW, Hardi SS, et al: Behavioral therapies in historical perspective, in Comprehensive Textbook of Psychotherapy: Theory and Practice. Edited by Bongar BM, Beutler LE. New York, Oxford University Press, 1995, pp 64–83

Marlatt GA, Donovan D: Relapse Prevention: Maintenance Strategies in the Treatment of Addictions, 2nd Edition. New York, Guilford, 2005

Monti PM, Abrams DB, Kadden RM, et al: Treating Alcohol Dependence: A Coping Skills Training Guide in the Treatment of Alcoholism. New York, Guilford, 1989

Sholomskas DE, Syracuse-Siewert G, Rounsaville BJ, et al: We don't train in vain: a dissemination trial of three strategies of training clinicians in cognitive-behavioral therapy. J Consult Clin Psychol 73:106–115, 2005 15709837

CHAPTER 27

Motivational Enhancement

27.1 A 46-year-old obese man with recently diagnosed hypertension, a 20-year history of a cocaine use disorder, and erectile dysfunction is evaluated in the emergency room for chest pain shortly after using $250 worth of cocaine intranasally. His symptoms rapidly resolve, and the evaluating physician attempts to counsel him about the dangers of ongoing cocaine use, offering a referral for substance abuse treatment. The patient appears disinterested, thanks the doctor for saving his life, and asks to be discharged, saying, "I just pushed it a little too far this time." In which of the "stages of change" does the patient appear to be regarding his cocaine use?

A. Precontemplation.
B. Contemplation.
C. Planning.
D. Action.
E. Maintenance.

The correct response is option A: Precontemplation.

Motivational interviewing is guided by assessment and awareness of where patients lie in the "stages of change" as described by DiClemente (2003), as different stages would suggest different therapeutic interventions (Table 27–1). Given this patient's presentation, characterized by disinterest and minimization, he would appear to be in the *precontemplation* stage (option A). Given his lack of ambivalence about substance abuse, he would not appear to be in the contemplation stage or in the preparation, action, or maintenance stages (options B, C, D, E). **(Understanding Motivation, pp. 398–400)**

27.2 Motivational interviewing (MI) and motivational enhancement therapy (MET) techniques could have adverse effects for which of the following patients?

A. An intravenous heroin user with no desire to stop using despite a recent diagnosis of endocarditis.
B. A two-pack-per-day smoker worried about the health effects of cigarettes but fearful of weight gain.
C. A 42-year old-woman with bipolar I disorder and several recent medical admissions for alcohol withdrawal.

TABLE 27–1. Stage tasks and motivational strategies

Stage of change	Description	Key tasks	Motivational strategies
Precontemplation	Not a problem Not interested	Interest Concern	**Engagement/evoking** Autonomy Listening OARS
Contemplation	Ambivalent Considering change	Risk-reward analysis Overcoming ambivalence Decision making	**Focusing/evoking** Double-sided reflections Values clarification Decisional balance OARS
Preparation	Getting ready for action	Acceptable, accessible, effective plan Commitment	**Evoking/planning** Commitment Client change plan Self-efficacy
Action	Stopping, modifying, or starting new behavior	Implementing and revising plan	**Planning/focusing** Revising plan Support Reinforcement
Maintenance	Sustaining change	Integrating change into lifestyle	**Sustained support** New sources of reinforcement Resolving associated problems

Note. For more detail on the strategies listed, see Miller and Rollnick 2013. OARS: O=Open-ended questions; A=Affirmations; R=Reflective listening; S=Summaries.

D. A 52-year-old man with a severe alcohol use disorder recently discharged from a detox unit who presents with his wife seeking observed disulfiram treatment.

E. A 45-year-old artist and daily marijuana user who insists he needs the drug to be creative.

The correct response is option D: A 52-year-old man with a severe alcohol use disorder recently discharged from a detox unit who presents with his wife seeking observed disulfiram treatment.

The MI/MET approaches as described in the OARS statements (**O**pen-ended questions, **A**ffirmations, **R**eflective listening, and **S**ummaries) are generally deployed in the setting of ambivalence about an ongoing behavior, and there is evidence to suggest that patients who are acting on plans to change their behavior or maintaining abstinence may not benefit from such an approach. The patient in option D is clearly motivated, given what appear to be a combination of internal and external contingencies and clear action plans, and attempts to remain neutral as regards his intended actions may be confusing or undermining of such goals. The patients in options A and E are in the precontemplation stage and are good candidates for MI/MET. The patients in options B and C are either ambivalent about substance use or continuing to use in a self-destructive way and thus would be appropriate for MI/MET. Co-occurring psychiatric disorders are not a contraindication for MI/MET approaches. **(Motivational Enhancement Interventions, pp. 400–401; Substance-Specific Reviews, pp. 401–405)**

27.3 A 36-year-old woman who uses vaporized marijuana five or six times per day presents to your office seeking treatment for anxiety after she quit her job due to "unmanageable stress." When asked about her substance abuse, she states that she would like to quit but fears that any new job she might get would require pre-employment drug testing and that she "cannot fathom" cutting down or stopping marijuana because her anxiety will "skyrocket." Which of the following intervention statements would be *best to make next*, in keeping with the principles of motivational interviewing?

A. "Many patients with drug addiction have a history of traumatic experiences. Have you ever witnessed a horrifying incident or been a victim of violence or abuse?"

B. "Perhaps you use marijuana because you cannot tolerate negative emotions."

C. "Marijuana can reduce motivation; it seems like it is really holding back your life."

D. "Clearly, marijuana is making your symptoms worse, but you still are resistant to stopping it. What do you make of that?"

E. "So you'd like to stop using because of how it is holding you back professionally, but you find yourself really paralyzed by anxiety, and marijuana seems to be the only thing you've tried that has ever helped with it?"

The correct response is option E: "So you'd like to stop using because of how it is holding you back professionally, but you find yourself really paralyzed by anx-

iety, and marijuana seems to be the only thing you've tried that has ever helped with it?"

Techniques used in motivational interviewing include complex reflections, use of summary statements to frame motivational messages, techniques to manage and roll with resistance, offering advice with permission, affirmation, building the patient's sense of self-efficacy, and assisting with creating a realistic change plan. Option E is an example of a summary statement that frames the patient's ambivalence in a nonjudgmental, empathic way and affirms the patient's current struggles while hinting at the negative role the drug use seems to play in his or her life. Summary statements are a core motivational interviewing (MI)/motivational enhancement therapy (MET) intervention. Option C is a reflection but is more judgmental and lacks the affirmation implicit in option E. Options B and D are excessively confrontational statements and may promote further resistance. Option A is a useful screening question about potential trauma history but is not an MI/ MET intervention. **(Motivational Enhancement Interventions, pp. 400–401)**

27.4   What is the most important difference between motivational enhancement (ME) and contingency management (CM) interventions for substance use disorders?

A. ME interventions do not provide rewards for abstinence from drugs or alcohol.
B. ME interventions are ineffective for opioid use disorders.
C. ME interventions seek to elaborate internal motivations or contingencies that are self-sustaining.
D. The benefits of ME interventions are relatively constant over time.
E. ME interventions are only effective for drug users in the precontemplation stage.

The correct response is option C: ME interventions seek to elaborate internal motivations or contingencies that are self-sustaining.

Contingency management uses behavioral reinforcement techniques (such as rewards for drug-free urines) to promote substitution of addictive behavior and to encourage abstinence. It is not psychotherapy and is a purely behavioral intervention, the effects of which generally do not long persist when those contingencies are removed (Benishek et al. 2014). Motivational enhancement seeks to elaborate internal contingencies that are being suppressed out of awareness or denied by the patient, and seeks to bring out emotions and cognitions relevant to the patient's substance use for examination in a judgment-free setting, with the goal of enacting long-term behavioral change (option C). Patients in the contemplation stage can benefit from ME treatment approaches (option E). ME interventions may have decreasing effects over time without further interventions or treatment (option D). ME treatment is effective for opiate use disorders (option B). Building awareness of contingencies is part of ME treatment even if it is not structured explicitly around external rewards (option A). **(Understanding Motivation, pp. 398–400; see also Chapter 29, Contingency Management)**

27.5   Screening, Brief Intervention, and Referral to Treatment (SBIRT) interventions for hazardous alcohol use may be *less* effective for which of the following subgroups of the general population?

A. Patients in a primary care clinic.
B. Women.
C. Dual-diagnosis patients.
D. Patients in general practice settings.
E. Adolescents.

The correct response is option B: Women.

There is significant evidence that SBIRT is effective for reducing risky drinking behavior and overall use for as long as 12 months both in primary care clinics and in general practice settings (options A, D), with adolescents (option E), and with patients with psychiatric disorders and co-occurring risky alcohol use (option C). A recent meta-analysis of 1-year outcomes of brief interventions in routine primary care found that such interventions were beneficial for men but not for women (option B) (Kaner et al. 2009), and more research is required on gender differences with SBIRT. **(Substance-Specific Reviews/Alcohol/Brief Interventions, p. 402)**

References

Benishek LA, Dugosh KL, Kirby KC, et al: Prize-based contingency management for the treatment of substance abusers: a meta-analysis. Addiction 109(9):1426–1436, 2014 24750232
DiClemente CC: Addiction and Change: How Addictions Develop and Addicted People Recover. New York, Guilford, 2003
Kaner EF, Dickinson HO, Beyer F, et al: The effectiveness of brief alcohol interventions in primary care settings: a systematic review. Drug Alcohol Rev 28:301–323, 2009 19489992

CHAPTER 28

Twelve-Step Facilitation

An Adaptation for Psychiatric Practitioners and Patients

28.1 A 35-year-old patient in treatment for social phobia recently reveals his long history of heavy alcohol use (as many as eight drinks per drinking day, 3–4 days per week). He started attending Alcoholics Anonymous (AA) meetings two or three times per week. He reports that he struggles to engage in the sessions and feels like the other attendees' problems are "way more serious" than the difficulties he has experienced as a result of drinking. What is the *best next step* to take with this patient?

   A. Start the patient on gabapentin to augment the pharmacological treatment of his social phobia.
   B. Confront the patient about his minimization of his alcoholism and how it reduces his chances for recovery.
   C. Re-explore the patient's current motivation to achieve sobriety and help to identify obstacles to feeling comfortable in the 12-step setting.
   D. Provide education about AA, including that participants are not required to speak during meetings.
   E. Emphasize the importance to the patient of identifying an AA sponsor to help him deal with the difficulties he is experiencing at meetings.

The correct response is option C: Re-explore the patient's current motivation to achieve sobriety and help to identify obstacles to feeling comfortable in the 12-step setting.

The overriding principle of 12-step facilitation (TSF) is to encourage patients to attend and make use of 12-step support group sessions. For this patient with an alcohol use disorder and co-occurring social phobia, anxiety may limit his ability to engage in sessions but may also conceal ambivalence about ceasing drinking. Option C is the correct answer because it opens the possibility of addressing anxiety symptoms should they be at issue here as well as exploring the status of the patient's motivation for sobriety. Starting the patient on gabapentin (option A) may be helpful for anxiety surrounding AA attendance but is premature without a more thorough exploration of the relevant issues. Confronting the patient about his alcoholism (option B) may push the patient away and reduce the likelihood that they will attend meetings, inconsistent with the principles of motivational interviewing that have been integrated into TSF. Providing education about AA (option D) is relevant, but without more exploration it may limit the patient's ability to make use of sessions by passively allowing him to minimize his participation; a better intervention might be to develop a script with the patient to say at meetings to limit anxiety. Obtaining a sponsor (option E) would likely benefit the patient, but the principles of TSF would involve both the clinician and the sponsor exploring issues to AA participation, rather than seeing the sponsor as someone who would handle such challenges alone. **(Role of the Therapist, pp. 417–418)**

28.2   A 22-year-old patient who identifies as an atheist has attended a few Alcoholics Anonymous (AA) meetings to address his severe alcohol abuse but is concerned about their incorporation of spirituality and use of the word "God," because he feels this is inconsistent with his own beliefs. What would be the best intervention to make next?

   A. "The experience from many years in AA is that without a spiritual awakening, people aren't really able to quit drinking for good."
   B. "If you feel that it is too big a stumbling block, we can try to find a meeting with people who have the same questions about this that you do."
   C. "This model has really worked for people; you should trust the people there who have been able to stop drinking."
   D. "It's not meant to be taken literally; think of it as a symbol for your struggle to quit drinking."
   E. "You seem resistant to thinking about what has been happening in your life in a different way even though you haven't been able to stop drinking on your own."

The correct response is option B: "If you feel that it is too big a stumbling block, we can try to find a meeting with people who have the same questions about this that you do."

Spirituality is considered a core component of AA and many other 12-step groups that have incorporated it into their models. The definition of what constitutes "spirituality" or a "higher power," or even "God," in the AA model may not match, however, with the beliefs or ideas of patients considering entering or participating in such groups. Particularly in large areas, there are many agnostic or atheist AA groups that the patient may find more accommodating, and many more with significant flexibility, and thus the physician would make the validating and educational statement in option B. Although the statement in option D may in some ways be consistent with this more flexible interpretation of the tenets of AA, it may serve to devalue this component of the 12-step ideology and thus is inconsistent with the broader goals of 12-step facilitation to encourage attendance and productive use of the concepts introduced in such meetings. Citing the necessity for a spiritual awakening (option A) is unsupported by data and may be unnecessarily provocative toward the patient in question. Options C and E may be valid observations under certain circumstances, but they do little to address the patient's discomfort with the vocabulary of AA at a time when he or she is not yet fully familiar with AA itself, and thus could push the patient away from further attendance. **(Core Elements of the TSF Manual/Spirituality, pp. 415–416)**

28.3   A 36-year-old woman with a severe alcohol use disorder and bipolar I disorder (three past hospitalizations for mania) has started attending Alcoholics Anonymous (AA) meetings. She is trying to identify a sponsor. Which of the following traits in a sponsor might be most beneficial for this patient?

   A. A sponsor with a co-occurring psychiatric disorder.
   B. A sponsor with many years of sobriety and experience in AA.
   C. A sponsor willing to regularly speak with you about the patient by phone.
   D. A sponsor with similar sociodemographic characteristics to the patient.
   E. A sponsor who continues to attend meetings at a high frequency.

The correct response is option A: A sponsor with a co-occurring psychiatric disorder.

The option of a sponsor can be pivotal in achieving success in 12-step group–based approaches to substance abuse treatment, and is a goal of 12-step facilitation techniques. For patients with substance abuse and co-occurring psychiatric illness, finding a sponsor with a similar dual-diagnosis history (option A) can be pivotal because there are AA meetings and attendees who are either unfamiliar with psychiatric illness or discourage the use of psychogenic medications, which could be very disruptive to this patient with serious mental illness. A sponsor with a history of psychiatric diagnosis and treatment will likely be more open to the unique needs of the patient in question. Options B, D, and E may be useful traits in a sponsor, especially considering the patient in question, but do not address the needs of the patient as specifically as option A. Communication between you and the patient's sponsor, if any, should be done with the patient present so as to maintain boundaries and respect the confidentiality of the patient's relationship with the sponsor (option C). **(Sponsors, p. 418)**

28.4   Which of the following is the primary goal of 12-step facilitation (TSF) for patients struggling with substance abuse?

   A. To explore past traumas that might affect current substance use.
   B. To replace 12-step group treatment for patients who cannot tolerate a group setting.
   C. To facilitate attendance and productive utilization of 12-step meetings.
   D. To illustrate the role of using substances in self-medicating psychiatric symptoms of participating patients.
   E. To address the shortcomings of the 12-step model as regards the management of co-occurring psychiatric illness.

The correct response is option C: To facilitate attendance and productive utilization of 12-step meetings.

The primary goal of TSF is to encourage attendance and productive use of 12-step meetings by supportive interventions, patient education, and reinforcement of key aspects of the content of 12-step group meetings (option C). Exploring the patient's history of trauma is not a core component of TSF (option A). TSF is intended as an adjunct to 12-step treatment that allows for continuity of care while meeting acute needs for substance abuse treatment; attending the meetings is essential to both the goals and practice of TSF (option B). Encouraging patients to conceptualize their use of substances as self-medication for psychiatric symptoms may be associated with poorer outcomes (option D). Addressing the shortcomings of the 12-step model as regards the management of co-occurring psychiatric illness may confuse the patient and imply that the clinician does not support their attendance of 12-step groups (option E). **(Introduction, pp. 411–412)**

28.5   A 44-year-old man with a 4-month history of depression and alcohol dependence has been attending Alcoholics Anonymous (AA) meetings two or three times per month. He stopped going to meetings, citing his continued drinking as evidence that "meetings don't work." What would be the most appropriate response to this patient?

A. "AA isn't for everybody; people tend to know soon whether it will work for them or not."
B. "This shows that you need more intensive treatment for your drinking."
C. "I won't continue to treat you if you don't make a commitment to abstinence."
D. "Maybe the real issue is your depression leading you to drink."
E. "You're right, you've continued to drink despite going to some meetings, but it seems like it has been difficult to attend meetings at the frequency that might really help you."

The correct response is option E: "You're right, you've continued to drink despite going to some meetings, but it seems like it has been difficult to attend meetings at the frequency that might really help you."

In this case, the patient has quickly concluded that 12-step meetings like AA "don't work," despite minimal attendance and exposure, and is resistant to returning. The statement in option E validates the patient's experience, and pairs that with a nonjudgmental confrontation that points out the contradictions of the patient's behavior and supports continued attendance, a main point of 12-step facilitation (TSF). The statement in option A does not support meeting attendance despite the significant evidence that these meetings are helpful in achieving abstinence and the wide variety in meeting types where almost all patients can feel comfortable. The statement in option B is premature and may serve to "write off" attending meetings, which would seem to contradict the goals of TSF. Option C could imperil the alliance between the patient and provider, the preservation of which is a component of TSF. The statement in option D may steer the patient away from acceptance of their substance abuse, could discourage further 12-step participation, and endorses self-medication as a root cause of substance abuse, a stance that may lead to a worse prognosis for substance abusing patients. Table 28–1 presents some common problems and offers solutions that may guide a clinician in his or her facilitation of AA participation. **(Role of the Therapist, pp. 419–420)**

TABLE 28–1. Engaging patients with Alcoholics Anonymous (AA) resistance

Problem	Solution
The patient has had previous bad experiences with treatment for alcohol dependence, and AA is guilty by association.	Explore these issues and interpret the resistance of guilt by association.
The patient has had a previous bad experience with AA directly (e.g., he or she might have met someone at a meeting and then drunk with him or her; the patient might have gone to a meeting and felt that he or she did not fit with the other attendees).	Explore what happened and the patient's role in this. Talk about matching meetings to the patient.
The patient has had a previous bad experience due to symptoms of co-occurring psychiatric problems (e.g., social phobia, paranoia).	Explore this, and explain that you will develop a strategy to deal with these symptoms. Explain to the patient that an AA meeting is about the safest place there is to exhibit symptoms publicly because it is a supportive and nonconfrontational environment.
The patient has had very little previous experience with AA, but stopped attending meetings, used alcohol or drugs, and concluded that meetings "don't work."	Explain that the patient's previous attendance and involvement was not an adequate "dose." Illustrate this point with the following analogies, selecting the analogy that the patient is most likely to hear or understand, given his or her clinical history: *Antibiotic model:* Would it be safe to conclude that an antibiotic was ineffective after taking only one-third of the dose for only one-third of the time prescribed? *Diabetes model:* Would it be safe to conclude that a diabetes treatment was ineffective after taking the medicine only half the time and eating chocolate cake between doses? *Bipolar model:* Would it be safe to conclude that a bipolar medication was ineffective after taking only one-third of the prescribed dose or skipping doses altogether for weeks at a time?

CHAPTER 29

Contingency Management

29.1 The parents of a 17-year-old high school student who lives with them want to address his marijuana use through contingency management (CM). Which CM intervention is most effective to help curb this patient's marijuana use?

A. Home drug testing and rewarding negative test results with gift certificates.
B. Drug testing in a specialized laboratory and rewarding negative test results with gift certificates.
C. Contingent upon positive test results, sending a deterrent letter to the patient's school stating that he will withdraw from school because he is a "junkie."
D. Paying $10 cash for every negative test result.
E. Confronting the patient about the negative consequences of his marijuana use.

The correct response is option A: Home drug testing and rewarding negative test results with gift certificates.

Immediate reward of negative test results is the most effective positive reinforcement of the target behavior and the most effective CM strategy to curb marijuana use (option A). Drug test results from a laboratory (option B) are less immediate and therefore less effective reinforcement targets. Although punishment of the undesired behavior (i.e., marijuana use) is effective (option C), withdrawing from school would remove the opportunity for the sober behavior of studying and the potential reward of academic success. Cash rewards (option D) are less appropriate than gift certificates in that they could be used to purchase marijuana. Confrontation (option E), even if contingent upon marijuana use, is not a CM intervention. **(Application of Behavioral Principles in Substance Abuse Treatment, p. 423; Reinforcement of Clinically Relevant Behaviors/Drug Abstinence/Voucher Reinforcement, pp. 425–426)**

29.2 What is an effective target of contingency management (CM) treatment as demonstrated by research studies?

A. Doing homework assignments in cognitive-behavioral therapy (CBT).
B. Looking for a job.
C. Finding a sober friend.
D. Entering treatment.
E. Going to an Alcoholics Anonymous meeting.

The correct response is option D: Entering treatment.

Paying cash rewards contingent upon attendance of one treatment session increased the probability that patients would enter treatment (option D). Although there are many potentially suitable target behaviors for CM, most have not been researched (options B, C, E). Indeed, not every potentially suitable target behavior proved to be effective in research studies. For example, Carroll et al. (2012) found that reinforcing completion of homework assignments did not improve treatment outcomes of CBT (option A). **(Reinforcement of Clinically Relevant Behaviors/ Treatment Attendance, pp. 423–425; Other Therapeutically Relevant Intervention Targets/Goal Attainment, p. 430)**

29.3   What learning principle best applies to contingency management (CM) interventions?

A. Intermittent reinforcement.
B. Negative reinforcement.
C. Positive reinforcement.
D. Aversive conditioning.
E. Response substitution.

The correct response is option C: Positive reinforcement.

CM interventions enhance positive consequences of drug abstinence (option C). Different schedules of reinforcement have shown effectiveness in CM interventions, including, but not limited to, intermittent reinforcement (option A). In CM interventions, reinforcement usually does not involve the removal of a negative consequence (option B), the contingency of a negative consequence to drug use (option D), or the training of a specific alternative sober response that is mutually exclusive with drug use (option E). **(Application of Behavioral Principles in Substance Abuse Treatment, p. 423)**

29.4   Which substance use disorder is most suitable for contingency management (CM) intervention?

A. Cocaine, because there currently is no specific pharmacotherapy.
B. Alcohol, because the monitored administration of disulfiram (Antabuse) introduces a specific contingency between drinking and an immediate negative consequence.
C. Nicotine, because in contrast to other substance use disorders, there are only limited immediate severe negative consequences to smoking cigarettes; introducing voucher incentives immediately contingent upon nonsmoking is therefore particularly effective in smoking cessation.
D. Marijuana, because the teenage onset of this disorder sets the particularly favorable stage for CM intervention of the patient's home and family milieu as settings of incentives of drug abstinence.
E. CM is an evidence-based effective treatment for a variety of substance use disorders, including stimulants, alcohol, nicotine, and marijuana.

The correct response is option E: CM is an evidence-based effective treatment for a variety of substance use disorders, including stimulants, alcohol, nicotine, and marijuana.

Abstinence incentives have been effectively used for treating stimulant, alcohol, tobacco, and marijuana users (options A, B, C, D) and have been found to be effective in drug users with a wide variety of demographic, psychosocial, and substance use characteristics (option E). **(Conclusion, pp. 435–436)**

29.5   A company decides to adopt a contingency management (CM) strategy to curb alcohol use among its employees. Given that most employees who drink alcohol also smoke cigarettes, which is the best target for the CM intervention?

   A. Alcohol, because there is no clinically significant relationship between alcohol use and smoking cigarettes.
   B. Abstinence from all substances to avoid *substitution,* namely, increased smoking to compensate for stopping drinking.
   C. Abstinence from all substances, which is the usual recommendation, despite lack of clear research evidence.
   D. Smoking, because smoking and drinking are related and smoking cessation is the easier-to-achieve goal given the current climate of laws against smoking and the presence of smoking detectors.
   E. CM interventions of substance use disorders are ineffective in company settings because of conflicting interests, including patient confidentiality and employees' fear of repercussion due to treatment failure.

The correct response is option C: Abstinence from all substances, which is the usual recommendation, despite lack of clear research evidence.

Abstinence from all drugs is the usual recommendation in CM interventions (option C). Dual drug targets make clinical sense and have evidence based effectiveness in CM interventions (options A, D). Interestingly, single drug targets have not resulted in detectable increases of nontarget drug use (i.e., "substitution; option B). CM studies have been successfully conducted with employees of companies (option E). **(Implementation Considerations/Number and Selection of Drug Targets, p. 431)**

References

Carroll KM, Nich C, Lapaglia DM, et al: Combining cognitive behavioral therapy and contingency management to enhance their effects in treating cannabis dependence: less can be more, more or less. Addiction 107(9):1650–1659, 2012 22404223

CHAPTER 30

Network Therapy

30.1 Which of the following is most likely to contribute to the effectiveness of network therapy in the treatment of substance use disorders?

A. Resolution of conflicts in the patient's interpersonal relationships.
B. Confrontation of the patient's addiction by concerned relatives and friends.
C. Education of network members about substance use disorders to better understand and help the patient.
D. Intervention by therapist and network members to facilitate treatment engagement.
E. The availability of greater social supports to the patient.

The correct response is option E: The availability of greater social supports to the patient.

Network therapy is an evidence-based and effective treatment for substance use disorders. The treatment draws on a group of family and friends of the patient to help the therapist to support the patient's abstinence (option E). The role of the network is to support, not to confront (option B), educate (option C), or stage an intervention (option D). In contrast to family therapy or group therapy, network members do not participate for their own treatment, but only the patient's (option A). **(Introduction, p. 441; Treatment Technique/Selection of Patients, p. 444)**

30.2 What psychotherapeutic treatment modality best characterizes network therapy?

A. Group therapy.
B. Family therapy.
C. Individual therapy.
D. Twelve-step facilitation.
E. Intervention.

The correct response is option C: Individual therapy.

In network therapy, a support group of family and peers attend individual therapy sessions of the patient and the therapist. The treatment draws on a group of family, friends, and relatives of the patient to help the individual therapist work with the patient toward the goal of abstinence (option C). During the network sessions, the members are therefore not in treatment themselves (options A, B, D). Although a network may be involved in an intervention, intervention is not the primary goal of network therapy (option E). **(Treatment Technique/The Network's Membership, pp. 444–445)**

30.3   What is a contraindication for network therapy for alcohol use disorder?

A. Unwillingness to stop drinking.
B. Inability to stop drinking.
C. Inability to comply with outpatient detoxification.
D. Simultaneous attendance of Alcoholics Anonymous meetings.
E. Unwillingness to accept reduced controlled drinking ("harm reduction") as treatment goal.

The correct response is option C: Inability to comply with outpatient detoxification.

Network therapy typically is an office-based, outpatient treatment for substance use disorders. Because alcohol withdrawal is potentially life threatening, failure to achieve detoxification on an outpatient basis (option C) mandates an inpatient setting of treatment. The treatment goal of network therapy is complete abstinence to be supported by the network members (option E). Network therapy is usually combined with other treatment modalities, including 12-step facilitation (option D). Unwillingness and inability to stop drinking are indications for network therapy (options A, B). **(Treatment Technique/Selection of Patients, p. 444)**

30.4   What is an important difference between network therapy and group therapy for substance use disorders?

A. Network members network outside therapy sessions; group members do not.
B. Groups, but not networks, have a therapist.
C. Group members use the group therapy sessions for their own treatment; network members do not use the network for their own treatment.
D. Group sessions take place in the therapist's office; network sessions take place in the patient's home.
E. Reduced controlled drinking (harm reduction) is a treatment goal in network therapy but not in group therapy.

The correct response is option C: Group members use the group therapy sessions for their own treatment; network members do not use the network for their own treatment.

Network members are not led to expect symptom relief or self-realization for themselves, unlike family members in family therapy or group members in group therapy (option C). Group members, just like network members, may meet outside sessions (option A). Groups have a group therapist; networks have the patient's individual therapist (option B). Group and network therapy sessions take place in the therapists' office (option D). Networks aim to support the patient in achieving complete abstinence; groups may aim for complete abstinence but also for harm reduction (option E). **(The Network's Task, p. 445)**

30.5   Which other treatment modality is not combined with network therapy?

A. Cognitive-behavioral therapy (CBT), because cognitive therapy is too technical for network members.
B. Contingency management (CM), because network members cannot be expected to provide incentives for abstinence to the patient.
C. Twelve-step facilitation (TSF), because this is self-help treatment rather than professional help.
D. An intervention, because the role of network members is to support the patient in achieving abstinence, not to confront the patient's unwillingness to go into treatment.
E. Motivational enhancement (ME), because network therapy is not effective if patients are ambivalent.

The correct response is option D: An intervention, because the role of network members is to support the patient in achieving abstinence, not to confront the patient's unwillingness to go into treatment.

Psychotherapeutic approaches have been found to yield improved outcomes when combined with certain addiction treatments, including CBT (option A), CM (option B), 12-step facilitation (option C), and ME (option E). In an intervention (option D), a number of people from the patient's family and close friends, who might otherwise constitute a network, confront the patient and threaten to withdraw support and personal contact if the patient does not agree to enter treatment. In network therapy, aggressive confrontation is not used. **(Treatment Technique/NT in Contrast to an Intervention, p. 451)**

CHAPTER 31

Group Therapy

31.1 Which of the following is true about group therapy in patients with substance use disorders (SUDs)?

A. Group therapy is primarily used in inpatient and residential settings.
B. Group therapy is only indicated for patients without co-occurring psychiatric disorders.
C. Group therapy may be problematic for use in managed care settings.
D. Group therapy is not helpful for the symptoms and adverse effects that are the consequences of substance abuse.
E. Group psychotherapy is the psychosocial treatment of choice for most patients with SUDs.

The correct response is option E: Group psychotherapy is the psychosocial treatment of choice for most patients with SUDs.

Because of its therapeutic effectiveness as well as its cost-effectiveness, group therapy plays an ever more important role as the psychosocial treatment of choice for most SUDs, including substance abuse and addiction (option E). Group psychotherapy can be used in a wide variety of treatment settings and can address many of the psychosocial factors involved in etiology of substance abuse (option A). It can also be used to treat symptoms and adverse effects that are the consequences of substance abuse and dependence, and can also treat co-occurring psychiatric disorders that are so common in individuals with SUDs (Flores and Brook 2011) (options B, D). The lower cost of group treatment is helpful in managed care settings (option C). **(Introduction, pp. 463–464)**

31.2 Which of the following is *not* true about the etiology and treatment of substance use disorders (SUDs)?

A. SUDs are rarely familial.
B. Cultural factors such as ethnic identification are important to address in treatment.
C. Substance abuse groups deal with many domains, including developmental, medical, and sociocultural.

267

D. The etiology of SUDs is multifactorial.

E. Group psychotherapy may include both cognitive-behavioral therapy (CBT) and relapse prevention.

The correct response is option A: SUDs are rarely familial.

Because the etiology of SUDs is multifactorial and SUDs affect a wide variety of organ systems, the treatment of SUDs is multidisciplinary, within a biopsychosocial framework that includes both medications and psychosocial interventions (option D). Substance abuse is often a familial disorder (option A), and family issues and cultural factors such as ethnic identification (Brook et al. 2003, 2006) are significant areas to address in group therapy (option B). Substance abuse groups address a variety of issues, such as developmental, familial, medical, sociocultural, environmental, intrapsychic, and interpersonal attachment issues (option C). A broad treatment approach using group psychotherapy can include CBT and relapse prevention and can permit group therapists to examine a variety of areas in the treatment of patients (Vannicelli 1995) (option E). **(Introduction, pp. 463–464)**

31.3 Which of the following statements is *not* true about patient selection for group therapy for substance use disorders (SUDs)?

A. Significant cognitive deficits are a contraindication.

B. Patients with severe antisocial personality disorder require a specialized group structure.

C. Preparatory sessions are not necessary before group entry to assess suitability.

D. In general, suicidal or homicidal patients are not suitable for group therapy.

E. Acute psychotic illness is a contraindication.

The correct response is option C: Preparatory sessions are not necessary before group entry to assess suitability.

Appropriate patient selection is extremely important for the therapeutic effectiveness and duration of the group. A number of types of patients are usually not suitable for group treatment, although they may be suited for specific groups under certain circumstances. These include patients who are acutely suicidal, homicidal, or acutely psychotic, as well as patients with serious organicity that limits their ability to take part in the group discussion (options A, D, E). In addition, those patients with severe antisocial personality disorder who might sell or provide substances of abuse to other group members need a special group structure (option B). Selection of group members also requires consideration of how the patient fits in with a particular group. Other considerations include each patient's ability to function with other people, as well as each patient's motivation, affective stability, impulse control, level of maturity, and phase of recovery. Before an individual is included in a group, preparatory sessions with the group leader are necessary to help assess the suitability of the prospective group member (option C). **(Specific Issues Related to Group Therapy for Substance Use Disorders, pp. 464–466)**

31.4 Which of the following statements about successful group leaders is *incorrect*?

A. Role of the group leader is active within the group process.
B. Successful leader attributes include compassion, empathy, and a sense of humor.
C. Most of group content is focused on early childhood-parental dynamics.
D. Leader techniques include supportive confrontation and the creation of an empathic holding environment.
E. Integrity and humility are critical leader attributes.

The correct response is option C: Most of group content is focused on early childhood-parental dynamics.

Grotjohn (1983) described attributes of successful group leaders; these include empathy, compassion, reliability, responsiveness, trustworthiness, a firm sense of identity, a sense of humor, and a feeling for others' human qualities (option B). Integrity and humility are also necessary attributes (option E). The role of the group therapist in the treatment of substance use should be an active one (option A). The therapist assists members in maintaining the group structure and adhering to the group contract by focusing on the here-and-now interactions in the group (option C). In this way, the therapist helps the group process and maintains the stability and cohesion of the group. One technique is the use of *supportive confrontation*, which allows for the use of an empathic "holding" environment to help group members explore painful feelings and self-destructive behaviors with understanding and support; group members can deal with loss of affective control without blame or shame (option D). **(Specific Issues Related to Group Therapy for Substance Use Disorders, pp. 464–466)**

31.5 Which of the following statements about different types of groups is *incorrect*?

A. Self-help and 12-step groups are a core part of group therapy for addiction.
B. Several models emphasize progression of group members from one phase of treatment to the next.
C. Groups often include a cognitive-behavioral focus.
D. Longer duration of groups predict increased abstinence.
E. Group therapy for substance use disorders (SUDs) is primarily employed in residential settings.

The correct response is option E: Group therapy for substance use disorders (SUDs) is primarily employed in residential settings.

A variety of group treatments may be used for patients with SUDs and co-occurring psychiatric disorders, including self-help groups, 12-step groups, groups based on interpersonal group psychotherapy, cognitive-behavioral therapy groups, psychodynamically focused groups based on the principles of modified dynamic group therapy, phase models of group treatment, relapse prevention groups, therapeutic community groups, and groups for adolescents who abuse substances (options A, C). Homogeneous groups treat specific patient populations and patients abusing specific drugs of abuse, and groups meet in a wide range of settings, including outpatient, inpatient, and partial hospitalization (Flores 2007) (option E). A number of treatment models emphasize the progression of group members from one phase of treatment to the next as they complete the tasks of each phase (option B). More effective treatment outcomes result from a longer duration in group treatment (option D). **(Introduction, pp. 463–464; Types of Group Treatments, pp. 466–474)**

References

Brook DW, Brook JS, Richter L, et al: Risk and protective factors of adolescent drug use: implications for prevention programs, in Handbook of Drug Abuse Prevention: Theory, Science, and Practice. Edited by Sloboda Z, Bukoski WJ. New York, Plenum, 2003, pp 265–287

Brook JS, Brook DW, Pahl K: The developmental context for adolescent substance abuse intervention, in Adolescent Substance Abuse: Research and Clinical Advances. Edited by Liddle HA, Rowe CA. New York, Cambridge University Press, 2006, pp 25–51

Flores PJ: Group Psychotherapy with Addicted Populations: An Integration of Twelve-Step and Psychodynamic Theory, 3rd Edition. New York, Haworth, 2007

Flores PJ, Brook DW: Group Psychotherapy Approaches to Addiction and Substance Abuse. New York, American Group Psychotherapy Association, 2011

Grotjohn M: The qualities of the group psychotherapist, in Comprehensive Group Psychotherapy. Edited by Kaplan HI, Sadock BJ. Baltimore, MD, Williams & Wilkins, 1983, pp 294–301

Vannicelli M: Group psychotherapy with substance abusers and family members, in Psychotherapy and Substance Abuse: A Practitioner's Handbook. Edited by Washton AM. New York, Guilford, 1995, pp 337–356

CHAPTER 32

Family Therapy

32.1 Several large-scale studies have determined which factor to be the predominant influence in getting individuals with substance use disorders to seek treatment?

A. Legal mandate.
B. Family pressure.
C. Primary medical doctor.
D. Pressure from employer.
E. Financial concerns.

The correct response is option B: Family pressure.

Although a confluence of factors can often contribute to an individual seeking treatment, such as legal mandate, medical concerns, or financial or employment concerns (options A, C, D, E), several large-scale studies have determined that family pressure is the predominant influence in getting individuals with substance use disorders to seek treatment (Stanton 2004). Hence, family members and significant others can be important resources for helping patients receive treatment (option B). **(Helping Individuals With Substance Use Disorders to Engage in Treatment or Self-Help, pp. 482–483)**

32.2 What family treatment model applies strategic-structural-behavioral–based (SSBB) methods with additional focus regarding systems external to the family, such as the school, legal, employment, mental health, and health system realms?

A. Multidimensional Family Therapy (MDFT).
B. Functional Family Therapy (FFT).
C. Transitional Family Therapy (TFT).
D. Brief Strategic Family Therapy (BSFT).
E. INternational CAnnabis Need for Treatment (INCANT).

The correct response is option A: Multidimensional Family Therapy (MDFT).

The MDFT model applies SSBB methods, with additional focus regarding systems external to the family, such as the school, legal, employment, mental health, and health system realms (option A). FFT (option B) was created by James F. Alexander and Bruce V. Parsons in the early 1970s and is strongly influenced by strategic and behavioral techniques. TFT (option C) is an SSBB with additional intergenerational aspects adapted from the work of pioneers like Murray Bowen and Ivan Boszormenyi-Nagy. BSFT involves conjoint sessions with family members and evolved as a model for treating adolescents who abuse substances, with a particular emphasis on working with minority populations (option D) (Szapocznik et al. 2012). Finally, INCANT (option E) is not a therapy but, rather, a large multinational multi-team randomized controlled trial to examine the efficacy of MDFT. **(Family/Couples Therapy Research and Components/Strategic-Structural-Behavioral–Based Therapies/Models, pp. 484, 488–491)**

32.3   In addition to supporting abstinence via a *daily sobriety contract,* what is the other main component of Behavioral Couples Therapy (BCT)?

     A. Focusing on systems external to the couple.
     B. Conducting therapy in the family home.
     C. Taking an intergenerational approach.
     D. Using relationship-focused interventions.
     E. Employing enactment (i.e., practicing a new behavior within session).

The correct response is option D: Using relationship-focused interventions.

There are two main components to BCT: one focuses on supporting abstinence via a *daily sobriety contract* in which the partners 1) commit to maintaining sobriety on a daily basis, 2) attend a 12-step program, and 3) engage in trust discussions whereby the patient states an intent to remain abstinent and the partner offers support. The other component pertains to engagement in *relationship-focused interventions* to increase positive feelings, shared activities, and constructive communication (option D). A focus on systems external to the couple (option A) is an approach used in Multidimensional Family Therapy. Option B, therapy conducted in the family home, is seen in Multisystemic Therapy. An *intergenerational approach* (option C) is used in Transitional Family Therapy. Finally, *enactment* (option E) is a term used to describe the restructuring process, in which a new pattern of behavior is actually practiced within session, rather than just being talked about. **(Family/Couples Therapy Research and Components/Behavioral Couples Therapy, pp. 491–492)**

32.4   In strategic-structural-behavioral–based (SSBB) models, the term *reframing* is used to describe what therapeutic process?

     A. Determining what resources may be called upon to effect positive change in a family.
     B. Altering family interactions to that keep the family and identified patient from making significant change.
     C. Practicing a new pattern of behavior within session.
     D. Forming therapeutic alliances.
     E. Redefining a problem or dysfunctional pattern in a more positive way.

The correct response is option E: Redefining a problem or dysfunctional pattern in a more positive way.

The *behavioral* aspects of SSBB therapies have social learning theory underpinnings. A key technique is *reframing*, whereby a problem or dysfunctional pattern is redefined in a more positive way, such as "we're all in this together" (option E). The *structural* aspects of the SSBB model emphasize three core strategies: *joining* (forming therapeutic alliances, option D), *family pattern diagnosis* (determining what family interactional problems have developed and what resources might be called upon to effect positive change, option A), and *restructuring* to alter family interactions that keep the family and identified patient "from making significant changes in their lives" (option B) (Rowe 2012). Option C, practicing a new pattern of behavior within a session, is a description of *enactment*. **(Family/Couples Therapy Research and Components/Strategic-Structural-Behavioral–Based Therapies/Models/Components and Outcome Studies, pp. 484, 488–490)**

32.5 The role of genetics is thought to be most pronounced in which substance use disorder?

A. Marijuana.
B. Opiates.
C. Alcohol.
D. Cocaine.
E. Amphetamines.

The correct response is option C: Alcohol.

There is good evidence that genetics can play a role both in the development of a substance use disorder and in the difficulties encountered in reversing the disorder. These effects appear to be greater for alcoholism (option C) than for other substance use disorders (options A, B, D, E). **(Common Family Patterns to Be Addressed in Treatment for Substance Abuse/Trauma, Life Events, and Identity Transmission, pp. 480–482)**

References

Rowe CL: Family therapy for drug abuse: review and updates 2003–2010. J Marital Fam Ther 38(1):59–81, 2012 22283381

Stanton MD: Getting reluctant substance abusers to engage in treatment/self-help: a review of outcomes and clinical options. J Marital Fam Ther 30(2):165–182, 2004 15114946

Szapocznik J, Schwartz SJ, Muir JA, et al: Brief strategic family therapy: an intervention to reduce adolescent risk behavior. Couple Family Psychol 1(2):134–145, 2012 23936750

CHAPTER 33

Inpatient Treatment

33.1 Why is it recommended that patients with co-occurring substance use disorders (SUDs) and psychiatric disorders receive treatment in an integrated inpatient setting?

A. There is less stigmatization.
B. It provides better cost containment.
C. It reduces treatment dropout rates.
D. It is generally more effective.
E. There are better patient satisfaction ratings.

The correct response is option D: It is generally more effective.

Recognition of the frequent comorbidity of SUDs and other psychiatric illnesses has led to the creation of numerous inpatient units that are devoted to the treatment of patients with co-occurring mental illnesses and SUDs. Integrated treatment is generally considered the optimal intervention for patients with co-occurring SUDs and mental health problems, and existing evidence suggests that inpatient programs providing greater integration of treatment are generally more effective for this population (Brunette et al. 2004). Although options A, B, C, and E may turn out to be true, it is option D that has been supported by evidence and that leads to this recommendation. **(Inpatient Treatment Settings, p. 500)**

33.2 What are the defining characteristics of the Minnesota Model?

A. Structured cognitive-behavioral therapy (CBT) and relapse prevention techniques.
B. A medical model of addiction and significant physician involvement.
C. Twelve-step philosophy and many counselors who are in recovery themselves.
D. An algorithm for medical detoxification of alcohol and opioid use disorders.
E. A contingency management (CM) program where patients earn increasing responsibility.

The correct response is option C: Twelve-step philosophy and many counselors who are in recovery themselves.

Minnesota Model treatment programs often feature a standardized, relatively fixed length of stay (commonly 4 weeks) and are based on principles of Alcoholics Anonymous and Narcotics Anonymous. These programs heavily employ recovering alcoholics and drug addicts as primary counselors. The Minnesota Model does not explicitly use CBT or relapse prevention techniques (option A), nor does it employ a medical model or significantly involve physicians (option B). It is not an algorithm for detoxification (option D), nor is it a contingency management program (option E). **(Minnesota Model, pp. 500–501)**

33.3   What is the evidence base regarding the outcome of inpatient treatment?

A. Several randomized controlled trials found abstinence rates of 50%–60%.
B. Several uncontrolled studies found abstinence rates ranging from 25% to 60%.
C. No randomized controlled studies have been done, and so no estimate can be made.
D. Several case-control cohorts found abstinence rates ranging from 25% to 60%.
E. Case reports and anecdotal data indicate abstinence rates ranging from 50% to 60%.

The correct response is option B: Several uncontrolled studies found abstinence rates ranging from 25% to 60%.

Several follow-up studies involving patients treated in treatment centers using the Minnesota Model have demonstrated abstinence rates of 50%–60% at 6–12 months after discharge. In a 1-year follow-up of patients treated in an integrated program for patients with substance use disorders and co-occurring psychiatric disorders, Moggi et al. (2002) reported an abstinence rate of 25%; this lower abstinence rate may, in part, reflect a more severe case mix, although programmatic factors cannot be excluded. Unfortunately, all of the studies mentioned here were uncontrolled and were therefore subject to the biases inherent in uncontrolled research. To date, there have been no randomized controlled trials to examine this issue (option A), but this does not prohibit the use of data from uncontrolled studies (option C). The study outcomes in options D and E have not been reported. **(Outcome of Inpatient Treatment/General Findings, p. 503)**

33.4   Studies have shown that individuals who are married, educated, employed full-time and who have strong family support tend to have a better prognosis after inpatient treatment. You are seeing a 24-year-old single female cocaine user who does not have good family support. She has been unable to stop using cocaine despite intensive outpatient treatment. How should her demographic data influence your decision to recommend an inpatient treatment setting?

A. Strongly—you should not recommend inpatient treatment because she is unlikely to have a good outcome.
B. Strongly—you should not recommend inpatient treatment because she lacks the social support necessary to ensure adherence to aftercare.

C. Strongly—you should not recommend inpatient treatment because she is young and therefore less likely to agree with the program's philosophy.
D. Not at all—you should recommend inpatient treatment because she has been unable to stop using in a less restrictive setting.
E. Not at all—you should recommend inpatient treatment because she does not have good family support.

The correct response is option D: Not at all—you should recommend inpatient treatment because she has been unable to stop using in a less restrictive setting.

Most studies of inpatient treatment have found that the following groups have a better prognosis: patients who are older, patients with more education, patients who are employed full-time, patients who are married, patients who abuse alcohol rather than other drugs, and patients whose families participate in treatment. Patients who have more social support for sobriety, who are confident in their ability to maintain sobriety, and who have greater motivation to change also appear less likely to resume use after discharge. Individuals with histories of injection drug use, antisocial personality disorder, cocaine dependence, and tobacco use tend to fare less well in inpatient treatment outcome studies. However, many of these same patient characteristics are associated with a favorable prognosis in other forms of SUD treatment.

The clinician must ultimately consider two major issues in deciding whether to hospitalize a patient: 1) the danger that the patient might imminently experience harm to self (e.g., as a result of withdrawal or suicidal ideation) or be dangerous to others and 2) the likelihood that the patient would achieve treatment success in a less restrictive environment. Given that the patient has clearly been unable to stop using in a less restrictive setting, demographic factors (options B, C, and E) should not deter you from referring her to an inpatient setting. Outcome for an individual cannot be predicted in advance, and even someone with a poor prognosis should not be denied the appropriate level of care (option A). **(Indications for Hospitalization, pp. 501–503; Outcome of Inpatient Treatment/Patient Characteristics in Inpatient Treatment Outcome Research, pp. 503–505)**

33.5   What has integrating employment into treatment, such as an employer mandating an employee to treatment, been shown to improve?

A. Substance-related outcomes.
B. Work-related outcomes.
C. Substance- and work-related outcomes.
D. Substance-related outcomes but not work-related outcomes.
E. Work-related outcomes but not substance-related outcomes.

The correct response is option C: Substance- and work-related outcomes.

The integration of employment into treatment is one component of inpatient treatment programs that has been found to improve both substance- and work-related outcomes. Specifically, having a workplace mandate a patient to substance use disorder treatment increases abstinence and inpatient treatment retention in addition to improving employment problems (option C). Although options A and B are correct, option C is the best answer. Options D and E are incorrect, since both substance-related and work-related outcomes have been shown to improve. **(Outcome of Inpatient Treatment/Program Characteristics in Inpatient Treatment Outcome Research, pp. 505–507)**

References

Brunette MF, Mueser KT, Drake RE: A review of research on residential programs for people with severe mental illness and co-occurring substance use disorders. Drug Alcohol Rev 23(4):471–481, 2004 15763752

Moggi F, Brodbeck J, Költzsch K, et al: One-year follow-up of dual diagnosis patients attending a 4-month integrated inpatient treatment. Eur Addict Res 8(1):30–37, 2002 11818691

CHAPTER 34

Therapeutic Communities

34.1 The therapeutic community (TC) approach has been summarized by the phrase "community as method." What does this mean?

A. Staff members act as "rational authorities" to establish standards for communal living and interdependence.
B. The primary therapeutic modality is group therapy sessions, which are led by staff and peers in recovery.
C. Individuals learn to use the activities and elements of the community as a vehicle for self-change.
D. A community of staff and peers creates a framework to transform negative conditioned responses into positive responses.
E. Individuals are provided with basic essentials and a social structure so they can concentrate on recovery.

The correct response is option C: Individuals learn to use the activities and elements of the community as a vehicle for self-change.

The TC approach can be summarized in the phrase "community as method" (De Leon 1997, 2000). Theoretical writings offer a definition of *community as method* as the *purposive* use of the community to teach individuals to *use* the community to change themselves (option C). The fundamental assumption underlying the TC approach is that individuals obtain maximum therapeutic and educational impact when they engage in and learn to use all of the activities and elements of the community as the tools for self-change. Thus, *community as method* means that the community itself provides a *context* of relationships and activities for social learning. Although staff members do act as "rational authorities" and help establish standards for living (option A), this does not describe the method of change that "community as method" is attempting to capture. Similarly, group therapy sessions (option B), along with provision of basic essentials and a social structure (option E), are all part of a TC, but these components do not explain how the community actually leads to change in an individual.

In the TC, learning occurs through participating in social interactions and program activities, and by taking on various social roles in the community. Therefore, it is not simply the transformation of negative conditioned responses (option D) that occurs, but rather a more complex form of social learning. **(The Therapeutic Community Perspective/View of Recovery/Social Learning, p. 513; The Therapeutic Community Approach/TC Program Model/Staff Members as Rational Authorities, p. 515)**

34.2 What are the four interrelated areas upon which the therapeutic community (TC) perspective is built?

A. Personhood, social learning theory, vocational therapy, and self-help groups.
B. Self-help groups, staff as role models, peer guidance, social hierarchy.
C. The social context, the family structure, the disease model, the moral model.
D. Personality structure, the substance use disorder, coping skills, social support.
E. The substance use disorder, the individual, the recovery process, right living.

The correct response is option E: The substance use disorder, the individual, the recovery process, right living.

The TC perspective consists of four interrelated views: those of the substance use disorder, the individual, the recovery process, and right living (option E). Although social learning theory, vocational therapy (work as therapy), self-help groups, role models, and social hierarchy (options A, B) are all components of a TC, they do not provide the foundation upon which the TC perspective is built. Option C lists various models in which addiction can be viewed, such as the disease model (found in medicine and Alcoholics Anonymous) and the moral model (found in the criminal justice system); however, most of these models do not directly inform the TC perspective, or even conflict with it. Option D describes components that are addressed or that compose a TC, but do not form the basis of the TC perspective (with the exception of substance use disorder). **(The Therapeutic Community Perspective, pp. 512–513)**

34.3 Both peers and staff can act as role models in a therapeutic community (TC). What are two main concepts that illustrate the therapeutic approach of these role models?

A. Role models organize therapeutic-educative activities and manage privileges.
B. Role models set expectations and assess how individuals are progressing.
C. Role models reinforce social hierarchy and act as one-on-one counselors.
D. Role models "act as if" and display responsible concern.
E. Role models confront individuals and mediate conflicts.

The correct response is option D: Role models "act as if" and display responsible concern.

Peers, serving as role models, and staff members, serving as role models and rational authorities, are the primary mediators of the recovery process. TC members who demonstrate the expected behaviors and reflect the values and teachings of the community are viewed as role models. TCs require multiple resident and staff role models to maintain the integrity of the community and ensure the spread of social learning effects. Two concepts illustrate the therapeutic significance of the role model in the TC: 1) *Role models "act as if."* The resident behaves as the person he or she should be, rather than as the person he or she has been. Despite resistances, perceptions, or feelings to the contrary, residents engage in the expected behaviors and consistently maintain the attitudes and values of the community. "Acting as if" is not merely an exercise in conformity; it is an essential mechanism for more complete psychological change (option D). 2) *Role models display responsible concern.* This concept is closely akin to the notion of being one's brother's or sister's keeper. Showing responsible concern involves willingness to confront others whose behavior is not in keeping with the TC's rules or the community's expectations for full participation. The other options are not main concepts of role models. **(The Therapeutic Community Approach/TC Program Model /Peers as Role Models, p. 515)**

34.4   What characteristics are commonly found in substance abusers enrolled in a therapeutic community (TC)?

A. Absence of conflict with family members.
B. Significant psychosocial dysfunction.
C. Some college education and a history of employment.
D. Relatively minor legal history.
E. Lack of psychiatric comorbidity.

The correct response is option B: Significant psychosocial dysfunction.

In many TC residents, vocational and educational problems are marked; middle-class, mainstream values are either missing or not sought. These residents usually emerge from a socially disadvantaged sector (option B). Although most adult admissions to TCs are voluntary, many of these patients come to treatment programs under various forms of perceived pressures originating from conflicts with family members or significant others, employment difficulties, or anticipated legal consequences (option A) (De Leon 1988; Joe et al. 1998; Melnick et al. 2014). Most patients have poor work histories and have engaged in criminal activities. Among adults who are admitted to TCs, fewer than one-third were employed full-time in the year before treatment, and more than two-thirds have been arrested (options C, D) (De Leon 1984; Hubbard et al. 1997; Simpson and Sells 1982). Approximately 25%–35% of adult admissions to community-based TCs have a legal status, in terms of being paroled, probated, or otherwise court-ordered to treatment. In diagnostic studies in which the Diagnostic Interview Schedule was used, nearly three-fourths of patients admitted to TCs had a non-drug-related psychiatric disorder in their lifetime in addition to substance-related problems (option E). **(The Therapeutic Community Perspective/View of the Individual, p. 512; Patients Admitted to Therapeutic Communities, pp. 521–523)**

34.5   What has been a consistent research finding among therapeutic community (TC) participants?

A. Longer retention in treatment is correlated with better posttreatment outcomes.
B. Treatment completion shows no improvement in employment.
C. Participation in a TC does not alter criminal activity.
D. TCs are an effective and cost-effective treatment for all substance abusers.
E. Enrollment alone in a TC is correlated with improved psychosocial functioning.

The correct response is option A: Longer retention in treatment is correlated with better posttreatment outcomes.

There is a consistent relationship between retention in treatment and positive post-treatment outcomes in TCs. Those who complete treatment show the best outcomes (option B), and the longer dropouts stay in treatment, the better the outcome (option A) (Barr 1986; De Leon et al. 1982; Holland 1983; Hubbard et al. 1989; Simpson and Curry 1997; Simpson and Sells 1982; Simpson et al. 1997; Substance Abuse and Mental Health Services Administration 1996). Enrollment alone is not enough, as it is the length of the time in the TC that is correlated with improved outcomes (option E). Similar findings have been obtained with the smaller number of controlled and comparative studies involving TC programs. Overall, the weight of the research evidence from multiple sources—multiprogram field effectiveness studies, single-program controlled studies, meta-analytic statistical surveys, and cost-benefit studies—is compelling in supporting the hypothesis that the TC is an effective and cost-effective treatment for *certain subgroups* of, but not all, substance abusers (option D). Findings are consistent in showing substantial improvements on separate outcome variables (i.e., drug use, criminality, and employment) and on composite indices for measuring individual success. Econometric evaluations have found a significant and positive cost-benefit outcome for TC, particularly associated with reduced criminal activity and gains in employment (options B, C) (De Leon 2010). **(Research: Effectiveness, p. 523)**

References

Barr H: Outcomes in drug abuse treatment in two modalities, in Therapeutic Communities for Addictions. Edited by De Leon G, Zeigenfuss JT. Springfield, IL, Charles C Thomas, 1986, pp 97–108

De Leon G: The Therapeutic Community: Study of Effectiveness (NIDA Treatment Research Monograph ADM-84-1286). Rockville, MD, National Institute on Drug Abuse, 1984

De Leon G: Legal pressure in therapeutic communities. NIDA Res Monogr 86:160–177, 1988 3140029

De Leon G (ed): Community as Method: Therapeutic Communities for Special Populations and Special Settings. Westport, CT, Greenwood, 1997

De Leon G: The Therapeutic Community: Theory, Model, and Method. New York, Springer, 2000

De Leon G: Is the Therapeutic Community an evidenced based treatment? What the evidence says. International Journal of Therapeutic Communities 31(2):104–128, 2010

De Leon G, Wexler HK, Jainchill N: The therapeutic community: success and improvement rates 5 years after treatment. Int J Addict 17(4):703–742, 1982 7107092

Holland S: Evaluating community based treatment programs: a model for strengthening inferences about effectiveness. International Journal of Therapeutic Communities 4(4):285–306, 1983

Hubbard RL, Marsden ME, Rachal JV, et al: Drug Abuse Treatment: A National Study of Effectiveness. Chapel Hill, NC, The University of North Carolina Press, 1989

Hubbard RL, Craddock SG, Flynn PM, et al: Overview of 1-year follow-up outcomes in the Drug Abuse Treatment Outcome Study (DATOS). Psychol Addict Behav 11(special issue):261–278, 1997

Joe GW, Simpson DD, Broome KM Effects of readiness for drug abuse treatment on client retention and assessment of process. Addiction 93(8):1177–1190, 1998 9813899

Melnick G, Hawke J, De Leon G: Motivation and readiness for drug treatment: differences by modality and special populations. J Addict Dis 33(2):134–147, 2014 24735224

Simpson DD, Curry SJ (eds): Special issue: Drug Abuse Treatment Outcome Study (DATOS). Psychol Addict Behav 11(4):211–337, 1997

Simpson DD, Sells SB: Effectiveness of treatment for drug abuse: an overview of the DARP research program. Adv Alcohol Subst Abuse 2(1):7–29, 1982

Simpson DD, Joe GW, Brown BS: Treatment retention and follow-up outcomes in DATOS. Psychol Addict Behav 11(special issue):294–307, 1997

Substance Abuse and Mental Health Services Administration: National Treatment Improvement Study (NTIES). Rockville, MD, Substance Abuse and Mental Health Services Administration, 1996

CHAPTER 35

Community-Based Treatment

35.1 A 22-year-old man is referred to the CPEP (comprehensive psychiatric emergency program) at 1 A.M. on Saturday morning by the emergency department attending after having been evaluated for right wrist pain. He fell down a flight of subway steps, fracturing his wrist. He states that he had gone out drinking that evening and "got wasted" after consuming about four beers and three shots of liquor over the course of the evening. He reports his tolerance was lower than he expected. He minimizes the extent of his injury because he has fractured his nondominant hand and reports that he typically doesn't drink this much and only "parties like this" about every other month. What is the *next best* clinical step regarding this patient's alcohol use?

A. Recommend inpatient detox because of his excessive consumption.
B. Assess for at-risk drinking behavior.
C. Assess for an alcohol use disorder.
D. Refer client to the closest Alcoholics Anonymous (AA) meeting held that Sunday morning in his neighborhood.
E. Provide patient with a follow-up appointment at an outpatient substance abuse clinic.

The correct response is option C: Assess for an alcohol use disorder.

The patient has provided enough information that assessing for at-risk drinking behavior is not necessary (option B). He exceeded the single-day safe limit (Table 35–1) of four standard drinks in the past year. Any number of days above the single-day safe limit constitutes a positive screen (option B). After assessing for at-risk drinking behavior, assessment of an alcohol use disorder will guide the clinician in deciding which brief intervention components to use (option C). Without assessing for an alcohol use disorder, there can be no guidance to determine components to use (options A, D, E). **(Community Intervention/Brief Intervention for Alcohol Misuse, pp. 531–532, 533)**

TABLE 35–1. Maximum safe drinking limits

Population	Single day	Per week
Men < 65 years	4 standard drinks	14 standard drinks
Women (all ages); men > 65 years	3 standard drinks	7 standard drinks

Source. Adapted from National Institutes of Health 2005.

35.2 What is an important first step in a brief intervention for at-risk drinkers who are ambivalent about stopping their use?

A. Admission to inpatient detox.
B. Insisting on attending specialized treatment.
C. Referral to 12-step recovery program.
D. Allying with the patient in setting goals and agreeing on a plan.
E. Referral to a 28-day alcohol rehabilitation center.

The correct response is option D: Allying with the patient in setting goals and agreeing on a plan.

The clinician should recommend abstinence for patients with alcohol use disorders and yet be willing to work with a patient on a plan to cut down drinking if the patient is not ready to commit to abstinence (Table 35–2). Detoxification, pharmacotherapy, referral to 12-step recovery, and referral to specialized treatment are appropriate considerations for patients with alcohol use disorders (options A, B, C, E). For at-risk drinkers (without an alcohol use disorder), the clinician should recommend cutting back to patterns within safe limits. The clinician then inquires whether the patient is interested in changing his or her drinking behavior. If so, the clinician allies with the patient in setting goals and agreeing on a plan (option D). The National Institutes of Health (2005) have created educational materials such as strategies for cutting down as well as flowcharts and scripts to walk the clinician through the brief intervention process. Follow-up improves effectiveness (Jonas et al. 2012) and is recommended whether or not the patient has agreed to change. **(Community Intervention/Brief Intervention for Alcohol Misuse, pp. 531–532, 533)**

35.3 What was the clinical significance of CASASARD?

A. Intensive case management (ICM) clients were significantly more likely to have completed treatment, be abstinent from substances, and be employed than those who received the usual screening and referral to treatment.
B. Drug courts showed significant reduction in drug and alcohol use and improved family relationships.
C. Brief motivational interviewing techniques increase tobacco quit rates 2%–8% as compared with brief advice.

TABLE 35–2. Components of brief intervention for alcohol misuse

Screening for at-risk drinking (e.g., single question or AUDIT)

Quantifying drinks per week

Assessing for alcohol use disorder

Expressing concern

Gauging readiness to change

Setting a goal

Agreeing on a plan

Providing educational materials

Follow-up with continued support

Note. AUDIT=Alcohol Use Disorders Identification Test (Babor et al. 2001).
Source. Adapted from National Institutes of Health 2005.

D. In substance-abusing individuals, approaches using therapeutic communities, psychosocial rehabilitation, 12-step program, and enhancement of supportive relationships are all successful.

E. Adding a family-based treatment component to a family treatment drug courts (FTDC) program has also been shown to improve the chances that an at-risk child will remain in the family.

The correct response is option A: Intensive case management (ICM) clients were significantly more likely to have completed treatment, be abstinent from substances, and be employed than those who received the usual screening and referral to treatment.

CASASARD is a model ICM program that provided substance-abusing women with longitudinal involvement with two case managers who performed a variety of functions At 24 months, ICM clients were significantly more likely to have completed treatment, be abstinent from substances, and be employed than those who received the usual screening and referral to treatment (option A). Data from the Multisite Adult Drug Court Evaluation showed significant reduction in drug and alcohol use and improved family relationships as a result of drug courts. These seven meta-analyses showed that drug courts decrease crime compared with judicial interventions. This evaluation was not related to CASASARD, a model ICM program (option B). According to Fiore and Baker (2011), 70% of smokers visit a primary care physician annually, and recording smoking as a vital sign identifies over 80% of smokers at an office visit. In the health care setting, brief motivational interviewing techniques increase quit rates from 2% to 8% as compared with brief advice (option C). In substance-abusing individuals, approaches using therapeutic communities, psychosocial rehabilitation, 12-step programs, and enhancement of supportive relationships are all successful (Hitchcock et al. 1995; Moos et al. 1999) (option D). Adding a family-based treatment component to an FTDC program has also been shown to improve the chances that an at-risk child will remain in the family (option E) (Oliveros and Kaufman 2011). **(Community Intervention/Tobacco Interventions, pp. 532–533; Interventions by Welfare Services/**

Disability and Public Support, p. 535; Child Protective Services, pp. 535–536; Interventions by the Judicial System, p. 538; Non-Hospital-Based Services/Community Residential Facilities, pp. 539–540)

35.4   An individual with severe alcohol disease and multiple DWIs (driving while intoxicated) has been referred to a drug treatment court. What outcome can this individual most likely expect?

A. Regularly scheduled weekly or twice-weekly urine drug screens.
B. Judicial hearings every 6 months.
C. Gifts for negative urine toxicologies.
D. Referral to a program expected to last 3–4 years.
E. An interlock device that must be worn to monitor blood alcohol concentration (BAC).

The correct response is option C: Gifts for negative urine toxicologies.

Drug court models typically last 12–18 months (option D) and can utilize positive reinforcement techniques (like gift cards) (option C). Urine toxicologies are random (option A), and judicial hearings are more frequent than every 6 months (option B). The interlock device is a breathalyzer built into the ignition system, requiring the operator to demonstrate a negative BAC (less than 0.02%–0.025%) prior to being able to drive. It is not a prerequisite that it must be worn. There are multiple sanctions that can be reserved for the repeat drunken driver (option E). **(Community Intervention/Interventions by Welfare Services/Interventions by the Judicial System/Drug Courts, pp. 537–538)**

35.5   You are evaluating a married 32-year-old woman, currently employed full-time as an administrative assistant for treatment services, after three of her close friends and supportive husband have called to express concern regarding her drug and alcohol use. She has cocaine and an alcohol use disorder. According to guidelines published by the American Society of Addiction Medicine, your patient requires intensive outpatient treatment. What type of service meets these criteria?

A. A program that requires 20 hours of intensive outpatient services.
B. A program that requires 9 hours of intensive outpatient services.
C. A partial hospitalization program, because she has both an alcohol use disorder and a cocaine use disorder.
D. Twelve-step recovery meetings without any other substance abuse treatment, because of her full-time employment.
E. A program with more immediate access to medical and psychiatric services.

The correct response is option B: A program that requires 9 hours of intensive outpatient services.

Guidelines published by the American Society of Addiction Medicine (2001; see also Mee-Lee et al. 2013) require 9 hours per week of structured programming for intensive outpatient programs (option B) and 20 hours per week for partial hospital programs (option A), which are described as also having more immediate access to medical and psychiatric services (option E). Thus, day or partial hospital programs may better serve patients who have a substantial need for comprehensive services. Neither a partial hospitalization program nor 12-step recovery meetings meet the criteria to be considered intensive outpatient treatment (options C, D). **(Non-Hospital-Based Services/Day Hospital and Intensive Outpatient Programs, p. 539)**

References

American Society of Addiction Medicine: Patient Placement Criteria for the Treatment of Substance-Related Disorders, 2nd Edition, Revised. Chevy Chase, MD, American Society of Addiction Medicine, 2001

Babor TF, Higgins-Biddle JC, Saunders JB, et al: AUDIT—The Alcohol Use Disorders Identification Test: Guidelines for Use in Primary Health Care (WHO Publ No PSA/92.4). Geneva, World Health Organization, 2001

Fiore MC, Baker TB: Clinical practice. Treating smokers in the health care setting. N Engl J Med 365(13):1222–1231, 2011 21991895

Hitchcock HC, Stainback RD, Roque GM: Effects of halfway house placement on retention of patients in substance abuse aftercare. Am J Drug Alcohol Abuse 21(3):379–390, 1995 7484986

Jonas DE, Garbutt JC, Amick HR, et al: Behavioral counseling after screening for alcohol misuse in primary care: a systematic review and meta-analysis for the U.S. Preventive Services Task Force. Ann Intern Med 157(9):645–654, 2012 23007881

Mee-Lee D, Shulman GD, Fishman MJ, et al (eds): The ASAM Criteria: Treatment Criteria for Addictive, Substance-Related, and Co-Occurring Conditions, 3rd Edition. Carson City, NV, The Change Companies, 2013

Moos RH, Moos BS, Andrassy JM: Outcomes of four treatment approaches in community residential programs for patients with substance use disorders. Psychiatr Serv 50(12):1577–1583, 1999 10577876

National Institutes of Health: Helping Patients Who Drink Too Much: A Clinician's Guide. Bethesda, MD, National Institutes of Health, 2005. Available at: http://pubs.niaaa.nih.gov/publications/Practitioner/CliniciansGuide2005/guide.pdf. Accessed January 14, 2015.

Oliveros A, Kaufman J: Addressing substance abuse treatment needs of parents involved with the child welfare system. Child Welfare 90(1):25–41, 2011 21950173

CHAPTER 36

History of Alcoholics Anonymous and the Experiences of Patients

36.1 As of 2011, what is the most common means of referral to Alcoholics Anonymous (AA)?

A. Self-referral.
B. Referral by a health care provider.
C. Referral by another AA member.
D. Referral by court order.
E. Referral by family.

The correct response is option B: Referral by a health care provider.

The 2011 membership survey (Alcoholics Anonymous 2012) documents increasing collaboration among physicians, other health care providers, and AA. Forty percent of members in the 2011 survey (Alcoholics Anonymous 2012) were referred by a health care provider (option B). Another 29% were self-motivated (option A), 34% were referred through an AA member (option C), 25% by family (option E), 12% by court order (option D), 4% by an employer or fellow employee, and 1% by clergy. **(AA Survey Data/Referral to AA, p. 552)**

36.2 According to the latest Alcoholics Anonymous (AA) survey, what is the most common length of sobriety among AA members?

A. Not sober and actively drinking.
B. Less than 1 year of sobriety.
C. 1–5 years of sobriety.
D. 5–10 years of sobriety.
E. More than 10 years of sobriety.

The correct response is option E: More than 10 years of sobriety.

According to the latest AA survey (Alcoholics Anonymous 2012), 27% of members report less than 1 year of sobriety (option B), 24% report 1–5 years (option C), 12% report 5–10 years (option D), and 36% report more than 10 years (option E). These data document that newcomers to AA can expect to meet alcoholic persons with long-term sobriety. **(AA Survey Data/Length of Sobriety, p. 552)**

36.3 During an Alcoholics Anonymous (AA) meeting, a member tells his story to the group in attendance, putting emphasis on the effect of alcohol in his life, how he got sober, and what he is doing now to stay sober. What type of AA meeting was this member most likely attending?

A. Speaker meeting.
B. Step meeting.
C. Discussion meeting.
D. Open meeting.
E. Closed meeting.

The correct response is option A: Speaker meeting.

During a speaker meeting, a member tells his or her story to the group in attendance, putting emphasis on what happened (e.g., the effect of alcohol in that person's life), what was done about it (how the person got sober), and what the person is doing now to stay sober (option A). During step meetings (option B), one of the 12 steps is introduced by a group leader and discussed by the members. Discussion meetings (option C) involve a group discussion focused on a salient aspect of recovery. AA meetings may be open (option D) or closed (option E). An open meeting welcomes guests and those attempting to recover from alcoholism. Only those who consider themselves AA members or are contemplating membership should attend closed meetings. There is nothing in the scenario described above to suggest that the meeting is either open or closed. **(AA Program/Meetings, pp. 553–554)**

36.4 Which of the following is one of the 12 steps of Alcoholics Anonymous (AA)?

A. The only requirement for AA membership is a desire to stop drinking.
B. Anonymity is the spiritual foundation of all our traditions.
C. We admitted we were powerless over alcohol.
D. Our common welfare should come first.
E. Every AA group ought to be fully self-supporting.

The correct response is option C: We admitted we were powerless over alcohol.

The 12 steps (Table 36–1) and the 12 traditions (Table 36–2) summarize the principles of AA and are widely printed in formats ranging from wallet cards to placards. One gains sobriety, in part, by working through the 12 steps. The 12 traditions reinforce the integrity of the AA approach. Option C, "We admitted we were powerless over alcohol," is the first of the 12 *steps*. Options A, B, D, and E are all part of the 12 *traditions*. **(AA Program/The 12 Steps and 12 Traditions, p. 554; Table 36–3,**

TABLE 36–1. **The 12 steps of Alcoholics Anonymous (AA)**

1. We admitted we were powerless over alcohol—that our lives had become unmanageable.
2. Came to believe that a Power greater than ourselves could restore us to sanity.
3. Made a decision to turn our will and our lives over to the care of God as we understood Him.
4. Made a searching and fearless moral inventory of ourselves.
5. Admitted to God, to ourselves, and to another human being the exact nature of our wrongs.
6. Were entirely ready to have God remove all these defects of character.
7. Humbly asked Him to remove our shortcomings.
8. Made a list of all persons we had harmed, and became willing to make amends to them all.
9. Made direct amends to such people wherever possible, except when to do so would injure them or others.
10. Continued to take personal inventory and when we were wrong promptly admitted it.
11. Sought through prayer and meditation to improve our conscious contact with God, as we understood Him, praying only for knowledge of His will for us and the power to carry that out.
12. Having had a spiritual awakening as the result of these steps, we tried to carry this message to alcoholics, and to practice these principles in all our affairs.

Source. Alcoholics Anonymous: *Twelve Steps and Twelve Traditions.* New York, Alcoholics Anonymous World Services, 1978. The Twelve Steps and Twelve Traditions are reprinted with permission of Alcoholics Anonymous World Services, Inc. ("AAWS"). Permission to reprint the Twelve Steps and Twelve Traditions does not mean that AAWS has reviewed or approved the contents of this publication, or that A.A. necessarily agrees with the views expressed herein. A.A. is a program of recovery from alcoholism only—use of the Twelve Steps and Twelve Traditions in connection with programs and activities which are patterned after A.A., but which address other problems, or in any other non-A.A. context, does not imply otherwise.

The 12 steps of Alcoholics Anonymous [AA], p. 555; Table 36–4, The 12 traditions of Alcoholics Anonymous [AA], p. 556)

36.5   Which of the following is a common personal reaction to Alcoholics Anonymous (AA) that deters participation?

A. "I'm afraid I won't be able to get sober."
B. "I don't want to speak up in groups."
C. "I'd rather do this on my own."
D. "I can't identify with that group."
E. "I'm afraid of being judged."

The correct response is option D: "I can't identify with that group."

In addition to the craving or incentive to return to alcohol, many people encountering AA have personal reactions that deter their participation. The clinician should be alert to common responses and motivate the patient to overcome them. These include "I wasn't as bad as that" (patients often find differences between themselves and the people they meet at AA), "I can't identify with that group" (option D), "They're too religious" or "It's a cult," or "Someone tried to hit on me."

TABLE 36–2. The 12 traditions of Alcoholics Anonymous (AA)

1. Our common welfare should come first; personal recovery depends upon AA unity.
2. For our group purpose there is but one ultimate authority—a loving God as He may express Himself in our group conscience. Our leaders are but trusted servants; they do not govern.
3. The only requirement for AA membership is a desire to stop drinking.
4. Each group should be autonomous except in matters affecting other groups or AA as a whole.
5. Each group has but one primary purpose—to carry its message to the alcoholic who still suffers.
6. An AA group ought never endorse, finance, or lend the AA name to any related facility or outside enterprise, lest problems of money, property, and prestige divert us from our primary purpose.
7. Every AA group ought to be fully self-supporting, declining outside contributions.
8. Alcoholics Anonymous should remain forever nonprofessional, but our service centers may employ special workers.
9. AA, as such, ought never be organized; but we may create special service boards or committees directly responsible to those they serve.
10. Alcoholics Anonymous has no opinion on outside issues; hence the AA name ought never be drawn into public controversy.
11. Our public relations policy is based on attraction rather than promotion; we need always maintain personal anonymity at the level of press, radio, and films.
12. Anonymity is the spiritual foundation of all our traditions, ever reminding us to place principles before personalities.

Source. Alcoholics Anonymous: *Twelve Steps and Twelve Traditions.* New York, Alcoholics Anonymous World Services, 1978. The Twelve Steps and Twelve Traditions are reprinted with permission of Alcoholics Anonymous World Services, Inc. ("AAWS"). Permission to reprint the Twelve Steps and Twelve Traditions does not mean that AAWS has reviewed or approved the contents of this publication, or that A.A. necessarily agrees with the views expressed herein. A.A. is a program of recovery from alcoholism only—use of the Twelve Steps and Twelve Traditions in connection with programs and activities which are patterned after A.A., but which address other problems, or in any other non-A.A. context, does not imply otherwise.

Options A, B, C, and E are possible reactions to AA but are not the key objections that patients often have to AA that deter participation. **(Experiences of Patients, pp. 555–559)**

References

Alcoholics Anonymous: Alcoholics Anonymous Membership Survey 2011. New York, Alcoholics Anonymous World Services, 2012. Available at: http:// www.aa.org/pdf/products/p-48_membershipsurvey.pdf. Accessed January 20, 2015.

CHAPTER 37

Psychological Mechanisms in Alcoholics Anonymous

37.1   Which 12-step cognition at the end of 12-step therapy treatment significantly predicts increased abstinence at 12-month follow-up?

A. Powerlessness over alcohol.
B. Belief in loss of control over drinking.
C. Belief in a higher power.
D. Disease attribution.
E. Commitment to Alcoholics Anonymous (AA) and to abstinence.

The correct response is option E: Commitment to AA and to abstinence.

Morgenstern et al. (2002) investigated how effectively 12-step therapy promoted desired changes in 12-step cognitions by patients and, in turn, how these shifts in attitudes and beliefs predicted drinking at discharge and at 6- and 12-month follow-ups. The following 12-step cognitions at treatment discharge did not predict 12-month abstinence: powerless over alcohol, belief in a higher power, and disease attribution (options A, C, D). Loss of control over drinking is an example of a belief in powerlessness over alcohol (option B). Commitment to AA and to abstinence significantly predicted increased abstinence at both 6- and 12-month follow-ups (option E).

As noted by Morgenstern et al. (2002), commitment to abstinence is not unique to 12-step therapy, and AA referral across different kinds of therapy is common. In this light, it is unclear whether 12-step-specific cognitions (or more general shared psychological mechanisms) accounted for later abstinence. **(Specific Psychological Mechanisms/Cognitive-Based Psychological Processes, pp. 567–568)**

37.2   According to Project MATCH, how did the rates of abstinence at 12-month follow-up differ among patients assigned to cognitive-behavioral therapy (CBT), motivational enhancement therapy (MET), and 12-step facilitation (TSF)?

A. CBT clients reported the highest rate of abstinence.
B. MET clients reported the highest rate of abstinence.
C. TSF clients reported the highest rate of abstinence.

D. TSF clients reported higher rates of abstinence relative to CBT clients but not to MET clients.

E. None of the groups reported a significant higher rate of abstinence relative to the other two groups.

The correct response is option C: TSF clients reported the highest rate of abstinence.

Project MATCH (Tonigan 2005) was a large (N=1,726) randomized clinical trial that investigated whether different types of patients fared better in different types of alcoholism treatment, which included MET, CBT, and TSF.

On the basis of videotapes of client-therapist sessions, Tonigan (2005) reported that TSF therapists endorsed the goal of abstinence significantly more than CBT or MET therapists (option C, which is correct; options A, B, D, and E, which are incorrect). Although TSF clients reported significantly higher rates of abstinence at 12-month follow-up than did CBT and MET clients, Tonigan did not find that endorsement of abstinence among TSF patients accounted for this advantage. It appears, then, that although TS therapy differentially endorses the goal of abstinence, this increased emphasis does not produce or account for higher rates of abstinence among substance users receiving 12-step therapy. **(Specific Psychological Mechanisms/Cognitive-Based Psychological Processes, pp. 567–568)**

37.3 Which cognitive shift did patients who participated in 12-step therapy have in common with those who underwent cognitive-behavioral therapy (CBT) according to the Finney et al. (1998) study?

A. Endorsement of the disease model of alcoholism.
B. Alcoholic identity.
C. Goal of abstinence.
D. Self-efficacy to remain abstinent.
E. Increase in positive expectancies surrounding the use of substances.

The correct response is option D: Self-efficacy to remain abstinent.

Finney et al. (1998) investigated desired cognitive shifts among patients in 12-step therapy (n=970) relative to changes in patient cognitions in eclectic (n=1,067) and cognitive-behavioral (n=1,191) therapies in a Veterans Affairs hospital population. At discharge, all patients reported significant and relatively equal increases in self-efficacy to remain abstinent (option D) and decreases in positive expectancy surrounding the use of substances (option E). Finney and colleagues found significantly larger gains in endorsement of the disease model of alcoholism, alcoholic identity, and the goal of abstinence among patients receiving 12-step therapy (options A, B, C).

Although Finney and colleagues did not investigate relationships between intended and unintended cognitive shifts and substance use, this study raised the question of whether common, nonspecific therapeutic mechanisms operate in

12-step programs. **(Specific Psychological Mechanisms/Cognitive-Based Psychological Processes, pp. 567–568)**

37.4   Which specific psychological mechanism is one of the most important and well-studied causal mechanisms explaining substance use behavior change among 12-step program members?

A. Self-efficacy.
B. Acquiring a sponsor.
C. Spirituality.
D. Powerlessness over alcohol.
E. Motivation for drinking reduction.

The correct response is option A: Self-efficacy.

Self-efficacy, or confidence to remain abstinent, is an important causal mechanism explaining substance use behavior change and consistent predictor of clinical improvement (option A). To date, 11 studies have investigated Alcoholics Anonymous (AA) exposure and abstinence self-efficacy, and one firm conclusion is that 12-step members do experience increased self-efficacy to remain abstinent and that, in turn, such changes predict later drinking reduction.

Although acquiring a mentor or sponsor in AA as a guide to lead one through the 12 steps is predictive of increased abstinence, the act of acquiring a sponsor does not produce, in itself, increased abstinence (option B).

Strong evidence, across diverse measures of religiousness and spirituality, documents spiritual increases among AA members. A meta-analysis of six well-conducted studies on spirituality by the chapter authors suggests that there is a significant weighted effect between 12-step attendance and later increases in abstinence. The salutary direct effect of AA on abstinence, however, is not uniform across studies and ranged from nonsignificant to highly significant (option C). Frequency of AA attendance and later gains in spiritual practices were positively and significantly related as well. Finally, the chapter authors found gains in spiritual practices when combined across studies to be a significant predictor of later abstinence, although the magnitude of this action varied significantly across the six studies.

Outwardly, self-efficacy to remain abstinent and self-control over alcohol would appear to be positively associated and at odds with AA prescriptions about powerlessness over alcohol. Current speculation is that increased self-efficacy and powerlessness over alcohol may be reconciled by AA members acknowledging a loss of control after taking the first drink of alcohol but having some personal control and/or responsibility in taking the first drink (option D).

Surprisingly few studies have investigated how AA attendance and engagement may mobilize and sustain motivation for abstinence in spite of the centrality of motivation for drinking reduction (option E). **(Definitions, Context, and Moderators for Understanding AA-Related Psychological Processes, pp. 565–566; Specific Psychological Mechanisms/Confidence to Remain Abstinent, pp. 568–569; Spirituality, pp. 569–571)**

37.5   Increased Alcoholics Anonymous (AA) attendance has been associated with reduction in which of the following negative affect states?

A. Anger.
B. Resentment.
C. Depression.
D. Selfishness.
E. Narcissism.

The correct response is option C: Depression.

Negative mood states are assigned high priority as relapse precipitants in the core AA literature. Anger, resentment, and selfishness, for example, are specifically identified in the core AA literature as reasons for relapse; therefore, substantial emphasis is placed in AA on reducing or moderating those emotional states through the practice of prescribed activities. Kelly et al. (2010a) examined how changes in depression may account for AA-related benefit in the Project MATCH outpatient and aftercare samples. Findings about depression were complex and require careful consideration. As predicted, high levels of AA attendance were associated with decreased depression in both study arms (option C). Likewise, reduced depression was predictive of increased abstinence as well as reductions in drinking intensity in the aftercare and outpatient samples. Changes in depression associated with AA attendance during follow-up statistically mediated the direct effect of AA attendance on later drinking. Unfortunately, all of these paths became nonsignificant after concurrent alcohol use during follow-up was included in the models. Essentially, it appears that AA attendance predicted increased abstinence, which in turn led to reductions in depression. The relationship between AA attendance and resentment has not been specifically examined in the preliminary studies cited in the text (option B).

Within the context of Project MATCH, Kelly et al. (2010b) investigated the proposition that increased AA attendance among outpatient and aftercare clients would lead to reductions in anger, which would in turn predict increased abstinence. Although self-reported anger "marginally" predicted later drinking, especially drinking intensity, reductions in anger were found to be unrelated to the extent that AA meetings were attended (option A).

Tonigan et al. (2013) investigated how, if at all, AA participation produced reductions in selfishness, which in turn was predicted to increase abstinence. The Narcissistic Personality Inventory (NPI) was used to assess selfishness. AA attendance was unrelated to later NPI scores, which remained elevated through the 9-month study. Second, the proxy of selfishness, the NPI, was not predictive of later alcohol or illicit drug use (options D, E). **(Specific Psychological Mechanisms/Negative Affect, pp. 571–573)**

37.6 Which of the following is *not* true of the research regarding Alcoholics Anonymous (AA) and spirituality?

A. In Project MATCH, 27.6% of outpatient clients who attended AA meetings during the 12 weeks of treatment reported having had a spiritual awakening as a result of their AA attendance.
B. Spirituality is uniformly discussed in mainstream AA meetings regardless of differences in perceived AA group social dynamics.
C. Spirituality is measured by asking only about the extent that God is discussed in meetings.
D. Exposure to AA is associated with increased spirituality.
E. Gains in spiritual practices among AA members are a significant predictor of later abstinence.

The correct response is option C: Spirituality is measured by asking only about the extent that God is discussed in meetings.

The core AA literature posits that an individual will have a spiritual awakening as a result of working the 12 steps and that continued practice of spiritual principles will lead to sustained abstinence. In a series of three studies, spirituality was uniformly discussed in mainstream AA meetings regardless of differences in perceived AA group social dynamics (option B). In each of these studies, *spirituality* was defined using items asking to what extent God, spirituality, or a higher power was discussed in meetings and to what extent prayer and meditation were discussed (option C). In project MATCH, 27.6% ($n = 108$) of the outpatient clients who attended AA during the 12 weeks of treatment also reported having had a spiritual awakening as a result of their AA attendance (option A). Strong evidence, across diverse measures of religiousness and spirituality, documents spiritual increases among AA members (option D). A meta-analysis of six well-conducted studies performed by the chapter authors found gains in spiritual practices when combined across studies to be a significant predictor of later abstinence (option E). **(Specific Psychological Mechanisms/Spirituality, pp. 569–571)**

37.7 A practitioner should consider *not* adopting which of the following measures in clinical practice with substance abusing patients?

A. Develop familiarity with the *Alcoholics Anonymous* text ("big book").
B. Experience firsthand the environment and fellowship of Alcoholics Anonymous (AA) by attending several closed meetings.
C. Routinely assess patients' prior experience with self-help groups.
D. Negotiate AA attendance at several meetings for some patients.
E. Develop strategies that entail arranging for a current AA member to speak with the patient and arrange to take the patient to a meeting.

The correct response is option B: Experience firsthand the environment and fellowship of Alcoholics Anonymous (AA) by attending several closed meetings.

For a foundation, practitioners should be familiar with the core AA literature and should experience firsthand the environment by attending several meetings. AA groups typically hold open as well as closed groups, and all interested individuals are welcome at open groups (option B). Probably the most relevant text is *Alcoholics Anonymous* (2001) (commonly referred to as the "big book") (option A). We recommend that clinicians routinely assess at intake patients' prior experiences with self-help groups (option C). For patients holding negative perceptions of self-help groups independent of any actual previous self-help group experiences, it often is helpful to negotiate attendance at several meetings so they can obtain that experience or reassess such involvement (option D). Some patients may be readily poised to attend and follow through with attendance. Other patients may need more encouragement or in some cases practical assistance in getting connected to AA. This need has led to the development of several helpful clinical strategies that entail arranging for a current AA member to speak with the patient and arrange to take the patient to the meeting or to meet the patient at the meeting to guide him or her through the meeting process (Option E). **(Clinical Recommendations, pp. 573–574)**

References

Alcoholics Anonymous: Alcoholics Anonymous, 4th Edition. New York, Alcoholics Anonymous World Services, 2001

Finney JW, Noyes CA, Coutts AI, et al: Evaluating substance abuse treatment process models, I: changes on proximal outcome variables during 12-step and cognitive-behavioral treatment. J Stud Alcohol 59(4):371–380, 1998 9647419

Kelly JF, Stout RL, Magill M, et al: Mechanisms of behavior change in alcoholics anonymous: does Alcoholics Anonymous lead to better alcohol use outcomes by reducing depression symptoms? Addiction 105(4):626–636, 2010a 20102345

Kelly JF, Stout RL, Tonigan JS, et al: Negative affect, relapse, and Alcoholics Anonymous (AA): does AA work by reducing anger? J Stud Alcohol Drugs 71(3):434–444, 2010b

Morgenstern J, Bux D, Labouvie E, et al: Examining mechanisms of action in 12step treatment: the role of 12-step cognitions. J Stud Alcohol 63(6):665–672, 2002 12529066

Tonigan JS: Examination of the active ingredients of twelve-step facilitation (TSF) in the Project MATCH outpatient sample. Alcohol Clin Exp Res 29:240–241, 2005

Tonigan JS, Rynes KN, McCrady BS: Spirituality as a change mechanism in 12-step programs: a replication, extension, and refinement. Subst Use Misuse 48(12):1161–1173, 2013 24041178

CHAPTER 38

Outcomes Research on Twelve-Step Programs

38.1 Which of the following statements regarding 12-step mutual-help organizations (MHOs) is true?

A. There is extensive randomized-control trial evidence to support their efficacy.
B. They extend the benefits of professionally delivered treatment for substance use disorders.
C. The magnitude of benefit is significantly lower than that achieved with professional intervention efforts.
D. People with dual diagnoses are unlikely to benefit from attendance.
E. They are most beneficial as a short-term adjunct to outpatient professional intervention efforts.

The correct response is option B: They extend the benefits of professionally delivered treatment for substance use disorders.

Twelve-step MHOs extend the benefits of professional delivered treatment for substance use disorders. Naturalistic studies support their role as an important adjunct to professional care, especially as continuing care, and in helping to protect against relapse (option B). Twelve-step MHOs are not ideally suited for efficacy research through randomized controlled trials, because real-world participation usually is self-initiated and voluntary (except when court mandated), and randomly assigning individuals to attend these groups (or not) would conflict with the purpose of the groups and the way they are typically used (option A). Twelve-step attendance provides recovery benefits that are on par with the magnitude of those seen with professional intervention efforts (option C). Patient subgroups, such as those with dual diagnoses, may benefit from participation in traditional MHOs, but these benefits may be enhanced by attending groups tailored to their specific needs (option D). Although even short-term attendance may provide some benefits, naturalistic studies suggest that 12-step groups can serve as an important adjunct to professional care, especially as continuing care (option E). **(Outcomes of 12-Step Programs: Efficacy and Effectiveness/Effectiveness Versus Efficacy, p. 580; Effectiveness Studies, pp. 580–581)**

38.2 Twelve-step facilitation is a professionally delivered intervention designed to support engagement with 12-step mutual-help organizations (MHOs) such as Alcoholics Anonymous (AA). Which of the following patient characteristics is most important to consider when deciding whether to provide a standard or intensive referral to a 12-step group?

A. Age.
B. Gender.
C. Spiritual beliefs.
D. Prior experience with 12-step groups.
E. Comorbid psychiatric diagnosis.

The correct response is option D: Prior experience with 12-step programs.

Studies of which intensity of referral is most likely to benefit patients have reported that individuals with prior AA experience tend to have better outcomes when given brief advice, whereas outcomes among those with no or limited AA experience tend to be better (e.g., greater attendance rates) when more intensive referrals are provided (option D). Patient age, gender, spiritual beliefs (or lack thereof), and presence of dual diagnosis all are important for the clinician to take into account when recommending a particular 12-step program to an individual patient. The available empirical evidence suggests that, in general, these patient subgroups can benefit from participation in traditional 12-step MHOs but that benefits may be enhanced by attending groups that are more tailored to their specific needs (options A, B, C, E). **(Outcomes of 12-Step Programs: Efficacy and Effectiveness/Effectiveness Studies, pp. 580–581; Efficacy Studies: 12-Step Facilitation, pp. 582–584)**

38.3 Which cognitive 12-step mutual-help organization (MHO) mechanism of change is most strongly associated with recovery in adolescents?

A. Enhanced self-efficacy.
B. Identifying coping strategies.
C. Motivation for abstinence.
D. Increased religiosity.
E. Reduction in anger.

The correct response is option C: Motivation for abstinence.

MHOs, including Alcoholics Anonymous (AA), work both through mechanisms similar to those operating in professional treatment, including cognitive, affective, and social network mechanisms, and through mechanisms more specific to MHOs, such as 12-step activities and spiritual mechanisms. Both single- and multiple-mediator studies have been conducted to determine the relative importance of these factors in explaining AA's effects, as well as in identifying specific interventions that may be of special benefit to particular patient subgroups. Self-efficacy, coping strategies, and motivation for abstinence all are cognitive MHO mechanisms. Research in adolescents has found that motivation for abstinence mediates both the effect of early AA attendance after inpatient treatment and subsequent substance use outcomes (option C). Self-efficacy and coping were not found to mediate these effects in adolescents (options A, B). Increased religiosity falls in the spiritual, rather than cognitive, mechanism category and is associated with better outcomes among patients with the most severe alcohol impairments (option D). It has been hypothesized that 12-step groups exert their effects through mitigating unpleasant affective states, such as anger and depression. Affective (rather than cognitive) strategies aimed at reducing anger have not been found to mediate the relationship between AA attendance and improved drinking outcomes (option E). **(Psychology and Mechanisms of 12-Step Programs/Research on Mechanisms, p. 586)**

38.4 Twelve-step mutual-help organization (MHO) participation has been associated with which of the following?

A. Increased health care costs.
B. Increased patient reliance on professional services.
C. An abstinence rate one-third lower than that achieved by patients treated in cognitive-behavioral therapy (CBT) programs.
D. Improved outcomes in adults, but not in adolescents.
E. Helping individuals change their social networks in support of recovery.

The correct response is option E: Helping individuals change their social networks in support of recovery.

MHOs, such as Alcoholics Anonymous (AA), work through mechanisms similar to those operating in professional treatment but work most powerfully by helping individuals change their social networks in support of recovery (option E). Mutual-help groups can be attended for as long as necessary at little or no cost (option A). Research has shown that involvement in 12-step organizations can reduce the need for more costly professional treatments while simultaneously improving outcomes (option B). Patients treated in 12-step–oriented professional treatment programs have been shown to have a roughly one-third *higher* rate of abstinence than those treated in CBT programs (option C). Adolescents attending 12-step programs have been shown to achieve similar benefits to those found in adult participants, including improved substance use outcomes and lower overall medical costs (option D). **(Outcomes of 12-Step Programs: Efficacy and Effectiveness/Enhancing Outcomes and Reducing Health Care Costs, pp. 581–582)**

38.5 A 56-year-old man is convicted of driving under the influence and ordered to attend Alcoholics Anonymous (AA) as a requirement of sentencing. He drinks 7–10 alcoholic beverages per week and has no prior arrests for driving while intoxicated. Which of the following aspects of AA is most likely to be helpful to this person's recovery?

A. Increase in spiritual practices.
B. Increased confidence in ability to abstain in high-risk social situations in which alcohol is present.

C. Decreasing self-efficacy.

D. Increased ability to cope with negative affect.

E. Helping patients maintain current social networks.

The correct response is option B: Increased confidence in ability to abstain in high-risk social situations in which alcohol is present.

Among patients with more severe alcohol impairment, AA has been found to mobilize increases in spiritual practices, leading to better outcomes. The alcohol use history provided suggests a moderate, rather than severe, pattern of usage (option A). Research by Kelly and Hoeppner (2013) found that AA affected outcomes in men by increasing confidence in their ability to abstain in high-risk situations in which alcohol was present (option B). This is an example of increased, rather than decreased, self-efficacy (option C). AA also helped participants to change their social networks (helping individuals drop heavy drinkers and adopt abstainers) (option C). The results also suggested that AA tended to benefit women more by helping them enhance their confidence in coping with negative affect (option D). AA also helped participants to change their social networks (helping individuals drop heavy drinkers and adopt abstainers) (option E). **(Psychology and Mechanisms of 12-Step Programs/Comparing Mediators, pp. 588–589)**

References

Kelly JF, Hoeppner BB: Does Alcoholics Anonymous work differently for men and women? A moderated multiple-mediation analysis in a large clinical sample. Drug Alcohol Depend 130(1–3):186–193, 2013 23206376

CHAPTER 39

Women and Addiction

39.1 How prevalent are substance use disorders (SUDs) in women as compared with men?

A. The prevalence of SUDs is the same for men and women.
B. The prevalence of SUDs is higher in women as compared with men.
C. The prevalence of SUDs is higher in men as compared with women.
D. The prevalence of SUDs is higher in men only for certain substances.
E. The prevalence of SUDs is higher in women only for certain substances.

The correct response is option C: The prevalence of SUDs is higher in men as compared with women.

The prevalence of SUDs in men (10.4%) was significantly higher than that in women (5.7%) (option C) (Substance Abuse and Mental Health Administration 2012). In addition, the prevalence of current illicit drug use among men (11.1%) was significantly greater than the prevalence among women (6.5%) (options A, B, E). Compared with women, men were more likely to use marijuana (9.3 vs. 4.9%), cocaine (0.7% vs. 0.4%), prescription drugs (2.6% vs. 2.2%), and hallucinogens (0.5% vs. 0.3%) and to have higher rates of current alcohol use (56.8% vs. 47.1%) and tobacco use (32.3% vs. 21.1%) (option D). **(Epidemiology, pp. 597–598)**

39.2 Which psychiatric comorbidity is more likely to occur in men with substance use disorders (SUDs) than in women?

A. Anxiety.
B. Depression.
C. Eating disorders.
D. Borderline personality disorder.
E. Attention-deficit/hyperactivity disorder.

The correct response is option E: Attention-deficit/hyperactivity disorder.

Patterns of comorbid psychiatric disorders in men and women with SUDs parallel those found in the general population, with higher rates of anxiety, depression, eating disorders, and borderline personality disorder (options A, B, C, D) in women and higher rates of antisocial personality disorder and attention-deficit/hyperactivity disorder in men. **(Gender Differences in Co-Occurring Psychiatric Disorders, pp. 598–599)**

39.3   What is the "telescoping" effect of substance use disorders (SUDs) in women?

    A. Women have significantly more medical, psychiatric, and adverse social consequences as a result of their addiction.
    B. Women advance more slowly than men from initial substance use to regular substance use.
    C. Women have generally fewer years and smaller quantities of use at treatment entry and therefore have less severe disorders.
    D. Women appear less vulnerable than men to the development of adverse medical consequences of addiction.
    E. Women and men have very similar courses of SUD illness progression.

The correct response is option A: Women have significantly more medical, psychiatric, and adverse social consequences as a result of their addiction.

One consistent finding in studies focused on gender differences in SUDs is the increased vulnerability of women to the development of adverse medical and psychosocial consequences of addiction (option A). For example, it appears that women advance more rapidly than men from initial to regular use, and to first treatment episode (options B, E). Specifically, although women have fewer years and smaller quantities of use at treatment entry, their substance use severity is generally equivalent to that of men (option C), with women having significantly more medical, psychiatric, and adverse social consequences as a result of their addiction (Hernandez-Avila et al. 2004; Randall et al. 1999) (option D). This has been called the "telescoping" of SUDs in women, and it is thought that both biological and psychosocial factors contribute. **(Gender Differences in Course of Illness, pp. 599–600)**

39.4   What is the relationship between temporal onset of substance use disorders (SUDs) and comorbid psychiatric disorders in women?

    A. Women rarely have a primary mental health disorder that precedes the onset of an SUD.
    B. Women with major depressive disorder are less likely than men to develop alcohol dependence.
    C. Women usually develop SUD and other psychiatric disorders concurrently.
    D. Women receiving treatment for SUDs are likely to have histories of physical or sexual abuse.
    E. Women with eating disorders are unlikely to go to develop a SUD.

The correct response is option D: Women receiving treatment for SUDs are likely to have histories of physical or sexual abuse.

Gender differences in the temporal onset of SUDs and comorbid psychiatric disorders have also been observed. Specifically, women more often than men have a primary mental health disorder that precedes the onset of an SUD (options A, C). This suggests that there could be differences in the etiological relationship of substance use and comorbid psychiatric conditions between men and women (Kessler 2004). An epidemiological study exploring gender differences in the onset of major depression and alcohol dependence found that women with depression were more than seven times more likely than women without depression to have alcohol dependence at a 2-year follow-up point (option B) (Gilman and Abraham 2001). A number of studies have found that over 50% of women receiving treatment for an SUD have histories of physical and/or sexual abuse, and a high percentage have symptoms that meet criteria for posttraumatic stress disorder (PTSD) (option D) (Brady et al. 2004; Greenfield et al. 2010). Finally, eating disorders, such as anorexia nervosa, bulimia nervosa, and binge-eating disorder, are two to three times more common in women than in men and are particularly common in women with SUDs (option E). **(Gender Differences in Co-Occurring Psychiatric Disorders, pp. 598–599)**

39.5   What is an important consideration in the treatment of women with substance use disorders (SUDs)?

A. Women-focused treatments have better outcomes.
B. Pharmacological treatments lead to better outcomes in women.
C. Addressing psychiatric comorbidities leads to better outcomes.
D. Pregnant women should not receive pharmacological treatments.
E. Sociocultural factors are not frequently barriers to treatment.

The correct response is option C: Addressing psychiatric comorbidities leads to better outcomes.

Although women are often underrepresented in SUD treatment programs, most studies demonstrate that retention in treatment and relapse rates of women are comparable to those of men (Greenfield et al. 2007). Sociocultural factors (e.g., shame, lack of spousal/family support) can be significant barriers to women seeking treatment for SUDs (option E). Whether single-gender treatment is associated with better outcomes is an open question (option A). Treatment programs that pay special attention to psychiatric comorbidity, family and parenting issues, victimization, and gender-specific barriers to treatment are likely to be more successful for women (option C). Gender differences in the neurobiology of SUDs and the potential impact of hormones on the effects of substances of abuse and relapse suggest that there may be gender differences in response to pharmacotherapeutic treatment. However, there is a paucity of clinical research exploring gender differences in response to pharmacological agents currently used in the treatment of SUDs (option B). Psychosocial and pharmacological interventions may be helpful in reducing substance use and associated issues among pregnant and postpartum substance-dependent women (option D). **(Treatment, pp. 601–603)**

References

Brady KT, Back SE, Coffey SF: Substance abuse and posttraumatic stress disorder. Curr Dir Psychol Sci 13(5):206–209, 2004

Gilman SE, Abraham HD: A longitudinal study of the order of onset of alcohol dependence and major depression. Drug Alcohol Depend 63(3):277–286, 2001 11418232

Greenfield SF, Brooks AJ, Gordon SM, et al: Substance abuse treatment entry, retention, and outcome in women: a review of the literature. Drug Alcohol Depend 86(1):1–21, 2007 16759822

Greenfield SF, Back SE, Lawson K, et al: Substance abuse in women. Psychiatr Clin North Am 33(2):339–355, 2010 20385341

Hernandez-Avila CA, Rounsaville BJ, Kranzler HR: Opioid-, cannabis- and alcohol-dependent women show more rapid progression to substance abuse treatment. Drug Alcohol Depend 74(3):265–272, 2004 15194204

Kessler RC: The epidemiology of dual diagnosis. Biol Psychiatry 56(10):730–737, 2004 15556117

Randall CL, Roberts JS, Del Boca FK, et al: Telescoping of landmark events associated with drinking: a gender comparison. J Stud Alcohol 60(2):252–260, 1999 10091964

Substance Abuse and Mental Health Services Administration: Results from the 2011 National Survey on Drug Use and Health: Mental Health Findings (HHS Publication No. (SMA) 12–4725). Rockville, MD, Substance Abuse and Mental Health Services Administration, 2012

CHAPTER 40

Perinatal Substance Use Disorders

40.1   Which common psychiatric disorder or medical condition has the highest prevalence rate during pregnancy?

A. Depression.
B. Gestational diabetes.
C. Preeclampsia.
D. Tobacco use.
E. Alcohol use.

The correct response is option D: Tobacco use.

Tobacco use and alcohol use occur at higher rates than do preeclampsia (option C) and gestational diabetes (option B). The most recent National Survey on Drug Use and Health (Substance Abuse and Mental Health Services Administration 2012) indicates that of pregnant women in the preceding month, 15.9% smoked cigarettes (option D), 8.5% reported current alcohol use (option E), 2.7% reported binge drinking, and 5.9% used illicit drugs. The rate of depression was found to be 13% (option A). **(Introduction, pp. 607–608; Figure 40–1: Prevalence of selected disorders in pregnant women, 2010–2011, p. 608)**

40.2   Among all drugs of misuse, which ones have the most conclusive evidence indicating that prenatal exposure results in negative maternal, fetal, and later development outcomes?

A. Alcohol and tobacco.
B. Cannabinoids and cannabis.
C. Hallucinogens and cocaine.
D. Inhalants and amphetamines.
E. Illicit and prescription opioids.

The correct response is option A: Alcohol and tobacco.

Of substances used during pregnancy (Table 40–1) (options B, C, D, E), alcohol and tobacco (Option A) have the most striking data to support their negative consequences to the child following prenatal exposure. For example, effects of prenatal exposure to alcohol include miscarriage; premature delivery; mental retardation; learning, emotional, and behavioral problems; and physical defects of the heart, face, and other organs (Substance Abuse and Mental Health Services Administration 2005). Prenatal tobacco exposure appears to increase the risks of prematurity and low birth weight, which are risk factors for mortality, morbidity, and later developmental problems (Clark and Nakad 2011). Women who have other substance use disorders also frequently use these two substances. (**Substances of Use and Abuse, pp. 610–623**)

40.3 What treatment is recommended, because of its efficacy and safety profile, for treatment of nicotine use disorder in pregnant women?

A. Nicotine replacement transdermal (NRT) patch.
B. Voucher-based reinforcement therapy.
C. Nicotine replacement inhalers.
D. Bupropion.
E. Varenicline.

The correct response is option B: Voucher-based reinforcement therapy.

Preclinical data have shown that nicotine is harmful to the developing fetus; all but one of the NRT products are placed in U.S. Food and Drug Administration (FDA) Pregnancy Category D, indicating that there is evidence of human fetal risk (options A, C). The only exception is nicotine gum, which is placed in Category C. To date, there is no clear and consistent evidence that NRT is efficacious for smoking cessation in pregnancy (Clark and Nakad 2011). Bupropion (option D) is an antidepressant and was developed as a non-nicotine aid for smoking cessation in a sustained-release formulation. Bupropion is included in FDA Pregnancy Category C. Varenicline, an FDA Pregnancy Category C medication, seems to be associated with greater smoking abstinence rates, as well as greater reductions in smoking cravings and subjective withdrawal, than NRT. Currently, no data are available on the effect of prenatal varenicline exposure on fetal or child development. Therefore, varenicline is contraindicated for use during pregnancy and lactation until evidence of its safety in pregnant and nursing women is available (option E). Taken together, data on the safety and efficacy of all these smoking cessation medications are largely lacking. One of the most promising interventions for smoking cessation during pregnancy is voucher-based reinforcement therapy that is delivered contingent on verification of smoking abstinence (option B). Although this intervention has shown efficacy in reducing smoking and improving fetal growth (e.g., Higgins et al. 2010), more widespread larger trials are needed. (**Maternal Treatment for Substance Use Disorders/Tobacco Use Disorder, pp. 623, 627**)

TABLE 40–1. Teratological, fetal, neonatal, and developmental effects associated with common drugs of use during the perinatal period

Substance	Teratological	Fetal	Neonatal	Developmental
			Effects	
Caffeine	None known with any certainty.	Possible increased risk of spontaneous abortion with daily ingestion of greater than 150 mg. Association between moderate caffeine consumption and fetal growth not demonstrated.	Conflicting findings regarding the relationship between caffeine ingestion and birth weight. Relationship between caffeine ingestion and risk for growth restriction or preterm birth not demonstrated.	Relationship between caffeine ingestion and any adverse outcome (e.g., conduct disorders, autism, mental retardation, anxiety disorders, cognitive impairment, behavior disorders) not demonstrated.
Tobacco	Multiple studies suggesting increased risk of cleft lip/palate, clubfoot, craniosynostosis, and limb reduction, urinary tract, and cardiac defects; however, large-scale epidemiological studies would suggest no such increased risk.	Multiple studies suggesting increased risk of ectopic pregnancy, spontaneous abortion, placenta previa, placental abruption, intrauterine growth restriction, premature rupture of membranes, preterm birth, and stillbirth.	Multiple studies indicating increased likelihood of lower Apgar scores, low birth weight, smaller head circumference, and shorter length. Multiple studies indicate an increased risk of heart, respiratory, and ear problems. Multiple studies suggesting increased risk of sudden infant death syndrome (SIDS).	Multiple studies indicating increased risk of a variety of childhood cancers. Multiple studies suggest increased likelihood of ischemic heart disease, hypertension, diabetes, lung disease, and cerebrovascular accidents in adults. Multiple studies suggest increased likelihood of a wide range of cognitive deficits and social problems.

TABLE 40–1. Teratological, fetal, neonatal, and developmental effects associated with common drugs of use during the perinatal period *(continued)*

Substance	Teratological	Fetal	Neonatal	Developmental
			Effects	
Alcohol	*Fetal alcohol spectrum disorder* (FASD), describing a wide range of physical, intellectual, and behavioral problems that result from prenatal exposure to alcohol. These problems are expressed in the infant and child in a multiplicity of possible ways, and range in their impact from mild to severe. Three types have been identified, which vary based on their expression: *Fetal alcohol syndrome* (FAS), representing the most severe form of FASD, can be expressed as any one or more of: • Fetal death • Growth restrictions (e.g., head size and height) • Facial malformations (e.g., small eyes, thin upper lip, midfacial hypoplasia)		Multiple studies indicating prematurity, low birth weight, and small for gestational age, and negative motor function outcomes in the absence of FASD.	Multiple studies indicating that children exposed in utero to maternal alcohol consumption are at increased risk for problems both during childhood and in adulthood, including a failure to achieve in school, poor social relations, greater likelihood of substance use disorders, psychiatric disorders, and legal problems.

TABLE 40–1. Teratological, fetal, neonatal, and developmental effects associated with common drugs of use during the perinatal period (continued)

Substance		Effects		
	Teratological	Fetal	Neonatal	Developmental
Alcohol *(continued)*	*Fetal alcohol syndrome (FAS) (continued)* • Visual impairments • Hearing impairments • Neurodevelopmental abnormalities (learning, memory, and attention problems) • Problems with social relationships *Alcohol-related neurodevelopmental disorder (ARND)*, resulting in impairments in learning, memory, attention, judgment, and/or impulse control. *Alcohol-related birth defects (ARBD)*, resulting in problems with the heart, kidneys, bones, and/or audition.			

TABLE 40–1. Teratological, fetal, neonatal, and developmental effects associated with common drugs of use during the perinatal period *(continued)*

Substance	Effects			
	Teratological	Fetal	Neonatal	Developmental
Cannabis and cannabinoids	None known with any certainty.	Reports of no identified fetal effects. Reports of: problems with embryonic implantation, suppression of ovulation, intrauterine growth restriction, and decreased uteroplacental perfusion; increases risk of complications during delivery, including delayed onset of respiration.	Multiple reports of low birth weight, shorter length, and smaller head circumference; with some reports of failure to find physical birth parameter anomalies. Reports of deficits in neurobehavior shortly after birth, including poor autonomic control. Single report of congenital abnormalities following high prenatal exposure to cannabis.	Possible impaired on short-term memory, abstract/visual reasoning, and verbal outcomes in children of mothers who regularly used cannabis. Possible problems with school achievement; negative effects on problem solving, memory, attention, planning at age 16, as well as delays in cognitive development. Longer-term studies report the greater likelihood of depression at age 10 and use of drugs at ages 16–21, problems with impulsivity at age 16, as well as multiple reports of increased hyperactivity, inattention, and impulsive symptoms, and increased delinquency and externalizing behavioral problems.

TABLE 40–1. Teratological, fetal, neonatal, and developmental effects associated with common drugs of use during the perinatal period *(continued)*

Substance	Teratological	Fetal	Neonatal	Developmental
			Effects	
Hallucinogens	None known with any certainty.	None known with any certainty.	Relationship between prenatal MDMA exposure and length of gestation, rate of prematurity, birth weight, length, or head circumference not demonstrated. Prenatal MDMA exposure associated with poorer motor performance and coordination and slowed and delayed movement responses at 4 months of age.	Dose-dependent relationship between prenatal MDMA exposure and motor development at 12 months of age, with motor development of infants with less exposure similar to that of nonexposed infants. Dose-dependent relationship between prenatal MDMA exposure and mental development at 12 months of age, with mental development of infants with less exposure similar to that of nonexposed infants.
Cocaine	None known with any certainty.	Possible increased risk of vaginal bleeding, intrauterine growth restriction, and premature separation of the placenta; greater risk of rupture of membranes, increased labor and delivery problems, preterm delivery, and stillbirth.	Multiple studies indicating increased likelihood of lower Apgar scores, low birth weight, smaller head circumference, and shorter length, although there are numerous studies that also fail to support such findings.	Multiple studies examining performance on the Brazelton or Bayley infant development measures, often, although by no means always, finding decrements in performance in infants and children with prenatal cocaine exposure.

TABLE 40–1. Teratological, fetal, neonatal, and developmental effects associated with common drugs of use during the perinatal period *(continued)*

Substance	Effects			
	Teratological	Fetal	Neonatal	Developmental
Cocaine *(continued)*		Possible higher mortality for infants who are of low birth weight. Greater likelihood of fetal distress, fetal growth defects, non-specific suppression of fetal T-lymphocyte response, and poor fetal neonatal profile, including differences in latency to arousal and number of stimuli needed until habituation. Possible increased risk of congenital abnormalities, although research has also failed to support this contention.	Multiple studies reporting increased likelihood of some form of respiratory distress at birth, although there is at least one finding to the contrary. Multiple studies reporting increased likelihood of a longer time in the hospital and/or a longer time in the NICU. Multiple studies reporting increased likelihood of greater neurobehavioral problems at birth and/or shortly after birth. Several studies reporting increased likelihood of various physical problems at birth, including heart problems and EEG abnormalities, and greater risk of ankyloglossia and of neonatal withdrawal syndrome.	Several studies reporting both expressive and receptive language difficulties associated with prenatal cocaine exposure. Multiple studies reporting increased likelihood of problems in maternal-child interaction, increased problems in dealing with frustration and stress, and greater problems in play, although at least one study failed to support such a contention.

TABLE 40–1. Teratological, fetal, neonatal, and developmental effects associated with common drugs of use during the perinatal period *(continued)*

	Effects		
Substance	Teratological	Fetal	Neonatal	Developmental
Inhalants	Possible renal-urinary and gastrointestinal defects; possible cardiac and limb abnormalities. *Fetal solvent syndrome*, characterized by a combination of morphological and behavioral anomalies, not all of which are necessarily present: large fontanelle, small palpebral fissures, a narrow bifrontal diameter, midface hypoplasia, ear abnormalities, hair pattern irregularities, micrognathia, thin upper lip, and down-turned corners of the mouth.	Possible excessive menstrual bleeding, dysmenorrhea, and reduced fecundity. Possible spontaneous abortion, preeclampsia, intrauterine growth restriction, and premature delivery.	Possible low birth weight, small for gestational age, and small-for-age head circumference.	Children born with fetal solvent syndrome are reported to experience longer-term developmental problems similar to those found with children born with FASD.

TABLE 40–1. Teratological, fetal, neonatal, and developmental effects associated with common drugs of use during the perinatal period *(continued)*

| Substance | Effects | | | |
	Teratological	Fetal	Neonatal	Developmental
Amphetamines/methamphetamines	Possible microcephaly, anophthalmia/microphthalmia/microtia, anotia/microtia, transposition of great arteries, single ventricle, ventricular septal defect, atrial septal defect, cleft palate alone, cleft lip with/without cleft palate, polydactyly, situs inversus, and trisomy 21.	None known with any certainty.	Possible low birth weight, shorter length, small for gestational age, and growth restriction in term infants; lower Apgar score; and increased risk of strokes and gastrointestinal difficulties. Possible reductions in brain volume, notably in the putamen, globus pallidus, and hippocampus. Possible problems with arousal and stress. Possible symptoms of agitation, vomit, and tachypnea.	Possible poorer visual-motor integration, sustained attention, and long-delay verbal memory. Possible decreased arousal, increased stress, and poor quality of movement with a dose-response relationship to methamphetamine use.

TABLE 40–1. Teratological, fetal, neonatal, and developmental effects associated with common drugs of use during the perinatal period *(continued)*

Substance			Effects	
	Teratological	Fetal	Neonatal	Developmental
Benzodiazepines	Multiple reports of an increased risk of cleft lip/palate, neural tube defects, and cardiovascular and genitourinary malformations. Multiple reports of no teratogenic effects.	Reports of increased risk for intrauterine growth restriction and preeclampsia, although there are also reports that fail to find such effects. Possible increased risk of complications during delivery, including increased bleeding during delivery, cesarean section, mild respiratory depression, and increased risk of preterm delivery.	Multiple reports of an increased risk of low birth weight, lower gestational age at delivery, lower Apgar score(s), and/or low infant birth weight, with multiple reports of failures to find such increased risks associated with prenatal benzodiazepine use, with conflicting reports due to the trimester of exposure and/or the amount of exposure, although definitive data in this regard are lacking. Two reports of an increased likelihood of a neonatal abstinence syndrome occurring after birth. Findings weakly suggest that this increased risk is associated with third trimester exposure to benzodiazepines. Multiple reports of prenatal benzodiazepine exposure in the context of co-occurring prenatal methadone exposure increasing the likelihood of methadone-associated neonatal abstinence syndrome, with two reports failing to find this effect.	Limited findings weakly suggesting no longer-term cognitive deficits associated with prenatal benzodiazepine exposure.

TABLE 40–1. Teratological, fetal, neonatal, and developmental effects associated with common drugs of use during the perinatal period *(continued)*

		Effects		
Substance	Teratological	Fetal	Neonatal	Developmental
Illicit opioids	Multiple studies reporting congenital abnormalities associated with exposure to illicit opioids with conflicting results, with some studies suggesting increased risks for various birth abnormalities, and others failing to find such relationships.	Possible increased risk of infertility with heroin use. Possible increased risk of spontaneous abortion and stillbirth in pregnant women who use heroin.	Multiple studies suggesting that neonates prenatally exposed to illicit opioids have poor physical birth parameters (weight, length, and head circumference) and/or are born prematurely, have lower Apgar scores and may be small for gestational age, and are at substantial risk for a neonatal abstinence syndrome. Multiple studies indicating increased likelihood of longer hospital stay and some form of special care nursery care.	None known with any certainty.
Prescription opioids	None known with any certainty.	None known with any certainty.	None known with any certainty.	None known with any certainty.

TABLE 40–1. Teratological, fetal, neonatal, and developmental effects associated with common drugs of use during the perinatal period *(continued)*

	Effects			
Substance	Teratological	Fetal	Neonatal	Developmental
Opioid agonist pharmaco-therapy	Single large-sample study suggesting increased like-lihood of occurrence of any congenital anomaly.	Depression of fetal activity, respiration, and heart rate.	Multiple studies suggesting that neonates prenatally exposed to opioid agonist medications have increased likelihood of adverse impact on physical birth parameters (weight, length and head circumference) and/or are born prematurely, have lower Apgar scores and may be small for gestational age, and are at substantial risk for a neonatal abstinence syndrome. These outcomes are relative to non-drug-exposed infants, and the role of environmental factors are often not examined.	A recent meta-analysis of data from children up to 5 years of age showed no significant impairments in the domains of cognitive, psychomotor, or observed behavioral outcomes for prenatally opioid-exposed infants and pre-school children compared with nonexposed infants and children.

Note.   Guidance regarding illicit opioids should be understood to be limited to heroin and opium. Prescription opioids should be understood to include the class of pain relievers such as oxycodone, and exclude methadone and buprenorphine.
EEG=electroencephalogram; MDMA=3,4-methylenedioxy-*N*-methylamphetamine (ecstasy); NICU=neonatal intensive care unit.
Source.   Copyright 2013, Hendrée E. Jones. Used with permission.

40.4   What is the appropriate recommendation to give to a pregnant woman using opioids regarding breastfeeding her baby?

    A. Women using opioids should try to stop using all substances cold turkey and not be placed on agonist therapy.

    B. Breastfeeding is prohibited for women using prescribed opioids.

    C. Breastfeeding is recommended for opioid-agonist–maintained women who are not using other drugs, unless there are medical contraindications.

    D. Pregnant women with opioid use disorders should be treated with the opioid antagonist naltrexone.

    E. Pregnant women with opioid use disorders are not eligible for treatment with buprenorphine.

The correct response is option C: Breastfeeding is recommended for opioid-agonist–maintained women who are not using other drugs, unless there are medical contraindications.

Breastfeeding in mothers who are using illicit opioids is not recommended. Unless there are specific medical contraindications, breastfeeding for nursing mothers who are maintained on prescription opioids is likely safe (option B). Breastfeeding is recommended for opioid agonist–maintained women who are HIV negative and not using other illicit drugs (option C). Under conditions in which medication-free and methadone treatment are both available, methadone is associated with longer treatment retention and less relapse (option A). Providing appropriate opioid agonist medication during pregnancy may attenuate adverse consequences of nonprescribed opioid use for mother, fetus, and neonate. The literature indicates that both methadone and buprenorphine have benefits for the mother, fetus, and newborn (option E). The largest randomized controlled trial on this topic showed no significant differences in maternal outcomes between the two medications (Jones et al. 2010); this study provided the most rigorous data available to date to support the relative safety and efficacy of methadone and of buprenorphine during pregnancy. Regarding naltrexone, there are some limited data from Australia to support its use in pregnant women (see Jones et al. 2013 for a review), yet conclusive findings regarding the relative safety and effectiveness of naltrexone during pregnancy are needed (option D). The effects on breast milk of common drugs of use during the postpartum period and current advice regarding breastfeeding are provided in Table 40–2. **(Maternal Treatment for Substance Use Disorders/Opioid Use Disorder, pp. 627–628)**

40.5   Exposure to which substance during pregnancy typically does *not* produce neonatal abstinence syndrome (NAS) or a formal withdrawal syndrome in newborns?

    A. Percocet.

    B. Methadone.

    C. Fluoxetine.

    D. Nicotine.

    E. Methamphetamine.

TABLE 40–2. Effects on breast milk of common drugs of use during the postpartum period and current advice regarding breastfeeding

Substance	Effect	Advice
Caffeine	Approximately 1% of maternal blood plasma level of caffeine is transferred to breast milk, with peak concentrations several hours after ingestion. However, an infant does not develop the ability to metabolize caffeine until 3–4 months of age; consequently, caffeine accumulates in an infant's system, rather than being excreted.	Caffeine equivalent to 1–2 cups of coffee a day is unlikely to cause any change in an infant's behavior, with amounts above this level sometimes associated with increased irritability and agitation, and problems sleeping. Nursing mothers should be reminded that caffeine is an ingredient in many consumer products, and thus labels should be read carefully with regard to caffeine content.
Tobacco	Concentrations of nicotine in breast milk of smoking women ranges between 1½ to 3 times the concentrations in maternal blood plasma. Maternal smoking negatively affects breast milk production, and the production of milk may be insufficient for the energy needs of the infant. There is also the issue of exposure to secondhand smoke that might occur for the neonate whose mother smokes while breastfeeding.	Current guidance from the American Academy of Pediatrics is that maternal smoking is not an "absolute contraindication" for breastfeeding.
Alcohol	Alcohol is not stored in breast milk. Rather, levels of alcohol in breast milk closely parallel maternal alcohol blood plasma levels. As a result, breast milk will contain alcohol as long as there is a non-negligible maternal blood alcohol level. Maternal blood levels, and hence breast milk levels, of alcohol peak 30–60 minutes following alcohol consumption, and decrease for the next 4–8 hours, with considerable individual differences in both peak levels and rate of decrease.	Nursing mothers should avoid breastfeeding for at least several hours after consumption of their last drink to allow elimination of all alcohol from their blood. Breast pumping will in no way reduce alcohol concentrations in breast milk.
Cannabis and cannabinoids	THC, the active metabolite in cannabis, has been found to be more concentrated in breast milk than in maternal blood plasma levels.	Breastfeeding should not be undertaken if the nursing mother begins or continues her cannabis use.

TABLE 40–2. Effects on breast milk of common drugs of use during the postpartum period and current advice regarding breastfeeding (*continued*)

Substance	Effect	Advice
Hallucinogens	Research on the transfer of hallucinogens from maternal blood plasma into breast milk is lacking; however, it is known that the molecular weights of LSD and MDMA, for example, are sufficiently low that they are likely to be passed into breast milk.	Use of hallucinogens by a nursing mother should be strongly discouraged.
Cocaine	Cocaine is found in breast milk. Any cocaine ingested by the neonate will be absorbed in the neonate's intestinal tract. There are a number of adverse physiological and behavioral signs and symptoms associated with neonatal cocaine ingestion, including increased heart rate and blood pressure, choking and vomiting, and irritability and agitation.	Nursing mothers who are using cocaine should refrain from breastfeeding.
Inhalants	A number of different inhalants have been found to occur in breast milk, at concentrations typically higher than found in maternal blood plasma levels.	Nursing mothers who are using inhalants should be strongly discouraged from breastfeeding.
Amphetamines/methamphetamines	Methamphetamine is estimated to be between three and eight times more concentrated in breast milk than in maternal blood plasma. Neonates exposed to such breast milk show a range of adverse behavioral effects following breastfeeding.	Nursing mothers who initiate or continue amphetamine or methamphetamine use should be discouraged from breastfeeding.
Benzodiazepines	There is some suggestion that benzodiazepines do transfer to maternal breast milk, although there is insufficient information regarding concentrations in either breast milk or infant blood plasma.	Nursing mothers currently using benzodiazepines, either illicitly or under medical supervision, should likely be discouraged from breastfeeding.

TABLE 40–2. Effects on breast milk of common drugs of use during the postpartum period and current advice regarding breastfeeding *(continued)*

Substance	Effect	Advice
Illicit opioids	Women who are currently using heroin and/or illicit prescription opioids and choose to breastfeed may expose their infants to levels of opioids that are sufficient to cause tremors, restlessness, vomiting, poor feeding, or even addiction.	Breastfeeding in mothers who are using illicit opioids is not recommended.
Prescription opioids	Excretion of hydromorphone into breast milk appears negligible.	Unless there are specific medical contraindications, breastfeeding for nursing mothers who are maintained on prescription opioids is likely relatively safe.
Opioid agonist pharmacotherapy	Concentrations of both methadone and buprenorphine in breast milk are quite low, and seemingly unrelated to maternal methadone dose.	Breastfeeding is recommended for opioid-agonist-maintained women who are HIV-negative and not using other illicit drugs.

Note. LSD=lysergic acid diethylamide; MDMA=3,4-methylenedioxy-*N*-methylamphetamine (ecstasy); THC=tetrahydrocannabinol.
Source. Copyright 2013, Hendrée E. Jones. Used with permission.

The correct response is option E: Methamphetamine.

Most infants prenatally exposed to opioids (e.g., heroin, oxycodone [OxyContin], acetaminophen/oxycodone [Percocet], methadone, buprenorphine) will exhibit neonatal abstinence syndrome signs and symptoms, with a high percentage requiring pharmacological intervention (options A, B). Nonopioid substances, notably benzodiazepines, nicotine (option D), selective serotonin reuptake inhibitors (option C), and alcohol, can also cause infant behaviors consistent with withdrawal and/or can exacerbate NAS. Cocaine and methamphetamines do not cause withdrawal, but infants prenatally exposed to these substances may exhibit behaviors similar to those of newborns experiencing NAS (option E). **(Neonatal Abstinence Syndrome, pp. 629–630)**

References

Clark SM, Nakad R: Pharmacotherapeutic management of nicotine dependence in pregnancy. Obstet Gynecol Clin North Am 38(2):297–311, 2011 21575802

Higgins ST, Bernstein IM, Washio Y, et al: Effects of smoking cessation with voucher-based contingency management on birth outcomes. Addiction 105(11):2023–2030, 2010 20840188

Jones HE, Kaltenbach K, Heil S, et al: Neonatal abstinence syndrome following methadone or buprenorphine exposure. N Engl J Med 363(24):2320–2331, 2010 21142534

Jones HE, Chisolm MS, Jansson LM, et al: Naltrexone in the treatment of opioid-dependent pregnant women: the case for a considered and measured approach to research. Addiction 108(2):233–247, 2013 22471668

Substance Abuse and Mental Health Services Administration: Alcohol Can Harm the Way Your Baby Learns and Behaves. Rockville, MD, US Government Printing Office, 2005

Substance Abuse and Mental Health Services Administration: Results from the 2011 National Survey on Drug Use and Health: Summary of National Findings, NSDUH Series H-44, HHS Publ No (SMA) 12–4713. Rockville, MD, Substance Abuse and Mental Health Services Administration, 2012

CHAPTER 41

Adolescent Substance Use Disorders: Epidemiology, Neurobiology, and Screening

41.1 Current use of which illicit substance has been increasing among adolescents, after a prior period of decline?

A. Cocaine.
B. Heroin.
C. Marijuana.
D. Nicotine.
E. Phencyclidine (PCP).

The correct response is option C: Marijuana.

Current use of illicit substances among adolescents has declined since 2002 for most substances, including cocaine (option A), heroin (option B), nicotine (option D), and PCP (option E) (Substance Abuse and Mental Health Services Administration 2012). The use of marijuana, however, has been rising after a period of gradual decline (option C). Several factors are believed to be contributing to the rise, including decline in perceived risk of marijuana use, decline in disapproval, perceived availability, parental involvement, and importance given to religious beliefs. **(Epidemiology, pp. 635–636)**

41.2 Developmental patterns in which brain regions lead to particular vulnerability for substance use disorders during adolescence?

A. Curvilinear development of the striatum.
B. Linear development of the striatum.
C. Curvilinear development in the prefrontal cortex.
D. Linear development of the sensory and motor cortices.
E. Neuronal pruning in the sensory and motor cortices.

The correct response is option A: Curvilinear development of the striatum.

Striatal development (associated with reactivity to motivational stimuli) occurs in curvilinear fashion (option A, not option B), whereas prefrontal development (associated with cognitive control) occurs in linear fashion (option B) over the course of adolescence (Casey and Jones 2010). Amid a developmental window in which motivational reactivity outpaces cognitive control, adolescents may be particularly prone to making high-risk choices, valuing immediate reward over long-term considerations. Development of the sensory and motor cortices (options D, E) does not play as significant a role in vulnerability for substance use disorders as does development of the striatum and prefrontal cortex. **(Neurobiology and Implications for Adverse Outcomes, pp. 636–637)**

41.3   Which of the following screening tools for substance use disorders has *low* sensitivity in adolescents?

A. Screening, brief intervention, and referral to treatment (SBIRT).
B. Alcohol Use Disorders Identification Test (AUDIT).
C. Problem Oriented Screening Instrument for Teenagers (POSIT).
D. CRAFFT (mnemonic acronym for key words **C**ar, **R**elax, **A**lone, **F**orget, **F**riends, and **T**rouble).
E. CAGE questionnaire.

The correct response is option E: CAGE questionnaire.

The SBIRT model (option A), AUDIT (option B), POSIT (option C), and CRAFFT (option D) have each been validated for use with adolescents. The CAGE (ever tried to **C**ut down, **A**nnoyed by others concern, had **G**uilt about drinking, or needed an **E**ye opener) questions have low sensitivity among teens (option E) and therefore are not generally recommended for use in this population. **(Screening and Assessment, pp. 637–639)**

41.4   What is the relationship between adolescent report of substance use, parental report, and urine drug screens?

A. Greater than 95% of youths reporting no cannabis use will have negative urine toxicology.
B. Less than 50% of youths reporting cannabis use have positive urine toxicology.
C. Greater than 99% of teens reporting cannabis use will have positive urine toxicology.
D. Parent reports are more consistent with results of urine toxicology than youth reports.
E. Greater than 50% of youths reporting no cannabis use will have positive urine toxicology.

The correct response is option A: Greater than 95% of youths reporting no cannabis use will have negative urine toxicology.

Gignac et al. (2005) found that 97% of youths reporting no cannabis use had a negative urine drug test (option A, not option E), whereas 79% of those reporting cannabis use had a positive urine drug test (options B, C). Parental report was comparatively less consistent with urine testing than youth report (option D). **(Screening and Assessment, pp. 637–639)**

41.5 Which of the following questions is included in the CRAFFT screening interview for substance use disorders in teens?

A. Have you ever been in a car crash when the driver was intoxicated?
B. Do you ever use alcohol or drugs to relax, feel better about yourself, or fit in?
C. Do you use alcohol or drugs at social gatherings or parties?
D. Are you concerned that anyone in your family is using too much alcohol or drugs?
E. Did you ever forget to do something after using alcohol or drugs?

The correct response is option B: Do you ever use alcohol or drugs to relax, feel better about yourself, or fit in?

The CRAFFT was specifically designed for adolescents; its name is a mnemonic acronym for the key words in the questions included in part B of the screening instrument (**C**ar, **R**elax, **A**lone, **F**orget, **F**riends, and **T**rouble)). The CRAFFT is designed to be administered orally, similar to the CAGE questionnaire commonly used in adults; however, the CAGE has been shown to have low sensitivity in the adolescent population. Additional CRAFFT questions include the following: have you ever ridden in a car driven by someone (including yourself) who was "high" or had been using alcohol or drugs (vs. been in a car crash) (option A); do you ever use alcohol or drugs while you are by yourself or alone (vs. at social gatherings) (option C); do your family or friends ever tell you that you should cut down on your drinking or drug use (vs. concern that others in your family are using too much) (option D); do you ever forget things you did while using alcohol or drugs (vs. forget to do something after using alcohol or drugs) (option E). **(Figure 41–1, The CRAFFT Screening Interview, p. 638)**

References

Casey BJ, Jones RM: Neurobiology of the adolescent brain and behavior: implications for substance use disorders. J Am Acad Child Adolesc Psychiatry 49(12):1189–1201, quiz 1285, 2010 21093769

Gignac M, Wilens TE, Biederman J, et al: Assessing cannabis use in adolescents and young adults: what do urine screen and parental report tell you? J Child Adolesc Psychopharmacol 15(5):742–750, 2005 16262591

Substance Abuse and Mental Health Services Administration: Results from the 2011 National Survey on Drug Use and Health: Summary of National Findings, NSDUH Series H-44, HHS Publ No (SMA) 12–4713. Rockville MD, Substance Abuse and Mental Health Services Administration, 2012

CHAPTER 42

Adolescent Substance Use Disorders: Transition to Substance Abuse, Prevention, and Treatment

42.1 What percentage of adolescents who use cannabis progress to use of additional illicit substances?

A. 5%.
B. 10%.
C. 25%.
D. 50%.
E. 66%.

The correct response is option C: 25%.

The frequently-cited "gateway theory" of drug use, developed by Kandel (1982), proposed at least four distinct developmental stages of drug use: 1) beer or wine consumption, 2) cigarette smoking or hard liquor consumption, 3) marijuana use, and 4) other illicit drug use. According to Kandel, approximately one-quarter (26%) of teens who use marijuana progress to the next stage of further illicit drug use (option C), compared with only 4% who have never used marijuana. **(Initiation of Substance Use and Transition to a Disorder, pp. 642–643)**

42.2 Drug abuse prevention programs that limit drug use during which developmental period are most likely to lead to long-term beneficial effects?

A. 10–13 years.
B. 14–17 years.
C. 18–21 years.
D. 22–25 years.
E. 26–29 years.

The correct response is option C: 18–21 years.

Programs aimed at reducing risk factors during adolescence may have more beneficial long-term effects if they can limit drug use during the peak lifetime use period, ages 18–21 years (option C). Drug abuse prevention programs may have beneficial effects during early adolescence (option A) and mid-adolescence (option B), as well as young adulthood (options D, E), but programs that limit drug use during the peak years of use are most likely to lead to long-term effects. **(Initiation of Substance Use and Transition to a Disorder, pp. 642–643)**

42.3   What strategy has been shown to be most effective in reducing alcohol and drug consumption in teens?

A. Enhancing public advisory campaigns.
B. Increasing cost.
C. Intensifying legal consequences.
D. Mandating school-based educational programs.
E. Implementing self-esteem building programs.

The correct response is option B: Increasing cost.

Reducing demand (as opposed to supply reduction strategies) is an integral component of prevention of drug and alcohol use in adolescents. Alcohol consumption in youths decreased when the cost of alcoholic beverages increased (option B). Public advisory campaigns have not been associated with decreased alcohol and drug consumption (option A). Increasing the legal drinking age was associated with decreased consumption among teens; however, there is no evidence that harsher legal consequences decrease consumption (option C). Educational programs to increase knowledge of consequences of drug use (option D), and self-esteem building and responsible decision-making programs (option E), have been found to be ineffective in preventing drug use. **(Prevention, pp. 644–645)**

42.4   Of the treatment modalities studied for substance use disorders in the Cannabis Youth Treatment Study (Dennis et al. 2004), which modality was associated with a significantly different outcome than the other modalities?

A. Motivational enhancement was found to be effective only when followed by 10 cognitive-behavioral therapy (CBT) sessions.
B. Individual CBT without a family psychoeducational intervention was ineffective.
C. The 12-session individual community reinforcement approach led to no significant reduction in rates of cannabis abuse.
D. The 12-week family therapy was the only condition that was followed by sustained results.
E. Multidimensional family therapy was almost three times more expensive than the other treatment modalities included in the study.

The correct response is option E: Multidimensional family therapy was almost three times more expensive than the other treatment modalities included in the study.

The Cannabis Youth Treatment study (Dennis et al. 2004) has been the largest ($N=600$), most methodologically rigorous multisite randomized controlled trial to date to address outcomes of different treatment modalities on substance use patterns in teens. Participants were randomly assigned to one of five arms: 1) motivational enhancement therapy (MET) plus three CBT sessions, 2) MET plus 10 CBT sessions, 3) MET plus 10 CBT plus family psychoeducational intervention, 4) 12-week individual adolescent community reinforcement approach, and 5) 12-week family therapy condition. All five interventions produced significant reductions in cannabis use and negative consequences of use at 3 months (options A, B, C), with reductions sustained at 12-month follow-up (option D). Multidimensional family therapy was almost three times more expensive than any of the MET/CBT variants, making it the least cost-effective of the modalities studied (option E). **(Treatment and Aftercare, pp. 645–648)**

42.5 What is a limiting factor in most studies on treatment outcomes in substance use disorders in teens?

A. Treatment outcomes tend to focus on completion of programs rather than maintenance of gains.
B. Treatment outcomes are limited by lack of appropriate research participants.
C. Treatment outcomes are limited by difficulty consenting minors to participate in research.
D. Low relapse rates lead to low power in treatment outcome studies.
E. Poor availability of effective interventions for the adolescent population limit treatment outcome studies.

The correct response is option A: Treatment outcomes tend to focus on completion of programs rather than maintenance of gains.

Rather than focus on providing additional follow-up status about maintenance of treatment gains, most studies on treatment outcomes for adolescents with substance use disorders have focused on completion of treatment (option A). Relapse rates are high and are not a limiting factor in studies (option D). Substance use disorders are prevalent in teens (option B), and although research with minors requires additional consenting of parents, this is not a major limiting factor in research (option C). Many effective interventions are available for study (option E). **(Treatment and Aftercare, pp. 645–647)**

42.6 What is the primary rationale for determining whether to include aftercare in the treatment plan for adolescents following the completion of a substance abuse treatment program?

A. Aftercare interventions do not affect outcomes if the treatment program was effective.
B. Multiple aftercare personal sessions are required to maximize treatment outcomes.
C. Poor treatment responders are unlikely to benefit from further aftercare interventions.
D. Brief phone aftercare intervention is as efficacious as individual aftercare sessions.
E. Targeting aftercare to teens who relapse is an economical strategy to ration limited resources.

The correct response is option D: Brief phone aftercare intervention is as efficacious as individual aftercare sessions.

Aftercare has been shown to be more efficacious than no aftercare following treatment for substance use disorders in teens (option A). Brief phone intervention (option D) was shown to be as efficacious as a personal session (option B) for aftercare outcomes. Poor responders should be followed up in an effort to reengage in treatment (option C). Waiting for teens to relapse or failing to engage poor responders is a major public health concern and is more expensive than providing follow-up and aftercare (option E). **(Treatment and Aftercare, pp. 645–648)**

References

Dennis M, Godley SH, Diamond G, et al: The Cannabis Youth Treatment (CYT) Study: main findings from two randomized trials. J Subst Abuse Treat 27(3):197–213, 2004 15501373
Kandel DB: Epidemiological and psychosocial perspective on adolescent drug use. J Am Acad Child Adolesc Psychiatry 21(4):328–347, 1982

CHAPTER 43

Psychiatric Consultation in Pain and Addiction

43.1   Which of the following risk assessment screeners is most helpful in predicting which patients will ultimately be discharged form opioid treatment because of aberrant drug-related behaviors?

A. Screener and Opioid Assessment for Patients With Pain—Revised (SOAPP-R).
B. Pain Medication Questionnaire (PMQ).
C. Opioid Risk Tool (ORT).
D. Semistructured clinical interview by a psychologist trained in assessing aberrant behavior in the chronic pain patient.
E. DSM criteria for substance use disorder.

The correct response is option D: Semistructured clinical interview by a psychologist trained in assessing aberrant behavior in the chronic pain patient.

It has been shown that currently available risk assessment screeners fall well short of their goals of accurately predicting who will ultimately misuse prescribed opioid medications. Jones et al. (2012) assessed patients using the SOAPP-R, the PMQ, the ORT, and a semi-structured clinical interview by a psychologist trained in assessing aberrant behavior in the chronic pain patient. The SOAPP-R is a paper-and-pencil tool to facilitate assessment and planning for chronic pain patients being considered for long-term opioid therapy (option A). The PMQ is a tool for ongoing assessment of aberrant behavior associated with chronic prescription opioid use (option B). The ORT is a five-question screening tool to assess risk of developing aberrant behavior with prescription opioid use (option C). The semi-structured clinical interview was found to be most capable of predicting which patients would ultimately be discharged from opioid treatment because of aberrant drug-related behaviors (option D). When assessed for validity as a useful clinical screening tool, not one of these methods, including the psychological assessment, reached the requisite value for clinical usefulness (Jones et al. 2012). DSM (option E), while helpful in diagnosing substance use disorder, is not a risk assessment tool. Ultimately, clinicians will have to select best screening tools based on the patient population they serve. **(Introduction, pp. 651–652)**

43.2 A chronic pain management specialist discovers that his patient is chewing controlled-release morphine. Which of the following is the most likely explanation for this behavior?

A. The patient is experiencing inadequate pain relief.
B. The patient is abusing the morphine for reasons other than pain relief.
C. The patient has run out of medication and is trying to make his pills last longer by breaking them into smaller pieces.
D. The patient is borrowing medication from someone else.
E. The patient is attempting to justify the continued use of morphine to his physician.

The correct response is option B: The patient is abusing the morphine for reasons other than pain relief.

When a patient compromises a controlled-release delivery system by chewing the medication, the probability that this represents simple inadequate pain relief diminishes (option B is correct and option A is incorrect). If a patient is parenterally misusing an oral medication, the behavior can easily be seen as inappropriate and almost certainly represents a primary substance use disorder. When a patient runs out of medication early (option C), claims to have lost a prescription, or "borrows" medication from someone else (option D), the patient is exhibiting forms of aberrant behavior. There may, however, be legitimate explanations for these behaviors in the context of inadequate symptom control. The consultant is faced with the challenge of separating the possible "motive" from the abnormal "behavior" when assessing the presence or absence of a concurrent substance use disorder (Gourlay and Heit 2008). Option E does not explain why a patient would be chewing rather than swallowing the medication. **(Complexity of Differential Diagnosis for Aberrant Behavior, p. 656)**

43.3 A psychiatrist is treating a patient with chronic back pain, which is treated by a pain practitioner with opioids. The psychiatrist prescribes benzodiazepines on an as-needed basis for anxiety. The psychiatrist drafts a treatment agreement with the patient stating that requests for benzodiazepine refills may not occur over the phone. Which of the following terms best describes this therapeutic technique?

A. Interval dispensing.
B. Risk assessment.
C. Boundary setting.
D. Contingency dispensing.
E. Collaboration with pain practitioner.

The correct response is option C: Boundary setting.

The diagnosis of an addictive disorder is often best made prospectively, over time. It is important, however, that the patient is given clear boundaries (option C) from the outset (option C) in order to identify aberrant drug-related behaviors, should they occur (Gourlay et al. 2005). In many respects, it is easier to identify aberrant behavior than it is to interpret the meaning behind it (Gourlay and Heit 2008). Even more challenging is the identification and implementation of boundaries "after the fact." It is much easier to relax overly tight limits, as the patient's initial risk assessment is either confirmed or refuted, than it is to try and tighten up boundaries that should have been more explicit from the start (option B). In a perfect world, these boundary issues are formally dealt with before the first prescription for a controlled substance is written, but this is often not the case, especially in a consultative practice where the genesis of the referral is commonly based on some form of problematic behavior.

One of the more controversial recommendations in most current chronic pain management guidelines is the use of various monitoring tools recommended for the safe prescription of controlled substances. Interval dispensing (option A), contingency dispensing (option D), pill counts, and even the use of urine drug testing have all been seen, at one time or other, as evidence of a fundamental mistrust of the patient (Fishman 2005). Interval dispensing manages risk by reducing the total number of medication doses a patient is responsible for at any given time (option A). For example, a patient may see the prescriber once a month and receive four appropriately dated and signed prescriptions that can be filled only at weekly intervals. This is not to be confused with postdating a prescription, which is illegal under current federal and state regulation. Contingency dispensing (option D) involves the linking of prescription medication to some specific behavior. For example, a patient may be required to bring a medication to the prescriber for a pill count prior to receipt of the next prescription. Of all the risk management tools, urine drug testing is likely to be the most misunderstood. While collaboration with a patient's pain practitioner (option E) can be helpful in the identification and management of abberant drug-related behaviors, it is not specifically described in this clinical example. **(Importance of Boundary Setting and Universal Precautions, p. 654; Patient Monitoring, p. 656)**

43.4   Which of the following is a common feature in the care of patients who are ultimately referred to a mental health professional for assessment of aberrant drug-related behavior?

A. A clear pain diagnosis with workable pain differential.
B. Formal risk assessment, including detailed personal and family drug and alcohol history.
C. Presence of numerous prior treatment agreements.
D. Problems with limits and boundary settings associated with the original prescription of controlled substances.
E. Lack of patient concern around symptom relief.

The correct response is option D: Problems with limits and boundary settings associated with the original prescription of controlled substances.

Many patients who are referred to a mental health professional for assessment of aberrant drug-related behavior are confused as to the reason for the referral. A patient's and prescriber's perceptions around the patient's drug use may be at odds with each other. The patient's focus often is around symptom relief at all costs ("If you had my pain, you'd increase the dose, too") (option E is thus incorrect). The consultant, however, may be the first to identify significant problems with limits and boundary settings associated with the original prescription of controlled substances (option D). The *absence* of 1) a clear pain diagnosis with workable pain differential (option A); 2) formal risk assessment including detailed personal and family drug and alcohol history (option B); and 3) treatment agreements are common with referrals of this sort (option C). **(Importance of Boundary Setting and Universal Precautions, p. 654)**

43.5   Which of the following is an appropriate action for the prescriber to take when a patient disagrees about the quantity of controlled substances to be dispensed?

A. Clear communication and documentation of the prescriber's reasoning.
B. Prescription of whatever the patient requests in order to reduce discomfort at all costs.
C. Revision of the treatment agreement in order to facilitate the patient's request.
D. Immediate and complete elimination of the use of controlled substances.
E. Omission of this disagreement from the medical record in order to protect the patient from legal ramifications.

The correct response is option A: Clear communication and documentation of the prescriber's reasoning.

Miscommunication between prescriber and patient may underpin many of the conflicts that arise during a trial of opioid therapy, especially when a decision is made to call the trial a failure and discontinue the drug. Therefore, a treatment agreement, either formally written or simply documented as a discussion between the patient and prescriber in the patient's medical record, can go a long way toward clarifying the expectations that the patient may reasonably have of the prescriber and that the prescriber will have of the patient regarding the treatment of chronic pain (Heit and Gourlay 2010). Rights and responsibilities, for the most part, are bidirectional. In patient-centered medicine, the responsibilities are more evenly shared between the clinician or clinical team and the patient, who ideally plays the dominant role in his or her own care. When the patient and prescriber disagree regarding the decision whether to prescribe controlled substances, the quantity to be dispensed, or the frequency, the "power" (and responsibility) ultimately resides with the trained health practitioner. If the prescriber truly believes that in the interest of safety, he or she must limit or eliminate the use of controlled substances in a patient's care, then the prescriber must do so. There should be documentation and clear communication of these reasons to the patient, and the discussion should be recorded in the medical record. Although every reasonable step should be taken to reduce any potential discomfort caused by this course of action, patient safety must never be compromised. **(Application of a Universal Precautions Approach to Chronic Pain, p. 655)**

References

Fishman SM: Trust and pharmaco-vigilance in pain medicine. Pain Med 6(5):392, discussion 396, 2005 16266361

Gourlay DL, Heit HA: Pain and addiction: managing risk through comprehensive care. J Addict Dis 27(3):23–30, 2008 18956526

Gourlay DL, Heit HA, Almahrezi A: Universal precautions in pain medicine: a rational approach to the treatment of chronic pain. Pain Med 6(2):107–112, 2005 15773874

Heit HA, Gourlay DL: Tackling the difficult problem of prescription opioid misuse. Ann Intern Med 152(11):747–748, 2010 20513831

Jones T, Moore T, Levy JL, et al: A comparison of various risk screening methods in predicting discharge from opioid treatment. Clin J Pain 28(2):93–100, 2012 21750461

CHAPTER 44

Prevention of Prescription Drug Abuse

44.1   Which prescription drug or class of drugs was most abused among twelfth-grade students?

A. Adderall.
B. Vicodin.
C. Dextromethorphan-containing cough medications.
D. Tranquilizers.
E. Sedatives.

The correct response is option A: Adderall.

Past-year prevalence rates in 2012 document that prescription drugs are among the most abused illicit substances among twelfth-grade students, with 7.6% reporting abuse of Adderall (option A), 7.5% Vicodin (option B), 5.6% dextromethorphan-containing cough medications (option C), 5.3% tranquilizers (option D), and 4.5% sedatives (option E) (Johnston et al. 2013). **(Introduction, pp. 659–660; Figure 44–2, Past-year pharmaceutical drugs abused among twelfth-grade students in the United States in 2012, p. 661)**

44.2   Which class of prescription drugs is most commonly abused among persons age 12 and older?

A. Analgesics.
B. Tranquilizers.
C. Stimulants.
D. Sedatives.
E. Cough medications.

The correct response is option A: Analgesics.

According to the National Household Survey on Drug Abuse (Substance Abuse and Mental Health Services Administration 2012), approximately 14.7 million persons, or 5.7% of the U.S. population ages 12 and older, abused prescription drugs in 2011. In this survey, the most commonly abused drugs were analgesics (4.3%) (option A), followed by tranquilizers (2.0%), stimulants (1.0%), and sedatives (0.2%) (options B, C, D, E) **(Introduction, pp. 659–660; Figure 44–1, Past-year nonmedical use of prescription psychotherapeutic drugs among persons ages 12 and older in the household population of the United States, by drug type, p. 660; General Issues/Epidemiology of Prescription Drug Abuse, pp. 662–663)**

44.3   In which age group are females more likely to have abused prescription drugs relative to males?

A. Adolescents (ages 12–17).
B. Young adults (ages 12–25).
C. Adults (ages 26–45).
D. Middle-aged adults (ages 45–65).
E. Older adults (ages 65 and older).

The correct response is option: A: Adolescents (ages 12–17).

The National Household Survey on Drug Abuse (Substance Abuse and Mental Health Services Administration 2012) found that, in general, males had higher rates of abuse, with an important exception that adolescent females (ages 12–17) were more likely than males to have abused prescription drugs (7.5% vs. 6.5%) (option A). Higher rates by younger females for extramedical use of prescription drugs, especially opioids, have been documented in school- and college-based studies, in which self-treatment of medical conditions is endorsed particularly commonly among younger women (options B, C, D, E). **(General Issues/Epidemiology of Prescription Drug Abuse, p. 662)**

44.4   What is the strongest predictor of opioid misuse in chronic pain patients?

A. Age.
B. Gender.
C. Disability.
D. Measures of socioeconomic status.
E. Previous alcohol or cocaine abuse.

The correct response is option E: Previous alcohol or cocaine abuse.

Patients with chronic pain are frequently prescribed opioids, and this exposure is associated with risk of opioid misuse. In one study of chronic pain patients who were treated with opioids ($N=196$), the strongest predictors of misuse were self-reported histories of alcohol or cocaine abuse, or previous criminal-drug or alcohol-related convictions (Ives et al. 2006) (option E). Age was also predictive, but the effect was not large (option A). Gender (option B), race, literacy, disability (option C), and measures of socioeconomic status (option D) were not associated with misuse. In addition, no relationship between pain scores and misuse was found. **(Opioids [Analgesics], p. 664/Epidemiology of Prescription Opioids, p. 664)**

44.5 In treatment samples studied, how do heroin abusers differ from prescription opioid abusers?

    A. Heroin abusers have higher levels of benzodiazepine use.
    B. Heroin abusers have higher levels of depression.
    C. Heroin abusers have lower levels of chronic pain.
    D. Heroin abusers are more likely to be involved in psychiatric treatment.
    E. Heroin abusers have fewer family problems and less income from illegal sources.

The correct response is option C: Heroin abusers have lower levels of chronic pain.

In a treatment sample in Canada ($N=679$), prescription opioid abusers had higher levels of use of benzodiazepines (option A), higher levels of depression (option B), and more reports of chronic pain (option C) than heroin abusers (Monga et al. 2007). In a study of patients admitted to methadone maintenance treatment, those who used prescription opioids only or initially were more likely to have ongoing pain problems and to be involved in psychiatric treatment (Brands et al. 2004) (option D). Furthermore, individuals addicted to prescription opioids appeared to be more stable than individuals addicted to heroin; the former reported fewer family and social problems and less income from illegal sources (option E). Thus, they may be particularly good candidates for treatment with an antagonist, such as naltrexone, and they may be particularly well suited for outpatient office treatment with buprenorphine (Fiellin 2006). **(Opioids [Analgesics]/Differences Between Prescription-Type Opioid and Heroin Abusers, p. 665)**

44.6 Which prescription stimulant is most commonly abused by students?

    A. Adderall.
    B. Ritalin.
    C. Concerta.
    D. Metadate.
    E. Strattera.

The correct response is option A: Adderall.

A study of students (Teter et al. 2006) found that three-fourths (75.8%) of the 269 past-year illicit users of prescription stimulants reported using an amphetamine-dextroamphetamine combination agent (e.g., Adderall) (option A) in the past year, and one-fourth (24.5%) reported using methylphenidate (e.g., Ritalin, Concerta, Metadate) (options B, C, D). **(Stimulants/Epidemiology of Prescription Stimulant Abuse, pp. 666–667)**

44.7   How do individuals who engage in nonmedical use of prescription stimulants differ from those who engage in nonprescription use of opioids?

A. Increased abuse of stimulants is associated with the increase in prescribing of stimulants, whereas increased abuse of opioids is not associated with increased prescribing of opioids.
B. There is a perception that because prescription stimulants are medical substances they are safe, whereas this perception does not exist for prescription opioids.
C. Abuse of prescription stimulants may be particularly apparent in friends and peers of persons with attention-deficit/hyperactivity disorder (ADHD), because of diversion, rather than in individuals with the disorder themselves, as occurs with opioids.
D. Abuse of prescription stimulants is concentrated in older adults, whereas abuse of prescription opioids is mostly concentrated in adolescents and young adults.
E. There are no gender differences associated with abuse of prescription stimulants, whereas there are well-documented gender differences in the abuse of opioids.

The correct response is option C: Abuse of prescription stimulants may be particularly apparent in friends and peers of persons with ADHD, because of diversion, rather than in individuals with the disorder themselves, as occurs with opioids.

Prescription drugs are "legal" compounds, manufactured and distributed by the medical system before diversion occurs. Thus, prescription drug abuse is inexorably linked to medical practice in ways quite different from most other drug abuse. This also means that prescription drug abuse engenders a false perception of being inherently less risky than abuse of "street drugs" (option B). Just as increased abuse of opioids is associated with increased prescribing of opioids in general, high rates of abuse of prescription stimulants may be related to recent increased in prescribing of these agents for ADHD (option A). One key difference is that the problems of abuse of prescription stimulants used to treat ADHD may be particularly apparent among friends and peers of persons with ADHD, because of diversion, rather than in the individuals with the disorder themselves, as occurs with opioids (Compton and Volkow 2006; Volkow and Swanson 2003) (option C). Amphetamines and other pharmaceutical stimulants have had a relatively high prevalence of use in the youth population for many years. Analgesic abuse is also mostly concentrated in adolescents and young adults (option D). Gender, race, literacy, disability, and measures of socioeconomic status were not associated with misuse of opiates. In the overall population studied in the National Survey on Drug Use and Health (Substance Abuse and Mental Health Services Administration 2012), gender differences were not found with regard to abuse of either prescription or nonprescription stimulants (option E). **(General Issues/Medical System Issues, p. 663; Opioids [Analgesics]/Epidemiology of Prescription Opioids, pp. 664–665; Stimulants, pp. 665–667)**

44.8   Which strategy to combat prescription drug abuse has the most limited data to suggest efficacy in reducing harm from prescription drug abuse?

A. Family-based drug abuse prevention approaches.
B. Treatment for addiction, such as buprenorphine for opioid addiction.
C. Community distribution of naloxone to high-risk individuals and interested friends and family members.
D. Take-back programs for patients to discard used prescriptions.
E. Controlled substance tracking and monitoring.

The correct response is option D: Take-back programs for patients to discard used prescriptions.

Strategies to address prescription drug abuse are multiple. Demonstrating the potential for broad-based prevention approaches, universal family-based drug abuse prevention approaches have been demonstrated to reduce prescription drug abuse (Spoth et al. 2013). These interventions target families are key agents to address a range of adolescent-onset risk behaviors and have been shown to impact prescription drug use (option A). Treatment for addiction, such as buprenorphine for opioid addiction, can also be used to address prescription drug addiction (Weiss et al. 2011) (option B). Recent work has demonstrated the cost-effectiveness of overdose intervention with naloxone administration for heroin abusers. Perhaps most compelling, Walley et al. (2013) have shown that community distribution of naloxone to high-risk individuals and interested family and friends is associated with lower levels of overdose (option C). Because increases in both the number of prescriptions and the doses of opioids prescribed seem to be significant contributors to the problem, education and enhanced prescription access to patient prescription records might be part of the solution. Rapid, automated access to state Prescription Drug Monitoring Program data can inform clinicians about other controlled substances that may have been prescribed to their patients. Such information can change prescribing practices and may reduce both inadvertent and intentional medication misuse (Gugelmann and Perrone 2011) (option E). Efforts are under way to provide easier ways for patients to discard partially used prescriptions. These take-back programs show promise in removing unwanted, abusable medications from the public (Kaye et al. 2010) and have an inherently practical appeal. However, limited empirical data address the effectiveness of take-back programs in reducing the rates of prescription drug abuse or in reducing the harms for such abuse (option D). **(General Strategies to Reduce Prescription Drug Abuse, pp. 668–670)**

References

Brands B, Blake J, Sproule B, et al: Prescription opioid abuse in patients presenting for methadone maintenance treatment. Drug Alcohol Depend 73(2):199–207, 2004 14725960
Compton WM, Volkow ND: Abuse of prescription drugs and the risk of addiction. Drug Alcohol Depend 83(suppl 1):S4–S7, 2006 16563663
Fiellin DA: Buprenorphine: effective treatment of opioid addiction starts in the office. Am Fam Physician 73(9):1513–1514, 2006 16719242

Gugelmann HM, Perrone J: Can prescription drug monitoring programs help limit opioid abuse? JAMA 306(20):2258–2259, 2011 22110107

Ives TJ, Chelminski PR, Hammett-Stabler CA, et al: Predictors of opioid misuse in patients with chronic pain: a prospective cohort study. BMC Health Serv Res 6:46, 2006 16595013

Johnston LD, O'Malley PM, Bachman JG, et al: Monitoring the Future National Results on Adolescent Drug Use: Overview of Key Findings, 2012. Ann Arbor, MI, Institute for Social Research, The University of Michigan, 2013. Available at: http://monitoringthefuture.org/pubs.html. Accessed February 28, 2013.

Kaye L, Crittenden J, Gressitt S, et al: Reducing Prescription Drug Misuse Through the Use of a Citizen Mail-Back Program in Maine: Safe Medicine Disposal Handbook and Summary Report. Bangor, University of Maine, 2010. Available at: http://www.safemeddisposal.com/documents/MailbackProgramReportFINAL.pdf. Accessed February 20, 2013.

Monga N, Rehm J, Fischer B, et al: Using latent class analysis (LCA) to analyze patterns of drug use in a population of illegal opioid users. Drug Alcohol Depend 88(1):1–8, 2007 17049753

Spoth R, Trudeau L, Shin C, et al: Longitudinal effects of universal preventive intervention on prescription drug misuse: three randomized controlled trials with late adolescents and young adults. Am J Public Health 103(4):665–672, 2013 23409883

Substance Abuse and Mental Health Services Administration: Results from the 2011 National Survey on Drug Use and Health. National Findings. Rockville, MD, Substance Abuse and Mental Health Services Administration, 2012

Teter CJ, McCabe SE, LaGrange K, et al: Illicit use of specific prescription stimulants among college students: prevalence, motives, and routes of administration. Pharmacotherapy 26(10):1501–1510, 2006 16999660

Volkow ND, Swanson JM: Variables that affect the clinical use and abuse of methylphenidate in the treatment of ADHD. Am J Psychiatry 160(11):1909–1918, 2003 14594733

Walley AY, Xuan Z, Hackman HH, et al: Opioid overdose rates and implementation of overdose education and nasal naloxone distribution in Massachusetts: interrupted time series analysis. BMJ 346:f174, 2013 23372174

Weiss RD, Potter JS, Fiellin DA, et al: Adjunctive counseling during brief and extended buprenorphine-naloxone treatment for prescription opioid dependence: a 2-phase randomized controlled trial. Arch Gen Psychiatry 68(12):1238–1246, 2011 22065255

CHAPTER 45

HIV/AIDS and Hepatitis C

45.1 Which of the following statements concerning the epidemiology of hepatitis C virus (HCV) is *incorrect*?

A. HCV prevalence is highest for those born between 1945 and 1965.
B. HCV is most efficiently transmitted through exposure to infected blood, either through unscreened donors or by drug injection.
C. Long-term injection drug–using individuals have a high prevalence of HCV infection.
D. Provision of both primary and secondary prevention efforts and improving linkage to care can reduce the burden of HCV infection.
E. HIV co-infection dramatically triples the risk of liver disease, liver failure, and liver-related deaths from HCV.

The correct response is option E: HIV co-infection triples the risk of liver disease, liver failure, and liver-related deaths from HCV.

In the United States, HCV prevalence is highest for those born between 1945 and 1965, at 3.25%, accounting for about three-fourths of all chronic HCV infections (Centers for Disease Control and Prevention 2012) (option A). HCV is most efficiently transmitted through exposure to infected blood, either through transfusion of blood from unscreened donors or through injection of drugs (option B). Of persons injecting drugs for at least 5 years, 60%–80% of are infected with HCV, compared with about 30% infected with HIV (option C). Because the highest incidence rates of HCV occur in those who were recently initiated injection drug users, providing primary and secondary prevention efforts and improving linkage to treatment services can help reduce the burden of HCV infection associated with injection drug use (Smith et al. 2012) (option D). HIV co-infection more than triples the risk for liver disease, liver failure, and liver-related death from HCV (option E). **(Epidemiology/Hepatitis C, pp. 678–679)**

45.2 Which of the following sources accounts for the majority of chronic infections from hepatitis C virus (HCV)?

A. Sexual transmission.
B. Unscreened blood product transfusion.

C. Perinatal exposure.

D. Injection drug use.

E. Occupational exposure.

The correct response is option D: Injection drug use.

Although less prevalent than infection due to drug injection, HCV infection can also result from occupational, perinatal, and sexual exposures (options A, C, E). HCV incidence has dropped sharply since effective safeguards for the blood supply were put into place (option B), and the most common route of transmission for new cases is now drug injection (option D). **(Epidemiology/Hepatitis C, pp. 678–679)**

45.3   Which of the following statements concerning primary prevention of new infections from either HIV or hepatitis C virus (HCV) is *not* true?

A. Community-based outreach can be an effective prevention strategy.

B. Substance abuse treatment constitutes an effective prevention technique.

C. Comprehensive prevention strategies include syringe programs.

D. Longer duration of exposure to methadone maintenance treatment (MMT) has not been associated with greater prevention benefits.

E. Substance abuse treatment that leads to reduced alcohol use is expected to have a role in secondary prevention of alcohol-related exacerbation of HIV and/or HCV infection.

The correct response is option D: Longer duration of exposure to methadone maintenance treatment (MMT) has not been associated with greater prevention benefits.

Efforts aim to achieve primary prevention of new infections by reducing risk behaviors associated with HIV and HCV, such as injection and risky sexual behavior (Table 45–1). Comprehensive HIV prevention strategies include community-based outreach, substance abuse treatment, and syringe programs (National Institute on Drug Abuse 2002) (options A, B, C). A meta-analysis of 12 studies that assessed the impact of MMT on the incidence of HIV found that MMT was associated with a 54% reduction in risk of HIV infection among people who inject drugs, with evidence for greater benefit associated with longer duration of exposure to MMT (MacArthur et al. 2012) (option D). In addition to preventing new cases of HIV infection, substance abuse treatment that leads to reduced alcohol use may also be expected to have a role in secondary prevention of alcohol-related exacerbation of HIV and HCV infection (option E) (Loftis et al. 2006). **(Prevention of HIV or Hepatitis C Transmission in Drug Users, pp. 680–681, 682)**

45.4   Which of the following antiretroviral medications used for HIV infection is associated with the adverse side effects of anxiety, depression, suicidal ideation, confusion, and hallucinations?

A. Efavirenz.

B. Zidovudine.

TABLE 45–1. HIV and hepatitis C virus (HCV) risk reduction interventions

HIV	HCV
Screening	
Recommended in all health care settings; separate consent not required, just general consent for medical care; annual screening for those at high risk; as part of routine panel for pregnant women	Should be offered to individuals • with HIV • with history of injection drug use • who had blood transfusion or organ transplant before 1992 • who received clotting factor concentrates before 1987 • who have been on long-term dialysis • who have liver disease
Routine screening leads to early detection; reduces perinatal transmission; increases likelihood of starting HIV treatment	
No adverse effects such as psychological deterioration or increased distress or suicide risk or worse outcome in drug abuse treatment	
Posttest counseling	
May increase seeking medical care early	Counseling to reduce risk of HCV transmission to others; counseling to limit alcohol intake
	Medical referral for evaluation and treatment options including antiviral medications and immunization with hepatitis A, hepatitis B, pneumococcal, and influenza vaccines
Education	
Aimed at reducing HIV/HCV infection; instruction regarding condom use, syringe access program, use of clean injection equipment; special populations, such as those with severe mental illness, may be at higher risk for HIV and in need of risk reduction education	Treatment options
	Factors affecting course of HCV infection, such as alcohol use and smoking
Small group interventions build social support and share information	
No one psychoeducational counseling method has been shown to be superior over others	
Counseling aimed at reduction of risky sexual behavior	
Education regarding condom use and safe sex practices; counseling about responsibility to adopt safer behaviors and disclosure of HIV status to partners; skills training to enhance partner communication and assist in negotiating safer sex	
Interventions that offered more education and skills training led to greater risk reduction	
Referrals to HIV testing and counseling and treatment for sexually transmitted diseases	

Source. Centers for Disease Control and Prevention, 2009; National Institute on Drug Abuse 2002.

C. Ritonavir.

D. Lopinavir.

E. Nevirapine.

The correct response is option A: Efavirenz.

Antiretrovirals used to treat HIV/AIDS can also produce psychiatric and neurologic adverse effects. Efavirenz, a nonnucleoside reverse transcriptase inhibitor (NNRTI), may be associated with anxiety, depression, suicidal ideation, confusion, and hallucinations (option A), whereas zidovudine, a nucleoside reverse transcriptase inhibitor, can induce mania as well as produce agitation and insomnia (option B). Buprenorphine has been associated with cognitive dysfunction and increased drowsiness in patients with HIV receiving treatment with the protease inhibitors atazanavir or a combination of atazanavir and ritonavir, which are associated with increases in buprenorphine exposure and delayed clearance (McCance-Katz et al. 2007) (option C). Although medications that affect methadone metabolism can cause opioid withdrawal symptoms (as seen with the NNRTIs efavirenz and nevirapine and with the protease inhibitor combination lopinavir/ritonavir), no such withdrawal was seen in buprenorphine-maintained individuals despite marked reductions in buprenorphine plasma concentrations (options D, E). **(Treatment, pp. 681, 683; Psychiatric Aspects of Substance Use Disorders in HIV and Hepatitis C/Psychiatric and Substance Use Disorders in HIV, pp. 683–684)**

45.5   Which of the following neuropsychiatric complications associated with hepatitis C virus (HCV) infection is most problematic in the management of HCV-infected patients?

A. Fatigue.

B. Lack of mental clarity.

C. Depression from chronic HCV.

D. Ribavirin-associated neuropsychiatric disturbance.

E. Interferon-alpha-associated neuropsychiatric disturbance.

The correct response is option E: Interferon-alpha-associated neuropsychiatric disturbance.

HCV infection is associated with direct neurocognitive effects as well as adverse effects due to the medications used for its treatment. Central nervous system (CNS) complications of HCV infection have been observed to manifest as neuropsychological symptoms such as fatigue, depression, and lack of mental clarity (Forton et al. 2005) (options A, B, C). As may be expected, impairments have been worse in HCV patients with HIV co-infection or with a history of substance use disorders. The causes of neurocognitive impairment in patients with chronic HCV are multifactorial, but a direct biological CNS effect of HCV is thought to be implicated (Forton et al. 2005). The most problematic neuropsychiatric disturbances associated with chronic HCV disease are directly related to treatment with interferon and, to a lesser degree, ribavirin, the two principal antiviral agents that are used in combination to treat HCV (option D). Antiviral therapy with interferon-alpha can cause severe cognitive impairment as well as a host of other psychiatric symptoms, including depression, irritability, anxiety, mania, and psychosis (option E). **(Psychiatric Aspects of Substance Use Disorders in HIV and Hepatitis C/Psychiatric and Substance Use Disorders in Hepatitis C, p. 684)**

References

Centers for Disease Control and Prevention: Recommendations for the identification of chronic hepatitis C virus infection among persons born during 1945–1965. MMWR Morb Mortal Wkly Rep 61(4):1–32, 2012

Forton DM, Allsop JM, Cox IJ, et al: A review of cognitive impairment and cerebral metabolite abnormalities in patients with hepatitis C infection. AIDS (London, England) 19 (suppl 3):S53–S63, 2005 16251829

Loftis JM, Matthews AM, Hauser P: Psychiatric and substance use disorders in individuals with hepatitis C: epidemiology and management. Drugs 66(2):155–174, 2006 16451091

MacArthur GJ, Minozzi S, Martin N, et al: Opiate substitution treatment and HIV transmission in people who inject drugs: systematic review and meta-analysis. BMJ 345:e5945, 2012 23038795

McCance-Katz EF, Moody DE, Morse GD, et al: Interaction between buprenorphine and atazanavir or atazanavir/ritonavir. Drug Alcohol Depend 91(2–3):269–278, 2007 17643869

National Institute on Drug Abuse: Principles of HIV Prevention in Drug-Using Populations: A Research-Based Guide (Publ No. 02-4733). Bethesda, MD, National Institute on Drug Abuse, 2002. Available at http://archives.drugabuse.gov/pdf/POHP.pdf. Accessed January 27, 2015.

Smith BD, Jorgensen C, Zibbell JE, et al: Centers for Disease Control and Prevention initiatives to prevent hepatitis C virus infection: a selective update. Clin Infect Dis 55 (suppl 1):S49–S53, 2012 22715214

CHAPTER 46

Substance Use Disorders Among Physicians

46.1   When a diagnosis of substance use disorder in a physician patient is being considered, which of the following is true?

A. Reports of alcohol on the breath cannot be related to diabetes mellitus.
B. Thyroid disease symptoms cannot be confused with substance use disorder symptoms.
C. Physicians cannot have attention-deficit/hyperactivity disorder (ADHD).
D. Psychiatric disorders such as bipolar disorder or depression should be on the differential diagnosis.
E. Physicians cannot have psychotic disorders.

The correct response is option D: Psychiatric disorders such as bipolar disorder or depression should be on the differential diagnosis.

A differential diagnosis should be considered before making a final diagnosis of a substance use disorder for a physician as with any patient. The differential should include diabetes mellitus (especially when there are reports of alcohol on the breath or other erratic behaviors) (option A), thyroid disease (option B), or other hormone irregularities. Psychiatric disorders such as ADHD (option C), bipolar disorder, and major depression (option D) should be considered as well. In addition, although rare, incipient psychosis should be considered in some patients (option E). **(Warning Signs and Symptoms, pp. 692–693; Confirming the Diagnosis, pp. 693–696)**

46.2   Which of the following is true of the presenting signs and symptoms of physician substance misuse?

A. The signs of substance misuse are always specific and therefore easily identified.
B. Changes in sleep cannot reflect substance misuse.
C. Changes in weight cannot reflect substance misuse.
D. Needle marks, bruises, or bandages can reflect substance misuse.
E. Physicians are not likely to conceal symptoms reflecting their substance misuse.

353

The correct response is option D: Needle marks, bruises, or bandages can reflect substance misuse.

Early attention to presenting signs and symptoms of physician substance abuse is important, even if many signs and symptoms are nonspecific (option A). The earliest signs may include disruptions of various sorts in personal and family life. Certain physical changes might also suggest a substance use problem. These signs include deterioration in physical appearance; visible weight changes (option C); excessive fatigue; significant changes in sleep patterns (including sleeping much more or much less than usual) (option B); arriving at work bleary-eyed; smelling of alcohol on duty; and the appearance of needle marks, bruises, or bandages (option D). Physicians can be quite savvy about concealing their substance use, so any of these signs noted can be subtle if present at all (option E). **(Warning Signs and Symptoms, pp. 692–693)**

46.3   Which of the following is true about the epidemiology of substance use among physicians in the United States?

A. The rate of substance use disorders is higher in the general population than among physicians.
B. Anesthesiologists and emergency medicine physicians are at higher risk for substance use disorders than other physicians.
C. Pediatricians and surgeons are at higher risk for substance use disorders than other physicians.
D. Anesthesiologists tend to use more benzodiazepines when misusing drugs than other types of substances.
E. Emergency medicine physicians tend to use more opioids when misusing drugs than other types of substances.

The correct response is option B: Anesthesiologists and emergency physicians are at higher risk for substance use disorders than other physicians.

Substance use disorder rates among U.S. physicians are similar to rates in the general population, with the lifetime prevalence of substance dependence generally reported to be between 10% and 12% (Flaherty and Richman 1993; McLellan et al. 2008) (option A). Anesthesiologists and emergency medicine physicians are at greater risk compared with physicians from other specialties for developing substance use disorders (Hughes et al. 1999; Knight et al. 2007; Mansky 1996) (option B). Surgeons and pediatricians report lower rates of substance use and tend to be underrepresented in state physician health monitoring programs (Hughes et al. 1999; Knight et al. 2007) (option C). Among physicians who misuse drugs, emergency medicine physicians tend to use more illicit drugs (option E), anesthesiologists tend to misuse opioids (option D), and psychiatrists are more likely to misuse benzodiazepines (Hughes et al. 1992). **(Epidemiology, pp. 691–692)**

46.4 The "FRAMER" acronym for the principles of directive interventions recommended for clinicians treating substance-misusing physicians includes which of following?

A. Always conduct interventions in public places.
B. Never include a second clinician when conducting an intervention.
C. Begin all interventions with a threat to take a way a clinician's medical license.
D. Do not conduct an intervention with a physician who is intoxicated.
E. Any intervention should be at least 3 months after a sentinel incident of substance misuse.

The correct response is option D: Do not conduct an intervention with a physician who is intoxicated.

"FRAMER" is the acronym for the principles of directive interventions used to best "frame" concerns about a colleague recommended for clinicians evaluating physicians for substance misuse (Table 46–1). The recommendations include arranging for an intervention in a private location (option A), and at the earliest possible time after a sentinel incident (option E), but not when the physician is intoxicated (Option D). **(Intervention, pp. 696–697)**

TABLE 46–1. Principles of directive interventions

F	Gather all of the FACTS.
R	Determine your RESPONSIBILITY for reporting; consult confidentially with medical and legal experts.
A	Bring in ANOTHER PERSON.
M	Begin the meeting with a MONOLOGUE in which you present the facts and summarize your responsibility.
E	Insist on a comprehensive, independent EVALUATION. Refrain from giving a diagnosis.
R	Insist on a REPORT BACK, and obtain signed releases allowing all parties to freely communicate.

46.5 Which of the following is accurate regarding the prognosis for physicians with substance use disorders?

A. Physicians treated for substance use disorder have a rate of treatment success of 10%.
B. Physicians treated for substance use disorders have a rate of treatment success comparable to that reported for general treatment populations.
C. The low cost of failure for physicians with substance use disorders may contribute to the treatment success rate.
D. The low reward for maintaining sobriety for physicians with substance use disorders may contribute to the treatment success rate.
E. Highly structured treatment and relapse prevention programs may explain the rates of treatment success for physicians with substance use disorders.

The correct response is option E: Highly structured treatment and relapse prevention programs may explain the rates of treatment success for physicians with substance use disorders.

Physicians treated and monitored for substance use disorders have high rates of success, generally in the 75%–80% range (McLellan et al. 2008) (option A). These rates are far higher than those reported for general treatment populations (Noda et al. 2001) (option B). High success rates may be attributed to the highly structured treatment programs than many physicians enter, as well as the early and aggressive interventions used to prevent relapse (option E). Other factors may include the high cost of failure (e.g., loss of medical license, loss of income) (option C) and the considerable reward for maintaining sobriety, such as the ability to continue in medical practice (option D). **(Prognosis, p. 700)**

46.6   Which of the following regarding treatment for physicians with substance use disorders is true?

A. Caduceus groups are designed specifically for spouses of physicians with substance use disorders.
B. Physicians are never referred to 12-step groups because of concerns of confidentiality.
C. Health insurance will always cover the cost of residential treatments for physicians with substance use disorders.
D. Treatment of physicians with substance use disorders is not supported by extensive research.
E. Physicians with substance use disorders are always treated as outpatients given the stigma of residential treatment.

The correct response is option D: Treatment of physicians with substance use disorders is not supported by extensive research.

Few scientific studies have been published on what kind of treatment is best for physicians with substance use disorders (option D). Many physicians with substance use disorders are referred to residential treatment programs for "professionals," lasting 2–4 months (option E). This practice is controversial because physicians may object to the high cost and disruption to family and professional life. Physicians in residential treatment will be medically stabilized first before beginning intensive psychosocial rehabilitation, which includes, among other components, individual and group therapy and 12-step interventions, including Caduceus group meetings, which are designed specifically for medical professionals (options A, B). Health insurance seldom covers more than a fraction of the cost of a residential program, and the programs' significant expense can be prohibitive for physicians in training or those whose substance use has taken a significant financial toll (option C). **(Initial Treatment, Aftercare, and Monitoring, pp. 697–698)**

References

Flaherty JA, Richman JA: Substance use and addiction among medical students, residents, and physicians. Psychiatr Clin North Am 16(1):189–197, 1993 8456044

Hughes PH, Brandenburg N, Baldwin DC Jr, et al: Prevalence of substance use among US physicians. JAMA 267(17):2333– 2339, 1992 [erratum in JAMA 268:2518, 1992] 1348789

Hughes PH, Storr CL, Brandenburg NA, et al: Physician substance use by medical specialty. J Addict Dis 18(2):23–37, 1999 10334373

Knight JR, Sanchez LT, Sherritt L, et al: Outcomes of a monitoring program for physicians with mental and behavioral health problems. J Psychiatr Pract 13(1):25–32, 2007 17242589

Mansky PA: Physician health programs and the potentially impaired physician with a substance use disorder. Psychiatr Serv 47(5):465–467, 1996 8740485

McLellan AT, Skipper GS, Campbell M, et al: Five year outcomes in a cohort study of physicians treated for substance use disorders in the United States. BMJ 337:a2038, 2008 18984632

Noda T, Imamichi H, Kawata A, et al: Long-term outcome in 306 males with alcoholism. Psychiatry Clin Neurosci 55(6):579– 586, 2001 11737790

CHAPTER 47

Substance Use Issues Among Lesbian, Gay, Bisexual, and Transgender People

47.1 Which of the following statements about substance use in gay men and lesbians is true?

A. Research has demonstrated a genetic link between substance use and homosexuality.
B. Homophobia and antigay bias have contributed to substance use in gay men and lesbians.
C. The process of coming out results in internalization and pride in one's identity and can decrease the likelihood of substance use.
D. Substance use facilitates a link between sexual activity and intimacy, especially in gay men.
E. Gay men and lesbians with internalized homophobia are more likely to seek treatment for their substance use than are gay men and lesbians without internalized homophobia.

The correct response is option B: Homophobia and antigay bias have contributed to substance use in gay men and lesbians.

A genetic link between substance use and homosexuality seems unlikely. Studies have suggested differing genetics of male and female homosexuality; however, rates of substance abuse in gay men and lesbians are the same (option A). Several factors contribute to the prominent role of substance use and abuse in gay men and lesbians, including biological factors, social factors, and the psychological effects of heterosexism and homophobia, both internal and external (option B). The internal state that accompanies internalized homophobia can include numerous feelings—including fear, anxiety, anger, guilt, and helplessness—that are similar to the internal state associated with substance abuse. External homophobia is better known as *antigay bias*. Identity development as a gay or lesbian person, as well as the concomitant coming-out process, is complex and spans the life cycle. Although intact identity and pride may result, the process of identity development can also be associated with a sense of real or perceived rejection, leading at times to dissociation and denial. Substances such as alcohol and drugs mimic these feelings and can contribute to symptom relief (option C). In gay men, sexual activity and intimacy are frequently detached; substance use further widens the split between these experiences (option D). It is often more difficult to treat substance use in gay men and lesbians who have had difficulty accepting their sexual orientation (option E). **(Factors That Contribute to Predisposition to Substance Use and Abuse, pp. 710–713)**

47.2   Which of the following is the optimal treatment approach for substance use in gay men and lesbians?

A. Clinicians should prescribe 12-step programs, such as Alcoholics Anonymous, as the optimal treatment for most gay men and lesbians with substance abuse problems.
B. Treatment should focus primarily on the substance of choice.
C. Abstinence, sobriety, and recovery are the primary focus of substance abuse treatment in gay men and lesbians.
D. Evaluation of internalized homophobia and the patient's state of self-acceptance is critical in effective treatment of substance abuse in gay men and lesbians.
E. Effective clinical treatment of substance abuse in gay men and lesbians requires that the men and women in question have publically "come out."

The correct response is option D: Evaluation of internalized homophobia and the patient's state of self-acceptance is critical in effective treatment of substance abuse in gay men and lesbians.

Certain guidelines of 12-step programs can pose difficulties for gay men and woman. Needing to avoid or give up old friends can be particularly challenging for gay men or lesbians with limited contact who relate to them as a gay person. Additionally, avoidance of bars and parties may be difficult if these are the only gay social outlets available. Twelve-step programs are often perceived as "religious," and this may pose problems for gay men or lesbians who have found their religious institutions to be hostile or condemning of homosexuality (option A). Although treatment inevitably takes into account the substance of choice, the focus must be on not only the recovery from substance abuse but also recovery from the consequences of homophobia; self-acceptance of sexual orientation is critical (option B). Although sobriety and recovery are the ultimate goals of treatment, other strategies, such as harm reduction and relapse prevention, are also important focuses (option C). Optimally, treatment of gay men and lesbians takes place in a gay-affirmative environment. A full assessment of the individual's background in terms of his or her coming out process, the extent of internalized homophobia, and available support networks is critical to treatment (option D). Exploration of these issues in the treatment setting does *not* require that the individual has come out publically (option E). **(Assessment, Intervention, and Treatment Considerations, p. 713)**

47.3 What best characterizes substance-associated risks faced by gay men and lesbians?

A. Domestic violence is often connected with substance use and is highly reported in the gay and lesbian communities.
B. Most gay men are unaware of safe sex practices and are especially unlikely to learn them if under the influence of substances.
C. Alcohol and drug use can significantly affect health maintenance in gay men and lesbians with HIV.
D. "Reparative therapies" describe attempts to treat substance use specifically associated with the gay and lesbian community.
E. "Survivor sex" details sex-for-pay encounters seen in homeless gay and lesbian youths and is rarely associated with drug or alcohol use.

The correct response is option C: Alcohol and drug use can significantly affect health maintenance in gay men and lesbians with HIV.

Domestic violence exists within gay couples but is often significantly underreported (option A). In most reviews of gay men and safer-sex practices, the majority of men who were knowledgeable about safer sex but failed to practice safer sex were under the influence of some substance at the time (Choi et al. 2005; Leigh and Stall 1993) (option B). Substance use can be a major complicating factor in health maintenance for HIV-infected people because it can interfere with taking a complex regimen of medications on a specific schedule (option C). "Reparative therapies" or "conversion" describes practices to change sexual orientation; no data support this type of intervention, and indeed it has been found to cause significant harm (option D). "Survivor sex" describes sex for money that has been associated with drug use in homeless gay youths (option E). **(Specific Issues Regarding Treatment and Recovery/HIV, AIDS, and Other Health Risks, pp. 714–715)**

47.4 Which of the following statements about suicidality in gay men and lesbians is true?

A. Suicidal thinking and attempts occur in gay men and lesbians at comparable rates with heterosexual individuals.
B. Suicidal thinking and attempts in gay men and lesbians occur less frequently than in heterosexual individuals.
C. Suicidal thinking and attempts in gay men and lesbians occur more frequently than in heterosexual individuals, but rates of mood disorders in gay men and lesbians are lower than in heterosexual individuals.
D. Suicidal thinking and attempts in gay men and lesbians occur more frequently than in heterosexual individuals, with increased suicidality in older individuals.
E. Suicidal thinking and attempts in gay men and lesbians occur more frequently than in heterosexual individuals, with increased suicidality in adolescents and young adults.

The correct response is option E: Suicidal thinking and attempts in gay men and lesbians occur more frequently than in heterosexual individuals, with increased suicidality in adolescents and young adults.

Suicidal thinking, attempts, and completed suicides are of major concern for all people who use substances, but the concern and risks are even higher for gay men and lesbians, especially for adolescents and young adults (option E, not option D). Studies of suicidality in gay men and lesbians found the incidence to be as high as three times the national average. According to Paul et al. (2002), up to 30% of gay and bisexual individuals may have made suicide attempts. Studies have also shown that lesbian, gay, bisexual, and transgender people have *higher* rates of mood disorders, which may be an additional risk factor for suicide (options A, B, C). Substance abuse raises the risk of suicide in general. **(Specific Issues Regarding Treatment and Recovery/Suicidality, p. 716)**

47.5   Which statement best characterizes the use of methamphetamine?

A. The use of methamphetamine has been linked to increased risk of contracting HIV.
B. Methamphetamine use/abuse is found almost exclusively in gay men.
C. Risk of methamphetamine use in the gay community is found equally among different racial and ethnic groups.
D. Most methamphetamine use among gay men occurs at home.
E. Methamphetamine use decreases social anxiety, facilitating increased sexual experiences.

The correct response is option A: The use of methamphetamine has been linked to increased risk of contracting HIV.

The use of methamphetamines has clearly been linked to a higher risk for HIV infection (Shoptaw and Reback 2006). Through the experience of heightened sexual feelings and duration of sexual activity, allowing some men to have sexual intercourse for several hours with multiple partners, methamphetamine use places patients at increased risk of exposure to HIV, especially with unprotected anal intercourse or injection drug use (option A). Although methamphetamine use poses numerous psychological and medical concerns for gay men, it is not a drug exclusive to the gay community (option B). Studies have shown that gay men at risk for methamphetamine use include specific populations not typically associated with excessive substance use, specifically Asian and Pacific Islanders (Choi et al. 2005) (option C). Methamphetamine use is highly associated with "circuit parties" or with men who have sought sexual encounters through the Internet (option D). Methamphetamine is highly associated with increased sexual activity, primarily because of its effects on heightening sexual feelings and prolonging duration of sexual activity (option E). **(Types of Substances Abused and Patterns of Abuse, pp. 717–718)**

References

Choi KH, Operario D, Gregorich SE, et al: Substance use, substance choice, and unprotected anal intercourse among young Asian American and Pacific Islander men who have sex with men. AIDS Educ Prev 17(5):418–429, 2005 16255638

Leigh BC, Stall R: Substance use and risky sexual behavior for exposure to HIV. Issues in methodology, interpretation, and prevention. Am Psychol 48(10):1035–1045, 1993 8256876

Paul JP, Catania J, Pollack L, et al: Suicide attempts among gay and bisexual men: lifetime prevalence and antecedents. Am J Public Health 92(8):1338–1345, 2002 12144994

Shoptaw S, Reback CJ: Associations between methamphetamine use and HIV among men who have sex with men: a model for guiding public policy. J Urban Health 83(6):1151–1157, 2006 17111217

CHAPTER 48

Minorities

48.1 A 25-year-old Asian American graduate student experiences severe flushing, nausea, and dysphoria after consuming two shots of whiskey. Which of the following genetic mechanisms is the most likely cause of his reaction?

A. Cytochrome P450 isoenzyme 1A2 ultrarapid metabolizer status.
B. Serotonin transporter gene polymorphism.
C. Aldehyde dehydrogenase (ALDH2) isoenzyme deficiency.
D. Tyrosine hydroxylase deficiency.
E. Methyl tetrahydrofolate reductase deficiency.

The correct response is option C: Aldehyde dehydrogenase (ALDH2) isoenzyme deficiency.

Up to 50% of Asians have a deficiency of the ALDH2 isoenzyme, which is responsible for metabolizing acetaldehyde. A deficiency in this enzyme may protect against excessive drinking behavior by causing an alcohol flush and dysphoric reaction (Wall et al. 1997). Options A, B, D, and E are not directly involved in alcohol metabolism. **(Cultural Risk Factors, pp. 730–731)**

48.2 Sacramental ingestion of peyote cactus in the Native American Church is an example of which of the following?

A. Generational change.
B. Norm conflict.
C. Inadequate ensocialization.
D. Culturally prescribed use.
E. Disenfranchised groups.

The correct response is option D: Culturally prescribed use.

Culturally prescribed use (option D), in which an individual must use a psychoactive substance under certain cultural circumstances, exists among many ethnic groups in the United States. Examples include consumption of wine at Jewish Passover Seders and peyote chewing at ceremonies of the Native American Church (La Barre 1964). Prescribed use serves religious and social ends. Duration of use and dosages are prescribed (options A, B, C, E), and failure to use the substance can be considered deviant. The other answers are examples of cultural risk factors for substance use. **(Ethnic Identity and Substance Use, pp. 729–730)**

48.3   Which of the following racial/ethnic groups has the highest alcoholic liver cirrhosis mortality rates?

A. White.
B. Black.
C. Hispanic.
D. Asian.
E. Pacific Islander.

The correct response is option C: Hispanic.

Hispanic people have the highest cirrhosis rates (option C), at 13 per 100,000 compared with 8.7 for African Americans (option B) and 6.8 for whites (option A) (Stinson et al. 2001). These highly variable rates probably reflect ethnic differences in health practices, health care disparities, and possibly genomic differences among ethnic groups. **(Medical Comorbidity and Culture, p. 732)**

48.4   A 19-year-old college freshman is brought to the local emergency department in an obtunded state. He had been at a frat party and consumed a case of beer in less than 2 hours. Which of the following cultural risk factors does his drinking represent?

A. Technological changes.
B. Pathogenic use patterns.
C. Inadequate ensocialization.
D. Disenfranchised groups.
E. Generational change.

The correct response is option B: Pathogenic use patterns.

Pathogenic use patterns (option B) can occur as a behavioral norm, especially in groups with norm conflict regarding substance use. An example of such a pathogenic use pattern is bingeing on alcohol. This pattern exists among some northern European groups, Native American tribes, island communities in the Pacific, and American college students. It is likely to lead to pathological use of alcohol among vulnerable persons. Lifetime risk of alcohol or opiate abuse can occur in up to half of the men and a quarter of the women in certain groups (Boehnlein et al. 1992–1993; Westermeyer 1982).

Technological changes (option A) can render a traditional use pattern unsafe. Particularly at risk are societies that formerly accepted very heavy intoxication at ceremonial times or that permitted alcohol or drug use during certain types of work. *Inadequate ensocialization* (option C) occurs if the society's norms regarding substances are not taught to children. Teaching occurs initially by role modeling and later through supervised use in ritual settings. *Disenfranchised groups* (option D) may play major roles in the drug trade. Funds raised through the drug trade have supported revolutionary and nationalistic movements, guerilla wars, and terrorism (Westermeyer 1982). *Generational change* (option E) can influence the forms of psychoactive substance use within a given culture. Secular use may replace ritual or ceremonial use, individual choice replaces group decision making, and untried patterns replace safe patterns that evolved over centuries. **(Cultural Risk Factors, pp. 730–731)**

48.5   By providing white and black addictions counselors with education about models of healing preferred by Native American patients receiving treatment in that program, which of the following perceived barriers to care can be ameliorated?

A. System barriers.
B. Family barriers.
C. Staff member barriers.
D. Patient barriers.
E. Community barriers.

The correct response is option C: Staff member barriers.

According to the 2000 U.S. census, individuals belonging to a racial or ethnic minority group represented approximately 30% of the population; this figure is expected to rise to approximately 50% by 2050. In recognition of growing diversity, the U.S. Department of Health and Human Services, Office of Minority Health, issued *National Standards for Culturally and Linguistically Appropriate Services in Health Care.* Acquiring an understanding of an individual's substance use disorder within the context of his or her cultural beliefs and attitudes may assist providers in delivering acceptable and more successful care (option C). Providing treatment that acknowledges the needs of minority patients is key to culturally competent care.

Perceived barriers to care can impede treatment seeking among minorities. In a community survey, Westermeyer et al. (2002) asked 543 Native American veterans about perceived barriers to mental health care in Department of Veterans Affairs (VA) settings. An item analysis found 24 barriers that fell into four general categories:

1. *System barriers* (option A). Problems using VA services; absence of VA outreach or services in Native American communities (2.0 barriers per veteran ± 1.4)
2. *Veteran barriers* (option D). Mistrust, lack of knowledge regarding VA, inadequate resources to access VA (e.g., telephone, transportation) (1.3 barriers per veteran ± 1.2)
3. *Staff member barriers* (option C). Staff's lack of familiarity or skill in providing care for Native American veterans (0.5 barriers per veteran ± 0.8)
4. *Family community barriers* (options B, E). Shame, stigma, not supporting veterans with mental health problems (0.04 barriers per veteran ± 0).

(Ethnicity and Treatment, pp. 734–735)

References

Boehnlein JK, Kinzei JD, Leung PK, et al: The natural history of medical and psychiatric disorders in an American Indian community. Cult Med Psychiatry 16(4):543–554, 1992–1993 1305532

La Barre W: The Peyote Cult. Hamden, CT, Shoe String Press, 1964

Stinson FS, Grant BF, Dufour MC: The critical dimension of ethnicity in liver cirrhosis mortality statistics. Alcohol Clin Exp Res 25(8):1181–1187, 2001 11505049

Wall TL, Peterson CM, Peterson KP, et al: Alcohol metabolism in Asian-American men with genetic polymorphisms of aldehyde dehydrogenase. Ann Intern Med 127(5):376–379, 1997 9273829

Westermeyer J: Poppies, Pipes and People: Opium and Its Use in Laos. Berkeley, University of California Press, 1982

Westermeyer J, Canive J, Thuras P, et al: Perceived barriers to VA mental health care among Upper Midwest American Indian veterans: description and associations. Med Care 40 (1, suppl):I62–I71, 2002 11789633

CHAPTER 49

Testing to Identify Recent Drug Use

49.1   What is most drug testing used to detect?

A. Recent use of drugs and alcohol.
B. Dependence.
C. Intoxication.
D. Impairment.
E. Addiction.

The correct response is option A: Recent use of drugs and alcohol.

Most drug testing retrospectively identifies the recent use of drugs and alcohol (option A). Drug tests cannot detect or measure drug-caused impairment (option D), physical dependence (option B), intoxication (option C), or addiction to alcohol or other drugs (option E) (DuPont 2000); these clinically important determinations rely, as does the diagnosis of addictive illness itself, primarily on clinical assessments, with the laboratory findings often providing complementary data (options B, C, D, E). **(Introduction, p. 741)**

49.2   A 25-year old man is pulled over while driving and found to have a blood alcohol concentration of 0.11. He pleads no contest to a charge of driving under the influence. As a condition of probation, he is required to abstain from alcohol use and to submit to follow-up testing. Which testing strategy is most appropriate for determining his abstinence from alcohol?

A. Blood alcohol level.
B. Urine alcohol level.
C. Urine test for ethyl glucuronide (EtG).
D. Saliva testing.
E. Breath alcohol testing.

The correct response is option C: Urine test for ethyl glucuronide (EtG).

EtG is a common and relatively stable metabolite of alcohol and generally is identifiable in urine 3–5 days after drinking, making urine testing for EtG useful in medical and criminal justice programs where abstinence is a program requirement (option C). Alcohol is eliminated from blood, urine, and breath within a few hours of consumption, and as such, direct alcohol tests by these methods (options A, B, E) are of limited value in programs where the standard involves complete abstinence. Saliva (oral fluid) testing may be helpful in assessing for very recent alcohol usage but is not used in monitoring for alcohol abstinence, because it has a common surveillance window of fewer than 48 hours (option D). See Table 49–1 for a summary of testing methods for drugs of abuse. **(Sample Selection: Blood, Urine, Hair, Oral Fluid, and Sweat, pp. 744–748, 750, 751–752; Alcohol Testing, pp. 749–750, 753)**

49.3   How are most drug and alcohol tests confirmed?

A. By the laboratory that conducted the test.
B. By a sample donor's admission of recent use.
C. By the manufacturer of the test kit.
D. By on-site (not laboratory based) confirmation tests.
E. By a certified medical review officer.

The correct response is option B: By a sample donor's admission of recent use.

Most drug and alcohol test results are confirmed by the sample donor's admission of recent use (option B). Although screening drug testing (e.g., workplace testing) can be done on site and does not require a clinical laboratory, confirmation tests are performed only in a laboratory (option D). Difficult and disputed cases may benefit from additional help in interpretation, including assistance from the laboratory that conducted the test (or the kit manufacturer for point-of-collection tests) and from a certified medical review officer (options A, C, E). **(Biology of Drug Tests, pp. 741–744; Sample Selection: Blood, Urine, Hair, Oral Fluid, and Sweat, pp. 744–748, 749, 750, 751–752; Dealing With Difficult Results, pp. 748–749)**

49.4   Which of the following tests for drugs of abuse is most vulnerable to cheating?

A. Blood.
B. Urine.
C. Hair.
D. Saliva.
E. Sweat patches.

The correct response is option B: Urine.

Chronic drug users are commonly motivated to purchase a wide variety of products designed to mask their drug use by creating false-negative findings. Because collection of urine involves privacy concerns, it is difficult in many settings to be sure that the named donor actually provided the sample being tested (option B). Although blood testing is intrusive, sample collection is not completed privately, and

TABLE 49–1. Comparison of blood, urine, hair, saliva, and sweat patch testing for drugs of abuse

Characteristic	Blood	Urine	Hair	Saliva	Sweat patch
Immunoassay screen	Yes	Yes	Yes	Yes	Yes
GC-MS confirmation option (laboratory-based)	Yes	Yes	Yes	Yes	Yes
Chain-of-custody option	Yes	Yes	Yes	Yes	Yes
Medical review officer option	Yes	Yes	Yes	Yes	Yes
Retest of same sample	Yes	Yes	Yes	Yes	Yes
Retain positive samples for retest option	Difficult	Possible	Easy	Difficult	Possible
Common surveillance window	<24 hours	1–3 days	≥7–90 days	<48 hours	1–21 days
Intrusiveness of collection	Severe	Moderate	None	Slight	Slight
Compatibility of new sample if original test disputed	No	No	Yes	No	No
Number of drugs screened	Unlimited[a]	Unlimited[b]	Large[c]	5+alcohol	5[d]
Cost/sample (DHHS-5)	$100–$200	$15–$40	$40–$80	$20–$60	≥$35
Test can distinguish between light, moderate, and heavy drug use	Yes (short term)	No	Yes (long term)	No	Yes (ongoing)
Test resistance to cheating	High	Low	High	High	High

TABLE 49–1. Comparison of blood, urine, hair, saliva, and sweat patch testing for drugs of abuse (continued)

Characteristic	Blood	Urine	Hair	Saliva	Sweat patch
Best application	Postaccident and overdose testing for alcohol and other drugs Blood alcohol concentration level	Reasonable-cause testing Frequent testing of high-risk groups such as those in posttreatment follow-up and the criminal justice system Unannounced, random tests with observed collection	Preemployment testing Random and periodic testing Testing to determine severity of drug use for referral to treatment Testing of subjects suspected of seeking to evade urine-test detection Opiate addicts claiming poppy seed false-positive	Post-accident and overdose testing for alcohol and other drugs Blood alcohol concentration level Reasonable-cause testing	Posttreatment testing Maintaining abstinence opiate addicts claiming poppy seed false positive Compliance testing in DOT and criminal justice applications

Note. DHHS-5=U.S. Department of Health and Human Services standard drug test panel; GC-MS=gas chromatography–mass spectrometry. Costs vary dramatically based on negotiated prices with laboratories for analysis and fees related to collection, administration, and reporting.

[a]Blood testing for alcohol is routine, costing about $25 per sample, but blood testing for drugs is done by only a few laboratories in the United States. Blood testing for drugs is relatively expensive, costing about $60 for each drug tested for.

[b]Urine tests for nonroutine drugs are available from most reference laboratories, and costs for broad screens are generally <$200.

[c]Hair testing is commonly performed for the NIDA-5 (cocaine, opiates, marijuana, amphetamines, and phencyclidine). However, a large number of drugs and metabolites can be detected, and routine, broad testing is performed in several toxicology reference laboratories. The cost of nonroutine testing of hair is <$500 in most cases.

[d]Commonly limited to the DHHS-5. Tests can also be performed for alcohol.

Source. Reprinted from DuPont RL, Goldberger BA, Gold MS, et al.: "The Science and Clinical Uses of Drug Testing," in *Principles of Addiction Medicine,* 5th Edition. Edited by Ries RK, Fiellin DA, Miller SC, et al. Philadelphia, PA, Lippincott Williams & Wilkins (in press). http://www.lww.com.

this makes it more difficult to cheat on this method of testing (option A). Saliva testing is only slightly intrusive and does not require private sample collection, and as such it has a higher resistance to cheating (option D). Hair testing is nonintrusive and difficult to cheat on and has the advantage of being able to identify chronic drug usage (option C). Once removed, sweat patches cannot be replaced without noticeable puckering at the edges of the device (option E). (See Table 49–1 for a summary of testing methods for drugs of abuse.) **(Biology of Drug Tests, pp. 741–744; Sample Selection: Blood, Urine, Hair, Oral Fluid, and Sweat, pp. 744–748)**

49.5   Which of the following is true of hair biomarker tests?

   A. Result in lower positive test rates for drug use versus urine testing.
   B. Can be used to distinguish between light, moderate, and heavy use of drugs and alcohol.
   C. Have a cost similar to drug urinalysis testing.
   D. May provide false-indicator results (e.g., positive tests for morphine after consumption of poppy seeds).
   E. Have a detection window of about 1–3 days.

The correct response is option B: Can be used to distinguish between light, moderate, and heavy use of drugs and alcohol.

Whereas urinalysis is subject to dilution related to fluid consumption and rapidly changing levels can arise in blood tests, hair biomarker tests can be used to distinguish between light, moderate, and heavy use of drugs and alcohol during the prior 90 days (option B). This critical quantitative estimation is more expensive than the simple positive or negative result from drug urinalyses (option C). When hair, urine, and oral fluid tests are performed at the same time on the same individuals, more positive results are found with hair testing and fewer with urine and oral fluid testing (option A). Hair testing typically is more expensive than urine testing, with an average cost of $40–$80 per test, versus a cost of $15–$40 per test for urine testing (option C). Urine testing has a common surveillance window of 1–3 days, as opposed to 7–90 days for hair testing (option E). Hair testing does not suffer from the evidentiary false-indicator issues associated with urine tests (option D). (See Table 49–1 for a summary of testing methods for drugs of abuse.) **(Sample Selection: Blood, Urine, Hair, Oral Fluid, and Sweat, pp. 744–748; Figure 49–1, Positivity rates for drug use with hair versus urine testing, general U.S. workforce, p. 749)**

References

DuPont RL: The Selfish Brain: Learning From Addiction. Washington, DC, American Psychiatric Press, 2000

CHAPTER 50

Medical Education on Addiction

50.1   Which of the following is a key element of successful change and enhancement to medical school substance abuse curricula?

A. Identify key faculty to champion change.
B. Engage medical students interested in learning.
C. Replace skills-based training with didactic training.
D. Increase curricula hours to incorporate substance abuse training.
E. Implement a single lecture on substance abuse training.

The correct response is option A: Identify key faculty to champion change.

For decades, calls have been made for improved integration of substance use curricula in medical school, preferably with an experiential component with direct patient contact (Burger and Spickard 1991; Pursch 1978) (Table 50–1). Dartmouth Medical School undertook a comprehensive and methodological approach to addiction medicine curriculum development by sorting content according to six competency domains established by the Liaison Committee on Medical Education, the nationally recognized accrediting authority (Seddon Savage, M.S., M.D., personal communication, May 23, 2007).

There are substantial barriers, including lack of curricular time (option D), interdepartmental coordination, treatment sites in which to provide relevant clinical experiences, and interested or qualified faculty. Burger and Spickard (1991) provide an approach to overcoming some of these barriers to improve substance abuse medical education (Table 50–2). Not surprisingly, identifying expert faculty (option A) poses a major challenge particularly during clinical training. Without supportive faculty and a "champion" to help initiate change, enhancements in existing medical school substance abuse curricula are particularly problematic.

During the 1980s, the medical literature began to contain reports describing substance use training initiatives. The programs usually were brief, consisting of lectures alone or a combination of didactic and experiential training often integrated within an ongoing clerkship (Polydorou et al. 2008). Some curricula incorporated group therapy participation, treatment program visits, Alcoholics Anonymous

TABLE 50–1. Curricular content based on Liaison Committee on Medical Education competency domains

Competency domain	Content
Knowledge	Understand the following:
	Epidemiology and etiology of substance use, misuse, and addiction.
	Chronic disease model of addiction.
	Diagnosis, intervention, referral, and treatment.
Skills for patient care	Apply appropriate prevention strategies during routine health maintenance.
	Implement screening, diagnosis, brief intervention, and referrals as indicated.
	Assess stages of change and use motivational interviewing strategies.
	Manage withdrawal syndromes and medical emergencies.
Interpersonal skills and communication	Use nonstigmatizing nomenclature and effective interviewing strategies.
	Engage families and significant others when appropriate.
	Recognize and address potential barriers to effective communication.
Professionalism	Use medical and public health approach to drug use and addiction.
	Effectively address substance use issues among colleagues.
	Practice self-awareness and self-care.
Practice-based learning and improvement	Access needed resources and information on substances and addiction.
	Know avenues for specialization and continuing education.
	Continuously improve motivational skills through practice.
Systems-based practice	Work cooperatively with available clinical and related systems, including integration into interdisciplinary teams.
	Understand medicolegal issues related to substance problems.
	Understand reimbursement issues affecting care of substance use disorders.

Source. Seddon Savage, M.S., M.D., Dartmouth Medical School, personal communication, June 25, 2014.

meeting attendance, and direct clinical experiences. Although student satisfaction with these earlier programs was high, outcomes were rarely formally assessed until later, when studies began demonstrating improved knowledge and development of more positive attitudes (Polydorou et al. 2008). Integrated experiential methods are potentially of great consequence in improving attitudes about treatment effectiveness (option E).

In support of interactive, skills-based training, a comprehensive review of tobacco intervention curricula in U.S. medical schools indicated that interactive ap-

TABLE 50–2. Recommendations for curricular change

Identify key faculty who will promote substance abuse education.

Obtain the endorsement of the medical school administration and department chairperson.

Involve student leaders to promote curriculum change.

Integrate substance abuse training in the ongoing curriculum to minimize the need for new curricular hours.

Integrate an evaluation component.

Make the evaluation fit the goals of the curriculum.

Support medical school faculty to independently develop their own course offerings.

Source. Adapted from Burger and Spickard 1991.

proaches incorporating standardized patients or role-playing are more effective than didactic methods alone (option C) (Spangler et al. 2002). Such approaches may be feasibly integrated into medical school curricula. While involving student leaders to promote curriculum change is recommended, engaging medical students interested in learning is not specifically recommended (option B). **(Integrating Substance Abuse Training in Medical School, pp. 758–761)**

50.2   The Substance Abuse and Mental Health Services Administration's Center for Substance Abuse Treatment (SAMHSA/CSAT) funded medical residency training program cooperative agreements to develop and implement training programs. Which of the following initiatives facilitates sustained practice change in graduating residents?

A. Brief educational half-day programs.
B. Longer clinical rotations in substance abuse treatment.
C. Role-play with supervising clinicians.
D. Feedback provision by simulated patients.
E. Skills-based sessions.

The correct response is option B: Longer clinical rotations in substance abuse treatment.

Combined, the aforementioned residency substance use education projects that assessed curricular impact demonstrate the short-term effectiveness of brief educational half-day (option A) or longer programs, particularly when coupled with skills-based sessions (option E), role-play (option C), or feedback provision by either supervising clinicians or simulated patients (option D). Longer clinical rotations might facilitate sustained practice change (option B). For example, family practice residents participating in a 3- to 4-week chemical dependency unit rotation had significantly greater documented substance use disorder recognition during the next year (Mulry et al. 1987). **(Integrating Substance Use Training During Residency/Residency Training Initiatives, pp. 761–762)**

50.3   The U.S. Drug Enforcement Administration approval to prescribe buprenorphine for opiate dependence and withdrawal requires additional training. Psychiatrists who have certification from which of the following boards are exempt from this exam?

A. American Osteopathic Association (AOA).
B. American Society of Addiction Medicine (ASAM).
C. American Board of Addiction Medicine (ABAM).
D. American Board of Pain Medicine (ABPM).
E. American Board of Internal Medicine.

The correct response is option C: American Board of Addiction Medicine (ABAM).

Physicians who have completed a general psychiatry residency can pursue further training in addiction psychiatry through a fellowship program. Currently, nearly 50 such fellowships accredited by the Accreditation Council for Graduate Medical Education (ACGME) exist in the United States. Fellowships typically divide trainee time between direct clinical care and academic activities. Some programs accept physicians who have completed residency in other fields (e.g., internal medicine, neurology). However, these trainees would not be eligible for the addiction psychiatry boards (option E).

The ABPN (American Board of Psychiatry and Neurology 2005) (option D) administers the addiction psychiatry boards and lists core competencies on its Web site (www.abpn.com). The first subspecialty certification examination (for what was then called Added Qualifications in Addiction Psychiatry) was given in 1993. Currently, more than 2,000 psychiatrists are certified in addiction psychiatry. Psychiatrists who complete an ACGME-accredited fellowship and receive ABPN certification in general psychiatry are eligible to sit for a subspecialty examination every 2 years. The 4-hour, multiple-choice examination covers addiction psychiatry topics such as evaluation and consultation, pharmacotherapy, pharmacology, psychosocial treatment, and the biological and behavioral aspects of practice.

ABPN addiction psychiatry certification is valid for 10 years. To maintain certification beyond 10 years, the American Board of Medical Specialties mandates participation in a Maintenance of Certification (MOC) program to document a commitment to lifelong learning and assessment of practice-based performance. The content and format of the recertification examination are similar to those of the certification examination.

The ABAM was founded in 2007 based on the work of committees appointed by the ASAM. ASAM offered a certification examination in addiction medicine from 1986 to 2008, after which the exam ownership and its accompanying question pool were transferred to ABAM (option B). The first ABAM examination was given in 2010. ABAM offers a certification path to physicians who have completed residency training in any medical specialty and have an additional year of clinical experience in treating substance use disorders. In addition to being eligible to sit for the ABAM boards through having a year of clinical experience, several 1- and 2-year fellowship training programs, accredited by the American Board of Addiction Medicine Foundation, are now available across the United States. To achieve MOC,

ABAM diplomates are required to complete 1) a yearly Lifelong Learning and Self-Assessment component, consisting of reviewing at least four journal articles (and subsequently passing a home multiple-choice examination); 2) a Cognitive Expertise part, by passing the recertification examination; and 3) a Practice Performance Assessment, to be phased in during 2014. The ABAM examination, like the ABPN examination, is offered every 2 years, with recertification required every 10 years. Both ABAM and ABPN certifications are widely recognized and accepted as evidence of expertise in substance abuse. Physicians who are certified by either ABAM or ABPN are exempt from taking a special training course before being approved by the U.S. Drug Enforcement Administration to prescribe buprenorphine to their patients (option C).

The AOA offers a Certification of Added Qualifications in addiction medicine (option A). The certification examination is available to osteopathic physicians who are certified in anesthesiology, family medicine, internal medicine, or psychiatry and neurology and who have either 1) completed 1 year of AOA training in addiction psychiatry or 2) fulfilled extensive work and continuing medical education (CME) requirements in addiction medicine. **(Postresidency Training/ Addiction Psychiatry Fellowships and Certification, pp. 762–763; Addiction Medicine Fellowships and Certification, p. 763)**

50.4   Identify an effective intervention that targets practicing physicians to improve their substance use practices below.

A. Continuing medical education (CME) programs using didactic sessions.
B. CD-ROM–based CME courses.
C. Online CME courses.
D. Augmentation of brief education training with system-based clinical prompt.
E. Recruitment of physicians to attend substance abuse CME programs.

The correct response is option D: Augmentation of brief education training with system-based clinical prompt.

A promising approach to improving clinician substance use practices is to augment brief educational training with system-based clinical innovations. One approach is to prompt clinicians in the actual clinical setting, such as through provision of chart-based reminders or computer-generated reports. Clinician prompts may improve primary care tobacco counseling and hopefully increase patient cessation rates (Unrod et al. 2007). Prompting primary care faculty and house staff with alcohol screening results and specific recommendations for intervention may improve physician counseling and, potentially, alcohol-related patient outcome (Saitz et al. 2003; Seale et al. 2006) (option D). In addition, coupling educational interventions and system-based prompts may improve the ability of primary care physicians to provide maintenance care for patients with alcohol use disorders in remission (Friedmann et al. 2006).

Practicing physicians who want to further their education and training in substance use disorders typically attend CME programs, a major means by which physicians stay up to date with medical information to improve practices and optimize patient care (Davis et al. 1999). el-Guebaly et al. (2000) reviewed 11 studies that assessed the outcome of CME programs devoted to teaching physicians about substance use disorders. Most programs tended to use a combination of didactic and interactive interventions (option A) to enhance screening, early intervention, and referral by primary care physicians, although a few included psychiatrists and obstetricians. Many studies found it difficult to recruit physicians for substance use CME programs (option E). The results of the studies examining the effect of these programs were often equivocal, but they suggested a need for educational reinforcement of training to improve CME impact (el-Guebaly et al. 2000).

With the passage of the Drug Addiction Treatment Act (DATA) in 2000 and the subsequent U.S. Food and Drug Administration approval of buprenorphine for treatment of opioid dependence, it became possible for physicians to provide office-based buprenorphine treatment. Under DATA, physicians without specialty substance abuse certification can qualify to prescribe buprenorphine by participating in 8 hours of CME training sponsored by designated medical societies, such as the ASAM, American Psychiatric Association (APA), and American Academy of Addiction Psychiatry. Training is based on national practice guidelines and has been delivered through in-person, online (option C), and CD-ROM courses (option B) during the past decade. Substance Abuse and Mental Health Services Administration's Center for Substance Abuse Treatment sponsored development and assessment of a combined online and in-person training curriculum (4 hours for each component), which was developed in collaboration with the APA (Gunderson et al. 2006). Physicians completing the program preferred the in-person training component, which incorporated an experiential small-group session with patients currently receiving buprenorphine maintenance treatment. **(Postresidency Training/Programs Targeting Physicians in Practice, pp. 764–765; Coupling Educational Interventions With Practice Prompts, p. 765; Opioid Risk Management and Opioid Dependence Treatment Education, pp. 765–766)**

50.5 Which of the following is an effective educational strategy to optimize substance use curriculum and expansion?

A. Prerecorded interviews.
B. Real patients.
C. Didactic lectures.
D. Virtual reality avatars.
E. Skills-based interactive curricula.

The correct response is option E: Skills-based interactive curricula.

On the basis of the findings of the studies described throughout the textbook chapter on which this study guide chapter is based that assessed the effects of various educational strategies, several observations may be made that could help optimize substance use curriculum development and expansion. These observations, summarized in Table 50–3, are briefly discussed in this section. Brief skills-based curricula can improve clinical knowledge, attitudes, and practices. Curricula should incorporate interactive sessions that are skills based (option E), such as small-group discussions or role-play, rather than solely using standard didactic programs (option C).

Attempts should be made to incorporate an experiential component if possible. Although experiential training ideally should take place in a substance use treatment setting, simulated patients (option D) also are an effective way to educate medical personnel about substance use, and the use of simulated patients has been rated favorably compared with prerecorded videotaped interview (option A) and even real patients (in one study teaching medical students about alcohol misuse) (option B) (Eagles et al. 2001). **(Observations About Effective Educational Strategies, pp. 766–767)**

TABLE 50–3. Observations about effective educational strategies

Brief skills-based curricula can improve physician knowledge, attitudes, and practices.

Skills-based interactive curricula are preferable to didactic methods.

Experiential training in a substance abuse treatment setting or with simulated patients is preferable.

Provision of feedback should be incorporated into training models.

Faculty role models are needed.

Clinic systems interventions such as physician prompts may improve practices.

Curricula are needed among many specialties at all levels of physician training.

References

American Board of Psychiatry and Neurology: Addiction Psychiatry Core Competencies Outline Version 3. Buffalo Grove, IL, American Board of Psychiatry and Neurology, 2005. Available at: http://www.abpn.com/downloads/ core_comp_outlines/core_AP_3.0.pdf. Accessed January 28, 2015.

Burger MC, Spickard WA: Integrating substance abuse education in the medical student curriculum. Am J Med Sci 302(3):181–184, 1991 1928229

Davis D, O'Brien MA, Freemantle N, et al: Impact of formal continuing medical education: do conferences, workshops, rounds, and other traditional continuing education activities change physician behavior or health care outcomes? JAMA 282(9):867–874, 1999 10478694

Eagles JM, Calder SA, Nicoll KS, et al: A comparison of real patients, simulated patients and videotaped interview in teaching medical students about alcohol misuse. Med Teach 23(5):490–493, 2001 12098371

el-Guebaly N, Toews J, Lockyer J, et al: Medical education in substance-related disorders: components and outcome. Addiction 95(6):949–957, 2000 10946443

Friedmann PD, Rose J, Hayaki J, et al: Training primary care clinicians in maintenance care for moderated alcohol use. J Gen Intern Med 21(12):1269–1275, 2006 16965560

Gunderson EW, Fiellin DA, Levin FR, et al: Evaluation of a combined online and in person training in the use of buprenorphine. Subst Abuse 27(3):39–45, 2006 17135179

Mulry JT, Brewer ML, Spencer DL: The effect of an inpatient chemical dependency rotation on residents' clinical behavior. Fam Med 19(4):276–280, 1987 3622974

Polydorou S, Gunderson EW, Levin FR: Training physicians to treat substance use disorders. Curr Psychiatry Rep 10(5):399–303, 2008 18803913

Pursch JA: Physicians' attitudinal changes in alcoholism. Alcohol Clin Exp Res 2(4):358–361, 1978 367205

Saitz R, Horton NJ, Sullivan LM, et al: Addressing alcohol problems in primary care: a cluster randomized, controlled trial of a systems intervention: the Screening and Intervention in Primary Care (SIP) study. Ann Intern Med 138(5):372–382, 2003 12614089

Seale JP, Shellenberger S, Tillery WK, et al: Implementing alcohol screening and intervention in a family medicine residency clinic. Subst Abus 26(1):23–31, 2006 16492660

Spangler JG, George G, Foley KL, et al: Tobacco intervention training: current efforts and gaps in US medical schools. JAMA 288(9):1102–1109, 2002 12204079

Unrod M, Smith M, Spring B, et al: Randomized controlled trial of a computer-based, tailored intervention to increase smoking cessation counseling by primary care physicians. J Gen Intern Med 22(4):478–484, 2007 17372796

CHAPTER 51

Prevention of Substance Abuse

51.1 In a study of LifeSkills Training (LST), a school-based, curriculum-driven program that uses social influences and social competency, the experimental groups were teachers who received annual provider training with ongoing consultation and teachers who received training via videotape without ongoing consultation, whereas the control arm comprised teachers representing a no-treatment control condition. Students who were exposed to 60% or more lessons were considered "high fidelity" and those receiving less than 60% lessons were considered "low fidelity." After 6 years, which of the following is a key finding?

A. No statistically significant differences in drug use between students whose teachers were personally trained and students whose teachers received training via videotape.
B. Statistically significant differences in drug use between students whose teachers were personally trained and students whose teachers received training via videotape.
C. No statistically significant differences on various measures of drug use between control students and high-fidelity students in the two experimental conditions.
D. Statistically significant differences between experimental students and control students classified as having low fidelity.
E. LST is efficacious for both students with good attendance and those with greater absenteeism.

The correct response is option A. No statistically significant differences in drug use between students whose teachers were personally trained and students whose teachers received training via videotape.

Botvin et al. (1995) reported 1) no statistically significant differences in drug use at 6 years between students whose teachers were personally trained and students whose teachers received training via videotape (option A, not option B) and 2) statistically significant effects on various measures of drug use between control students and high-fidelity students in the two experimental conditions (option C). Between one in four and one in three students in the two active arms of the study

383

were classified as having low fidelity to the program (i.e., chronic absenteeism). There were no statistically significant differences between experimental students and control students classified as having low fidelity (option D). LST seems to be efficacious for students with good attendance but not for those with greater absenteeism (option E). **(School-Based, Curriculum-Driven Drug Prevention Programming, pp. 771–774)**

51.2 Which of the following school-based, curriculum-driven drug prevention programs has the highest level of success in reducing substance abuse?

A. LifeSkills Training (LST).
B. Project ALERT.
C. Take Charge of Your Life (TCYL).
D. Hutchinson Smoking Prevention Program (HSPP).
E. Positive Action (PA).

The correct response is option E: Positive Action (PA).

PA significantly reduced developmental declines in the number of positive behaviors associated with social-emotional and character development in each of three trials (Beets et al. 2009; Snyder et al. 2010; Washburn et al. 2011) (option E). These effects were statistically significant at a moderate to strong level, confirming the effectiveness of PA. The PA findings reinforce the results of a meta-analysis of 213 school-based, universal, social and emotional learning programs involving more than 270,000 students in grades K–12 (Durlak et al. 2011). The principal outcome for schools is learning and achievement, a central outcome of PA and the programs reviewed by Durlak et al. (2011). These are outcomes largely ignored by other school-based, curriculum-driven programs.

The Project ALERT authors (Ellickson and Bell 1990) reported statistically significant effects for current and regular use of cigarettes and current use of marijuana, only modest effects for alcohol use, and no significant differences based on who delivered the intervention (similar to LST). The effects of interventions were no longer significantly different from those of the control condition by the last follow-up (option B). Using agricultural extension agents to deliver ALERT, St. Pierre et al. (2005) found no positive effects on substance use or the mediators and risk factors addressed by the curriculum. Ringwalt et al. (2009, 2010) also found no significant effects on drug use and putative mediators.

Given the large number of participants and the amount of funding to develop, deliver, and evaluate TCYL, the overall effects were disappointing. Hammond et al. (2008) reported that police officers are effective regarding implementation fidelity and adolescents are comfortable with and perceive police officers as credible instructors. Who delivers a drug prevention curriculum may be less important than more thorny conceptual and methodological issues. The disappointing TCYL findings may reflect theory failure (option C).

The HSPP focus was only on cigarette smoking. There were 46.75 hours of exposure units, compared with 15 or fewer in LST, ALERT, and TCYL. Implementation fidelity was high, and none of the control districts violated a commitment to remain intervention free during the 15-year trial. Retention in HSPP was 93% at 2 years beyond high school, compared with 60% for LST in the last year of high school. Unfortunately, there was less than one percentage point difference between the experimental and control students (reported by gender) in daily smoking in the twelfth grade (option D).

For LST, the authors (Botvin et al. 1995) reported 1) no statistically significant differences in drug use at 6 years between students whose teachers were personally trained and students whose teachers received training via videotape and 2) statistically significant effects on various measures of drug use between control students and high-fidelity students in the two experimental conditions. Between one in four and one in three students in the two active arms of the study were classified as having low fidelity to the program (i.e., chronic absenteeism). There were no statistically significant differences between experimental students and control students classified as having low fidelity. LST seems to be efficacious for students with good attendance but not for those with greater absenteeism (option A). **(School-Based, Curriculum-Driven Drug Prevention Programming, pp. 771–774)**

51.3   The Communities That Care (CTC) community-based and community-placed substance abuse prevention program focuses on "individual-level" changes using a risk-protective factors framework and measures. These risk factors are organized under four concepts: 1) community, 2) family, 3) school, and 4) peer-individual. The outcome variables are substance abuse, delinquency, teen pregnancy, school dropout, violence, depression, and anxiety. Hawkins et al. (2012) found that in communities with CTC, there were lower levels of target risk factors, less initiation of delinquent behavior, lower alcohol and cigarette use, lower prevalence of past-month cigarette use, and lower prevalence of past-year delinquency and violence. Which of the following items is one of the limitations to the CTC intervention?

A. Community-level responses to the CTC survey are used to "prioritize" risk factors to be addressed.
B. Only data from students followed from fifth through tenth grades in 24 small-to medium-sized communities are used to measure change in spite of the fact that each school contains multiple cohorts.
C. Substance use and other problem behaviors targeted by CTC may be expressed by students, who are embedded in "social networks" that are included in the CTC.
D. Students providing data from fifth through tenth grade undergo many changes, and life events are captured in frequent surveys.
E. The CTC survey measures capture dynamic aspects of the lives of the students and the events happening to the adults in their families that affect the students.

The correct response is option B: Only data from students followed from fifth through tenth grades in 24 small-to-medium-sized communities are used to measure change in spite of the fact that each school contains multiple cohorts.

CTC has a number of limitations. First, individual-level responses to the CTC survey are used to "prioritize" risk factors to be addressed (option A). This practice demonstrates reliance on etiological factors that reside "under the skin" rather than in community structural–level environmental contexts. Second, only data from students followed from fifth through tenth grades in 24 small- to medium-sized communities are used to measure change in spite of the fact that each school contains multiple cohorts (option B). Third, substance use and the other problem behaviors targeted by CTC may be expressed by students, but almost all of these individuals are embedded in a number of "social networks" (cliques, peer groups, school, and sports and other types of organizations inside and outside the school). Even so, social networks are ignored by CTC (Borgatti et al. 2009; Christakis and Fowler 2008) (option C). Fourth, students providing data undergo puberty and a host of other changes and experience a large variety of events from fifth through tenth grades. These events and responses to events cannot adequately be reflected in a cross-sectional survey that occurs infrequently (option D).

Simply put, the CTC survey's measure of risk and protective factors does not begin to capture the dynamic aspects of the lives of these young people and the events happening to adults in their families that affect the students (e.g., death, divorce, periods of unemployment, economic stability or instability, food insecurity) (option E). The CTC survey also does not adequately measure what is happing in the lives of these students when they are not in school—before and after school, on scheduled breaks, and during the summer. The so-called evidence-based programs by CTC to community boards have a relatively minimal number of exposures for the students to experience. **(Community-Based and Community-Placed Prevention/Community-Placed Coalitions, pp. 775–778)**

51.4   PROSPER, the PROmoting School-community-university Partnerships to Enhance Resilience community-placed coalition, involves a university-community partnership with many teams. It has demonstrated a slower growth in misuse of illicit substances for six and seventh graders who participate in a family- or school-based curriculum-driven program when they enter eleventh and twelfth grade. Which of the following is a limitation of the PROSPER program?

A. The reliance on only two cohorts of students followed longitudinally to assess community-level change.
B. The large number of exposure units for the school-and-family-oriented interventions.
C. The existence of a potential infrastructure for dissemination of prevention.
D. The family and consumer science agricultural extension agents that are an integral component of land-grant universities in the United States.
E. The evaluation was conducted in 28 matched-pair communities, 14 each in Iowa and Pennsylvania.

The correct response is option A: The reliance on only two cohorts of students followed longitudinally to assess community-level change.

The principal limitations of PROSPER are 1) its reliance on only two cohorts of students followed longitudinally to assess community-level change (option A) and 2) the relatively small number of exposure units for the school-and-family-oriented interventions (option B). A strength of the program is the existence of a potential infrastructure for dissemination of prevention (option C), the family and consumer science agricultural extension agents (option D) that are an integral component of land-grant universities in the United States.

The evaluation was conducted in 28 matched-pair communities, 14 each in Iowa and Pennsylvania, randomly assigned to either an experimental partnership intervention or usual programming (baseline $N=11,960$) The actual interventions occurred among two successive cohorts of sixth and seventh graders who received a family or a school-based curriculum-driven program (Option E). **(Community-Based and Community-Placed Prevention/Community-Placed Coalitions, pp. 775–778)**

51.5 Media campaigns have been used as a vector for prevention of substance abuse. Which of the following agency campaigns has demonstrated a dose-response relationship between exposure to media and decline in substance use?

A. National Youth Anti-Drug Media Campaign of the National Drug Control Policy (ONDCP).
B. Partnership for a Drug-Free America.
C. Tobacco industry-sponsored smoking prevention.
D. American Legacy Foundation.

The correct response is option D: American Legacy Foundation.

The *truth* campaign is a tobacco countermarketing campaign that has been extensively evaluated, initially in Florida with significant positive effects (Sly et al. 2001) and later as part of a national campaign directed by the American Legacy Foundation (option D). Farrelly et al. (2005) found a dose-response relationship between exposure to the *truth* antismoking ads and the prevalence of smoking among youths, estimating that the campaign accounted for about 22% of the 18%–25.3% decline in smoking prevalence that occurred nationally among youths between 1999 and 2002.

The National Youth Anti-Drug Media Campaign of the ONDCP has three goals: 1) to educate and enable America's youth to reject illegal drugs; 2) to prevent youth from initiating use of drugs, especially marijuana and inhalants; and 3) to convince occasional users of these and other drugs to stop using drugs. In an evaluation of the ONDCP antidrug campaign covering the period 1999 through June 2004 (Westat 2006), over 70% of parents and youths reported exposure to one or more of the media messages weekly. The recall of the ads increased substantially over the years of the campaign. Brand recognition of the campaign's theme was high. The campaign had favorable effects on three of four belief and behavior outcome measures (i.e., talking with children about drugs, doing fun activities, beliefs about monitoring). However, there was no evidence of effects on parental monitoring behavior until the last data collection of the campaign. Parental monitoring is a major protective factor regarding adolescent drug use. There was no evidence of effects on marijuana use by the early interventions or for the campaign as a whole. There were effects in an unfavorable direction. Higher exposure led to weaker antidrug norms, and there may have been a significant unfavorable effect of exposure to the marijuana initiative on initiation of marijuana use (option A).

Recall is one of the most important measures of effectiveness. The "This is your brain. This is your brain on drugs" public service announcement created by the Partnership for a Drug-Free America achieved high recall. Although this campaign is widely remembered, the effects on substance use were minimal (option B).

Wakefield et al. (2006) examined the effect of the tobacco industry–sponsored smoking prevention advertising using the Monitoring the Future surveys. They found no beneficial effects and the possibility of some harmful effects on youth in grades 10 and 12. Terry-McElrath et al. (2011) reported that exposure to antidrug advertising had some influence on attitudes, beliefs, and behaviors using Monitoring the Future data from 1995 to 2006 (option C). **(Media-Based Prevention, pp. 778–779)**

References

Beets MW, Flay BR, Vuchinich S, et al: Use of a social and character development program to prevent substance use, violent behaviors, and sexual activity among elementary-school students in Hawaii. Am J Public Health 99(8):1438–1445, 2009 19542037

Borgatti SP, Mehra A, Brass DJ, et al: Network analysis in the social sciences. Science 323(5916):892–895, 2009 19213908

Botvin GJ, Baker E, Dusenbury L, et al: Long-term follow-up results of a randomized drug abuse prevention trial in a white middle-class population. JAMA 273(14):1106–1112, 1995 7707598

Christakis NA, Fowler JH: The collective dynamics of smoking in a large social network. N Engl J Med 358(21):2249–2258, 2008 18499567

Durlak JA, Weissberg RP, Dymnicki AB, et al: The impact of enhancing students' social and emotional learning: a meta-analysis of school-based universal interventions. Child Dev 82(1):405–432, 2011 21291449

Ellickson PL, Bell RM: Drug prevention in junior high: a multi-site longitudinal test. Science 247(4948):1299–1305, 1990 2180065

Farrelly MC, Davis KC, Haviland ML, et al: Evidence of a dose-response relationship between "truth" antismoking ads and youth smoking prevalence. Am J Public Health 95(3):425–431, 2005 15727971

Hammond A, Sloboda Z, Tonkin P, et al: Do adolescents perceive police officers as credible instructors of substance abuse prevention programs? Health Educ Res 23(4):682–696, 2008 17947250

Hawkins JD, Oesterle S, Brown EC, et al: Sustained decreases in risk exposure and youth problem behaviors after installation of the Communities That Care prevention system in a randomized trial. Arch Pediatr Adolesc Med 166(2):141–148, 2012 21969362

Ringwalt CL, Clark HK, Hanley S, et al: Project ALERT: a cluster randomized trial. Arch Pediatr Adolesc Med 163(7):625–632, 2009 19581545

Ringwalt CL, Clark HK, Hanley S, et al: The effects of Project ALERT one year past curriculum completion. Prev Sci 11(2):172–184, 2010 20012199

Sly DF, Hopkins RS, Trapido E, et al: Influence of a counteradvertising media campaign on initiation of smoking: the Florida "truth" campaign. Am J Public Health 91(2):233–238, 2001 11211631

Snyder F, Vuchinich S, Acock A, et al: Impact of the Positive Action program on school-level indicators of academic achievement, absenteeism, and disciplinary outcomes: a matched-pair, cluster randomized, controlled trial. J Res Educ Eff 3(1):26–55, 2010 20414477

St Pierre TL, Osgood DW, Mincemoyer CC, et al: Results of an independent evaluation of Project ALERT delivered in schools by Cooperative Extension. Prev Sci 6(4):305–317, 2005 16160759

Terry-McElrath YM, Emery S, Szczypka G, et al: Potential exposure to anti-drug advertising and drug-related attitudes, beliefs, and behaviors among United States youth, 1995–2006. Addict Behav 36(1–2):116–124, 2011 20961691

Wakefield M, Terry-McElrath Y, Emery S, et al: Effect of televised, tobacco company-funded smoking prevention advertising on youth smoking-related beliefs, intentions, and behavior. Am J Public Health 96(12):2154–2160, 2006 17077405

Washburn IJ, Acock A, Vuchinich S, et al: Effects of a social-emotional and character development program on the trajectory of behaviors associated with social-emotional and character development: findings from three randomized trials. Prev Sci 12(3):314–323, 2011 21720782

Westat: Evaluation of the National Youth Antidrug Media Campaign. Rockville, MD, Westat, 2006

CHAPTER 52

Forensic Addiction Psychiatry

52.1   In which of the following scenarios is the psychiatrist serving as an expert witness, as opposed to a witness of facts?

A. The psychiatrist is subpoenaed to testify about a former patient's diagnoses.
B. The patient asks the psychiatrist to provide copies of treatment records for a disability hearing.
C. The psychiatrist is asked to testify about a current patient's adherence to treatment recommendations.
D. The psychiatrist is asked to provide an independent opinion regarding the role of substance use in a domestic violence dispute.
E. The psychiatrist is accused of medical malpractice and provides testimony regarding treatment rendered to a patient.

The correct response is option D: The psychiatrist is asked to provide an independent opinion regarding the role of substance use in a domestic violence dispute.

Professionals who testify in a deposition, hearing, or trial may do so as witnesses of facts or as experts. It is important to maintain the distinction between these roles, and one must think ahead about which role one is being asked to perform. A clinician who is asked to describe his or her patient or who is asked (perhaps via subpoena) to produce his or her records on the patient is serving as a fact witness. This is very different from the expert who, in cases of crime or litigation, has been asked to give an independent opinion related to the legal questions at hand. In the above question, only option D requires an independent opinion related to a legal question. The other options (A, B, C, E) involve provision of facts regarding diagnosis and treatment. **(Process of Forensic Psychiatry/Communicating Psychiatric Information to Legal Bodies/Fact Versus Expert Witness, pp. 784–785)**

52.2   Which of the following diagnoses carries the greatest risk of violence?

A. Schizophrenia.
B. Bipolar disorder.

C. Alcohol use disorder.

D. Co-occurring alcohol and cocaine use disorders.

E. Co-occurring schizophrenia and cocaine intoxication.

The correct response is option E: Co-occurring schizophrenia and cocaine intoxication.

There is a significant difference in the dangerousness associated with severe mental disorders when substance abuse enters the picture. Investigation, particularly the MacArthur Violence Risk Assessment Study, has shown that persons with co-occurring substance use and psychiatric disorders are more frequently violent than are persons in the general population who do not have a psychiatric or substance use diagnosis or persons who have severe mental illness alone (Steadman et al. 1998; Swartz et al. 1998). The most important findings over the past decade have shown that violence is not usually associated with major mental disorders that occur in isolation; perhaps only 4% of reported violence is the result of mental disorders (Swanson 1994). However, when these mentally ill patients use substances, the risks of violence increase dramatically (Steadman et al. 1998). Added to this risk is the finding that treatment noncompliance increases the risk of violence (Torrey 1994) and that treatment noncompliance increases with substance use (Swartz et al. 1998). Additionally, recent studies demonstrate that the intoxication phase tends to be more predictive of violence than the presence of a dependence diagnosis (Mulvey et al. 2006). Therefore, the correct answer is option E, which includes the presence of a major mental illness along with acute intoxication. The other options include single mental illnesses (options A, B) or substance use disorders rather than intoxication (options C, D). **(Process of Forensic Psychiatry/ Forensic Psychiatric Content: Areas of Forensic Addiction Expertise/Comorbid Substance Use and Psychiatric Disorders, p. 788; Alcohol, pp. 788–789)**

52.3 Under which of the following circumstances can intoxication be used as a defense against responsibility for a crime?

A. There was no intent to cause harm.

B. The individual was tricked into using a substance.

C. The crime is nonviolent.

D. The individual's presentation does not meet criteria for a substance use disorder.

E. Laboratory evidence supports the claim of intoxication.

The correct response is option B: The individual was tricked into using a substance.

In a few special situations, responsibility cannot be assigned to a criminal offender. These situations include "insanity," involuntary intoxication, and being otherwise incompetent (such as being a minor). Over time, case law and statutes have almost completely eliminated voluntary intoxication as a defense against responsibility for any crime; however, *involuntary intoxication* may be exculpatory. This term reflects situations in which intoxication occurs via trickery, under duress, or as a result of a previously unknown vulnerability to an atypical reaction to a substance or side effect of medication (Myers and Vondruska 1998) (option B). There are many examples of crimes in which intoxication would not be an appropriate defense, regardless of whether there was intent to cause harm (option A), a lack of violence (option C), lack of a substance use disorder diagnosis (option D), and laboratory evidence of intoxication (option E). For example, an individual with alcohol intoxication may have intended no harm, been stopped by police prior to causing any physical harm, not had a presentation that met criteria for an alcohol use disorder, and not tested positive for alcohol on breathalyzer, yet that individual would still be responsible for driving under the influence. **(Process of Forensic Psychiatry/Effect of Substance Use and Substance Use Disorders in the Criminal Process/Criminal Setting, pp. 790–791)**

52.4 When asked by a court to make recommendations for a parolee with a substance use disorder, an addiction psychiatrist should recommend treatment for at least what period of time?

A. 1 month.
B. 3 months.
C. 6 months.
D. 1 year.
E. 5 years.

The correct response is option D: 1 year.

When asked by a court to suggest a treatment plan for the parolee, the addiction psychiatrist should offer multiple modes of multidisciplinary treatment and surveillance. One should consider residential, group, or day treatment; medication management; and other treatments. The period of treatment should be for a minimum of 1 year (option D). Random screens are best done twice weekly. Attendance at activities should be required. The clinician should reevaluate at regular intervals. **(Process of Forensic Psychiatry/Effect of Substance Use and Substance Use Disorders in the Criminal Process/Nonincarceration Correctional Settings, pp. 793–794)**

52.5 A psychiatrist is asked to evaluate an individual who was arrested for murder while driving under the influence. The defendant caused a motor vehicle accident which led to the death of the other driver. At the time of the arrest, the individual was acutely intoxicated. In the forensic setting, which of the following requests is appropriate for the psychiatrist to answer?

A. To render an opinion about whether the defendant possessed the intent necessary for a charge of murder.
B. To conduct a complete psychiatric assessment in order to help the court better understand the defendant.
C. To render an opinion regarding the likelihood that the defendant will drive while under the influence in the future.

D. To render an opinion regarding the degree of dangerousness the defendant poses if released while awaiting trial.

E. Estimating the degree of violence possessed by the defendant when under the influence of alcohol.

The correct response is option A: To render an opinion about whether the defendant possessed the intent necessary for a charge of murder.

Various events in law enforcement or judicial settings call for decisions on how to proceed: whether to report an incident, whether to prosecute, what crime to prosecute, whether the defendant may stand trial, whether he or she can be held responsible, whether he or she had—or could have had—the requisite "evil mind" (*mens rea*) or intent for that crime (option A), what the punishment should be, and so forth. The opinion of the addiction expert may be helpful with any of these decisions. Thus, the correct answer is option A, which involves rendering an opinion about the defendant's intent. The other options are not appropriate requests in the forensic setting. Although courts or attorneys may ask for it, there is no such thing as a "complete psychiatric assessment" (option B). The expert psychiatrist must help the attorney or the court pose a specific question to be answered in his or her report and testimony. Every forensic psychiatry assessment must be done with a particular focus and a specific question in mind. Additionally, the court often asks the expert for predictions on the future or the degree of dangerousness. This reflects a problem for the psychiatrist in the courtroom—that although one may feel pressured to, one should refrain from making predictions (options C, D, E) that one cannot quantify or validate. **(Process of Forensic Psychiatry/Communicating Psychiatric Information to Legal Bodies/Clinical Assessments for Legal Bodies, pp. 784–787; Effect of Substance Use and Substance Use Disorders in the Criminal Process/Criminal Setting, pp. 790–791)**

References

Mulvey EP, Odgers C, Skeem J, et al: Substance use and community violence: a test of the relation at the daily level. J Consult Clin Psychol 74(4):743–754, 2006 16881782

Myers WC, Vondruska MA: Murder, minors, selective serotonin reuptake inhibitors, and the involuntary intoxication defense. J Am Acad Psychiatry Law 26(3):487–496, 1998 9785291

Steadman HJ, Mulvey EP, Monahan J, et al: Violence by people discharged from acute psychiatric inpatient facilities and by others in the same neighborhoods. Arch Gen Psychiatry 55(5):393–401, 1998 9596041

Swanson JW: Mental disorder, substance abuse, and community violence: an epidemiological approach, in Violence and Mental Disorder: Developments in Risk Assessment. Edited by Monahan J, Steadman HJ. Chicago, IL, University of Chicago Press, 1994, pp 101–136

Swartz MS, Swanson JW, Hiday VA, et al: Violence and severe mental illness: the effects of substance abuse and nonadherence to medication. Am J Psychiatry 155(2):226–231, 1998 9464202

Torrey EF: Violent behavior by individuals with serious mental illness. Hosp Community Psychiatry 45(7):653–662, 1994 7927289

CHAPTER 53

Substance Abuse and Mental Illness

53.1   Which of the following is most likely to co-occur with a substance use disorder (SUD)?

A. Schizophrenia.
B. Bipolar disorder.
C. Major depressive disorder.
D. Generalized anxiety disorder.
E. Posttraumatic stress disorder.

The correct response is option B: Bipolar disorder.

According to the Epidemiologic Catchment Area (ECA) study, bipolar spectrum disorders (option B) were the Axis I disorders most likely to co-occur with an SUD (excluding nicotine use disorders), with 56% of any bipolar diagnosis being associated with a lifetime SUD (Regier et al. 1990). The comorbidity rate was 61% for bipolar I disorder and 48% for bipolar II disorder; of the patients with bipolar I disorder, 46% had a lifetime rate of an alcohol use disorder and 41% had a lifetime history of a drug use disorder. The other disorders listed also co-occur with substance use disorders (options A, C, D, E), but none with a comorbidity rate as high as bipolar disorder. **(Epidemiology/Bipolar Disorder, p. 806)**

53.2   A 28-year-old patient is admitted to a psychiatric hospital with acute onset of paranoia, auditory hallucinations, and irritability. The patient admits to recent use of cocaine. Which of the following is *most* likely to help clarify whether the patient's psychosis is due to a substance-induced disorder or co-occurring schizophrenia and cocaine use disorder?

A. Administering urine toxicology on admission.
B. Making serial assessments of psychiatric symptoms over time.
C. Eliciting a family history of substance use disorders.
D. Using a structured diagnostic interview on admission.
E. Eliciting a history of prescriptions for antipsychotic medication.

The correct response is option B: Making serial assessments of psychiatric symptoms over time.

Although the task of making a definitive diagnosis or diagnoses is most complex when substance abuse, psychiatric illness, and medical illness all coexist, there are certain elements of assessment that are helpful in the diagnostic formulation (Table 53–1). Two significant factors that contribute to misdiagnoses are the use of single, cross-sectional assessments, especially in the acute setting, and the use of single sources of information. An optimal approach at making definitive diagnoses relies on using serial, longitudinal assessments (option B) as well as multiple sources to gather data, such as clinician-administered structured or semistructured interviews, self-report, collateral information, physical examination, and laboratory tests (Carey and Correia 1998). Although administering urine toxicology on admission (option A) is important in a comprehensive assessment, a single laboratory test cannot differentiate between substance-induced and co-occurring disorders. Similarly, use of a structured diagnostic interview may be helpful (option D), but it will need to be repeated longitudinally in order to clarify the diagnosis. Family history of substance use (option C), and personal history of prescriptions for antipsychotics (option E), although important in a comprehensive assessment, do not provide sufficient information to differentiate between substance-induced and co-occurring disorders. **(Diagnostic Assessment, pp. 807, 808–809)**

53.3   It is prudent to wait several months prior to making a formal diagnosis of a psychotic spectrum disorder when treating a patient with psychotic symptoms and use of which of the following substances?

A. Phencyclidine.
B. Cocaine.
C. Methamphetamine.
D. Marijuana.
E. Inhalants.

The correct response is option C: Methamphetamine.

To avoid overdiagnoses and overtreatment, it is important to know the optimal time of abstinence necessary before making a formal mental illness diagnosis. It is prudent to wait until an individual is no longer in active withdrawal before attempting to make a psychiatric diagnosis. Methamphetamine (option C) and chronic alcohol–induced psychoses also necessitate waiting up to several months before making the formal diagnosis of a psychotic spectrum illness. For most other substances of abuse (options A, B, D, E), a general rule of thumb is to wait 2–4 weeks after acute withdrawal before diagnosing a mental illness. **(Diagnostic Dilemmas and Pitfalls: Under- and Overdiagnosis, pp. 807, 809)**

53.4   Which of the following medications has the most evidence supporting its effectiveness in treating patients with co-occurring schizophrenia and substance use disorders?

TABLE 53–1. Diagnostic formulation

1. Substance abuse history
   - For all presenting substances, review the following: age at first use; pattern of use over time, including heavy/binge use, amount, frequency, route of use; subjective experience while using; problems related to use, including overdose and withdrawal syndromes; time of last use; and history of substance abuse treatment, including detoxification programs, inpatient rehabilitation programs, residential programs, outpatient programs, and methadone maintenance programs.

2. Family history
   - Include family's history of psychiatric/medical illnesses and substance use disorders.

3. Premorbid history
   - Consider age at onset and symptom pattern. For example, onset of dementia at age 30 in a patient with a history of inhalant dependence suggests a substance-induced dementia rather than co-occurring Alzheimer's disease, or premorbid paranoid personality traits suggest co-occurring schizophrenia in a patient who presents with psychosis in the setting of a cocaine-induced myocardial infarction.

4. Temporal history
   - Determine order of onset of substance use disorder versus psychiatric illness and/or medical illness, and assess the relationship between the three variables.

5. Controlling variables (i.e., periods of abstinence)
   - Determine whether patient has had continued presence of psychiatric or medical symptoms during significant periods of abstinence, which suggests dual or multiple diagnoses.

6. Typology of symptoms
   - Consider the types of symptoms. For example, with psychosis: most drugs of abuse induce only positive symptoms of psychosis, but the N-methyl-D-aspartate (NMDA) antagonist hallucinogens can occasionally induce all symptoms clusters of psychosis (i.e., positive, negative, and cognitive).

7. Severity of symptoms
   - Consider severity even during periods of active substance abuse. For example, severe anxiety during active use of constant dose/pattern and not in withdrawal suggests a co-occurring anxiety spectrum disorder, or malignant, labile hypertension in a patient with alcohol abuse who has three or four drinks per day suggests co-occurring hypertension.

8. Collateral history
   - Obtain history from family, friends, case managers, and treatment providers as warranted.

9. Physical examination
   - Look for classic symptoms of substance presentation (e.g., vertical, horizontal, rotary nystagmus with NMDA antagonist hallucinations; dry skin with anticholinergics; stigmata of cirrhosis seen in alcoholic persons).

10. Toxicology monitoring
    - Consider urine testing, which is the most common method.

11. Multiple sources of information
    - Use patient self-report, collateral information, physical examination, laboratory tests, and formal structured or semistructured measures such as the Structured Clinical Interview for DSM-IV (SCID-I) to enhance the reliability and validity of diagnoses.

TABLE 53–1. Diagnostic formulation *(continued)*

12. Serial, longitudinal assessments

- Increase reliability and validity of diagnoses through use of such assessments as opposed to relying on single assessments, especially those done in acute settings (e.g., when a patient is admitted to an inpatient dual-diagnosis unit while actively in withdrawal, psychotic, and suicidal).

13. Beware of making psychiatric diagnoses during periods of active withdrawal to avoid confusing withdrawal states with psychiatric symptoms.

    A. Haloperidol.
    B. Olanzapine.
    C. Fluphenazine.
    D. Clozapine.
    E. Risperidone.

The correct response is option D: Clozapine.

Of the second-generation antipsychotics (SGAs), clozapine (option D) is the most studied and promising medication to treat patients with schizophrenia and co-occurring SUDs, with case reports and correlational studies demonstrating a decrease in substance abuse for alcohol, nicotine, cocaine, and other drugs of abuse (Brunette et al. 2006). Typical neuroleptics (options A, C) have not been associated with decreases in substance abuse in this cohort of dually diagnosed patients, and there is some evidence that they may actually precipitate or increase substance abuse in individuals with co-occurring psychotic and addictive disorders (McEvoy et al. 1995; Stuyt et al. 2006; Voruganti et al. 1997). Evidence supporting the efficacy of other atypical antipsychotics in improving both psychiatric and substance abuse (alcohol or drug use disorder) outcomes in open-label and controlled trials is increasing, with the evidence most consistent for quetiapine (Brown et al. 2001; Potvin et al. 2004, 2006) and aripiprazole (Beresford et al. 2005; Brown et al. 2005) and mostly positive but mixed for olanzapine (option B) (Linszen and van Amelsvoort 2007; Noordsy et al. 2001a, 2001b; Sayers et al. 2005; Smelson et al. 2006) and risperidone (option E) (Green et al. 2003; Petrakis et al. 2006; Rubio et al. 2006b; Smelson et al. 2002). General principles of psychotropic interventions in the dually diagnosed are presented in Table 53–2. **(Treatment, pp. 809–810/Schizophrenia and SUDs/Medications, pp. 811–813)**

53.5   In a patient with co-occurring bipolar disorder and alcohol use disorder (AUD), which of the following medications has the most evidence to support its use in addressing both mood symptoms and drinking outcomes?

    A. Valproic acid.
    B. Lithium.
    C. Quetiapine.
    D. Aripiprazole.
    E. Lamotrigine.

TABLE 53–2. General principles of psychotropic interventions in the dually diagnosed

1. Keep in mind these general goals:
   - Acute stabilization of symptoms (mental illness/addictive behavior).
   - Achievement of remission (mental illness/addictive behavior): resolution of symptoms, return to baseline function, prophylaxis to avoid relapse, improvement of medication compliance, and improvement in quality of life.

2. Consider stage of motivational engagement (e.g., choosing agents to initiate abstinence versus maintaining abstinence; using abstinence-oriented approaches versus use/harm reduction approaches).

3. Treat both disorders (mental illness/substance use disorder) at the same time, early in the course of illness and aggressively; avoid undertreatment if possible, because failure to treat one disorder negatively affects the longitudinal course of the other.

4. Avoid overtreatment; make sure not to overdiagnose and overtreat, depending on the particular substance of abuse and its potential for substance-induced mental phenomena.

5. Choose a medication that has the potential to treat symptoms of both disorders (e.g., clozapine for treating both psychosis and substance use).

6. Choose a medication with a broad spectrum of activity across non–substance use disorders (e.g., bupropion for major depression and attention-deficit/hyperactivity disorder).

7. Start with a medication that has the least addictive liability if possible (e.g., selective serotonin reuptake inhibitors or buspirone before benzodiazepines in a patient with generalized anxiety disorder and alcohol use disorder).

8. Watch for potential toxicity, interactions with other medications, and interactions with active use of substances of abuse.

9. Closely monitor treatment adherence; involve family members and case managers as needed.

The correct response is option A: Valproic acid.

Indirect evidence suggesting that anticonvulsants (valproic acid [option A] or carbamazepine) should be selected over lithium (option B) as first-line agents includes the following: 1) substance abuse is a predictor of poor response to lithium and 2) mixed/rapid-cycling variants of bipolar disorder are more prevalent among patients with co-occurring substance use disorders (SUDs), and these variants are more likely to respond to anticonvulsants than to lithium (Brady et al. 2003). Additionally, evidence from a randomized controlled trial (RCT) and open-label trials support the efficacy of valproic acid in this population. Two small open-label trials demonstrated the efficacy of valproic acid in improving both mood symptoms and substance abuse in participants with co-occurring bipolar disorder and SUDs (Brady et al. 1995; Salloum et al. 2007). In an RCT, 59 patients with bipolar disorder and AUD received treatment as usual, with lithium carbonate and psychosocial interventions, and were randomly assigned to receive valproic acid or placebo. Although both groups had equal improvements in mood outcomes, the valproic acid group demonstrated improved drinking outcomes at follow-up (Salloum et al. 2005). Evidence for the other answer choices is less robust. Emerging evidence from small open label trials suggests that lamotrigine (option E) may be useful in reducing both mood symptoms and improving substance abuse outcomes (i.e., craving or substance use) among individuals with bipolar disorder and comorbid cocaine dependence (Brown et al. 2003, 2006) and alcohol dependence (Rubio et al. 2006a). There are also some data from open label trials that suggest the efficacy of second-generation antipsychotics—both quetiapine (option C) (Brown et al. 2002) and aripiprazole (option D) (Brown et al. 2005; Tolliver et al. 2007; Verduin et al. 2007)—in improving both affective symptoms and substance-related outcomes in patients with co-occurring bipolar disorder and SUDs. However, RCTs for quetiapine have not supported its efficacy for alcohol-related outcomes. (General principles of psychotropic interventions in the dually diagnosed are presented in Table 53–2.) **(Treatment/Bipolar Disorder and SUDs/Medication, pp. 813–814)**

References

Beresford TP, Clapp L, Martin B, et al: Aripiprazole in schizophrenia with cocaine dependence: a pilot study. J Clin Psychopharmacol 25(4):363–366, 2005 16012280

Brady KT, Sonne SC, Anton R, et al: Valproate in the treatment of acute bipolar affective episodes complicated by substance abuse: a pilot study. J Clin Psychiatry 56(3):118–121, 1995 7883730

Brady KT, Myrick H, Sonne S: Co-occurring addictive and affective disorders, in Principles of Addiction Medicine, 3rd Edition. Edited by Graham AW, Schultz TK, Mayo-Smith MF, et al. Chevy Chase, MD, American Society of Addiction Medicine, 2003, pp 1277–1286

Brown ES, Nejtec VA, Perantie DC: Quetiapine in psychiatric illness with comorbid stimulant abuse. Paper presented at the 40th Annual Meeting of the American College of Neuropsychopharmacology, Waikoloa, HI, December 9–13, 2001

Brown ES, Nejtek VA, Perantie DC, et al: Quetiapine in bipolar disorder and cocaine dependence. Bipolar Disord 4(6):406–411, 2002 12519101

Brown ES, Nejtek VA, Perantie DC, et al: Lamotrigine in patients with bipolar disorder and cocaine dependence. J Clin Psychiatry 64(2):197–201, 2003 12633129

Brown ES, Jeffress J, Liggin JD, et al: Switching outpatients with bipolar or schizoaffective disorders and substance abuse from their current antipsychotic to aripiprazole. J Clin Psychiatry 66(6):756–760, 2005 15960570

Brown ES, Perantie DC, Dhanani N, et al: Lamotrigine for bipolar disorder and comorbid cocaine dependence: a replication and extension study. J Affect Disord 93(1–3):219–222, 2006 16519947

Brunette MF, Drake RE, Xie H, et al: Clozapine use and relapses of substance use disorder among patients with co-occurring schizophrenia and substance use disorders. Schizophr Bull 32(4):637–643, 2006 16782758

Carey KB, Correia CJ: Severe mental illness and addictions: assessment considerations. Addict Behav 23(6):735–748, 1998 9801713

Green AI, Burgess ES, Dawson R, et al: Alcohol and cannabis use in schizophrenia: effects of clozapine vs. risperidone. Schizophr Res 60(1):81–85, 2003 12505141

Linszen D, van Amelsvoort T: Cannabis and psychosis: an update on course and biological plausible mechanisms. Curr Opin Psychiatry 20(2):116–120, 2007 17278907

McEvoy J, Freudenreich O, McGee M, et al: Clozapine decreases smoking in patients with chronic schizophrenia. Biol Psychiatry 37(8):550–552, 1995 7619979

Noordsy DL, O'Keefe C, Mueser KT, et al: Six-month outcomes for patients who switched to olanzapine treatment. Psychiatr Serv 52(4):501–507, 2001a 11274497

Noordsy DL, O'Keefe C, Mueser KT, et al: Switching to olanzapine in naturalistic community care. Paper presented at the 154th annual meeting of the American Psychiatric Association, New Orleans, LA, May 5–10, 2001b

Petrakis IL, Poling J, Levinson C, et al: Naltrexone and disulfiram in patients with alcohol dependence and comorbid posttraumatic stress disorder. Biol Psychiatry 60(7):777–783, 2006 17008146

Potvin S, Stip E, Roy JY: The effect of quetiapine on cannabis use in 8 psychosis patients with drug dependency. Can J Psychiatry 49(10):711, 2004 15560324

Potvin S, Stip E, Lipp O, et al: Quetiapine in patients with comorbid schizophrenia-spectrum and substance use disorders: an open-label trial. Curr Med Res Opin 22(7):1277–1285, 2006 16834826

Regier DA, Farmer ME, Rae DS, et al: Comorbidity of mental disorders with alcohol and other drug abuse. Results from the Epidemiologic Catchment Area (ECA) Study. JAMA 264(19):2511–2518, 1990 2232018

Rubio G, López-Muñoz F, Alamo C: Effects of lamotrigine in patients with bipolar disorder and alcohol dependence. Bipolar Disord 8(3):289–293, 2006a 16696832

Rubio G, Martínez I, Ponce G, et al: Long-acting injectable risperidone compared with zuclopenthixol in the treatment of schizophrenia with substance abuse comorbidity. Can J Psychiatry 51(8):531–539, 2006b 16933590

Salloum IM, Cornelius JR, Daley DC, et al: Efficacy of valproate maintenance in patients with bipolar disorder and alcoholism: a double-blind placebo-controlled study. Arch Gen Psychiatry 62(1):37–45, 2005 15630071

Salloum, IM, Douaihy A, Cornelius JR, et al: Divalproex utility in bipolar disorder with co-occurring cocaine dependence: a pilot study. Addict Behav 32(2):410–415, 2007 16814474

Sayers SL, Campbell EC, Kondrich J, et al: Cocaine abuse in schizophrenic patients treated with olanzapine versus haloperidol. J Nerv Ment Dis 193(6):379–386, 2005 15920378

Smelson DA, Losonczy MF, Davis CW, et al: Risperidone decreased craving and relapse in individuals with schizophrenia and cocaine dependence. Can J Psychiatry 47(7):671–675, 2002

Smelson DA, Ziedonis D, Williams J, et al: The efficacy of olanzapine for decreasing cue-elicited craving in individuals with schizophrenia and cocaine dependence: a preliminary report. J Clin Psychopharmacol 26(1):9–12, 2006 16415698

Stuyt EB, Sajbel TA, Allen MH: Differing effects of antipsychotic medications on substance abuse treatment patients with co-occurring psychotic and substance abuse disorders. Am J Addict 15(2):166–173, 2006 16595355

Tolliver BK, McRae AI, Verduin MI, et al: A Comparison of the efficacy of aripiprazole on psychiatric and substance use outcomes in bipolar and schizophrenic patients. Paper presented at the 69th Annual Meeting of the College of Problems of Drug Dependence, Quebec City, Quebec, June 12–17, 2007

Verduin MI, McRae AI, Tolliver BK, et al: Efficacy of Aripiprazole in Patients With Substance Use Disorders. Paper presented at the 69th Annual Meeting of the College on Problems of Drug Dependence, Quebec City, Quebec, June 12–17, 2007

Voruganti LNP, Heslegrave RJ, Awad AG: Neuroleptic dysphoria may be the missing link between schizophrenia and substance abuse. J Nerv Ment Dis 185(7):463–465, 1997 9240366